ABBREVIATIONS

Age

NB – newborn
A – adult
C – child

Time/Frequency

s – second
min – minute
h – hour
d – day
wk – week
mo – month
y – year
q.d. – every day
q.o.d. – every other day
b.i.d. – twice a day
t.i.d. – three times a day
q.i.d. – four times a day
q4–6h (for example) – every 4–6 hours
h.s. – hour of sleep (at bedtime)
a.c. – before meal
p.c. – after meal
a.m. – morning
p.m. – evening
PRN – whenever necessary

Routes

IM – intramuscularly
IO – intraosseous
IV – intravenously
PO – by mouth (oral)
PR – per rectum (rectally)
SC – subcutaneously
SL – sublingual
vag – vaginally

Drug Form

amp – ampule
amt – amount
cap – capsule/caplet
conc – concentration
elix – elixir
gt(t) – drop(s)
inf – infusion
inhal – inhalant

inj – injection
liq – liquid
ma – maintenance
max – maximum
oint – ointment
sol – solution
supp – suppository
susp – suspension
tab – tablet

Measurements

oz – ounce
lb – pound
in – inches
g – gram
mg – milligram
μ**m** – microgram
U – unit
mEq – milliequivalent
L – liter
mL – milliliter
dL – deciliter
kg – kilogram
m^2 – square meter
bpm – beats per minute
$\times$ – times per
$>$ – more than
$<$ – less than
$\geq$ – more than or equal to
$\leq$ – less than or equal to
$-$ – to (range of one value to another value)

Miscellaneous

Preg Cat – pregnancy category
t½ – half-life
UK – unknown
CSS – Controlled Substance Schedule
ACE – angiotensin-converting enzyme
ADD – attention deficit disorder
AMI – acute myocardial infarction

congestive heart failure
CNS – central nervous system
Cr cl – creatine clearance
D_5W – 5% dextrose in water
ECG – electrocardiogram; electrocardiographic; electrocardiography
ETT – endotracheal tube
GERD – gastroesophageal reflux disease
GI – gastrointestinal
GU – genitourinary
I – imipenem
ICP – increased intracranial pressure
IOP – increased ocular pressure
IPPB – intermittent positive pressure breathing
LD – loading dose
LR – lactated Ringer's
MAOIs – monoamine oxidase inhibitors
MDI – metered dose inhaler
NA – not applicable
NGT – nasogastric tube
NSAIDs – nonsteroidal anti-inflammatory drugs
NSS – normal saline solution
OTC – over-the-counter
PB – protein-binding
RBC(s) – red blood cell(s)
RD – respiratory distress
RDA – recommended daily allowance
SR – sustained release (tab/cap)
TDM – therapeutic drug monitoring
VS – vital signs

PHARMACOLOGY

**Pocket
Companion
for Nurses**

PHARMACOLOGY

Pocket Companion for Nurses

Evelyn R. Hayes, RN, PhD
Professor
College of Nursing
University of Delaware
Newark, Delaware

Joyce LeFever Kee, RN, MS
Associate Professor Emerita
College of Nursing
University of Delaware
Newark, Delaware

W.B. SAUNDERS COMPANY
A Division of Harcourt Brace & Company

Philadelphia London Toronto Montreal Sydney Tokyo

W.B. SAUNDERS COMPANY
A Division of Harcourt Brace & Company

The Curtis Center
Independence Square West
Philadelphia, Pennsylvania 19106

Library of Congress Cataloging-in-Publication Data

Hayes, Evelyn R.

    Pharmacology pocket companion for nurses / Evelyn R. Hayes,
Joyce LeFever Kee. — 1st ed.
       p.   cm.

    ISBN 0–7216–4732–4

    1. Pharmacology—Handbooks, manuals, etc.   2. Nursing—
Handbooks, manuals, etc.   I. Kee, Joyce LeFever.   II. Title.
    [DNLM: 1. Drugs—nurses' instruction—handbooks. 2. Drug
Therapy—nurses' instruction—handbooks. QV 39 H418p 1996]
RM301. 12.H39   1996
615'.1—dc20
DNLM/DLC   94-43775

PHARMACOLOGY
POCKET COMPANION FOR NURSES   ISBN 0–7216–4732–4
International Edition   ISBN 0–7216–6828–3

Printed in the United States of America.

Last digit is the print number: 9   8   7   6   5   4   3   2   1

CONSULTANTS

Michele Bockrath-Welch, RNC, MSN
Senior Clinical Scientist
Wyeth-Ayerst Laboratories
Philadelphia, Pennsylvania

Betty B. Laliberte, RN, MSN
Assistant Professor
School of Nursing
University of Connecticut
Storrs, Connecticut

Anne E. Lara, RN, MS, OCN, CS
Nurse Manager
Radiation Oncology
Medical Center of Delaware
Wilmington, Delaware

Linda Laskowski-Jones, RN, MS, CCRN, CEN
Trauma Nurse Specialist
Trauma Service
Medical Center of Delaware
Wilmington, Delaware

Lois W. Lowry, PhD, RN
Associate Professor
University of Southern Florida
Tampa, Florida

Nancy G. M. Miner, RNC, MSN
Director
Bridgeport Community Mental
Health Center
Bridgeport, Connecticut

Donna Obra, PharmD
Director of Medical Information
Zeneca Inc.
Wilmington, Delaware

Joseph Peoples, RPh
Clinical Pharmacist
Alfred I. Du Pont Institute
Wilmington, Delaware

Lisa Plowfield, PhD, RN
Assistant Professor
College of Nursing
University of Delaware
Newark, Delaware

Nancy Sharts-Hopko, PhD, RN
Associate Professor
Villanova University
Villanova, Pennsylvania

Robert Thornton, RPh, BSc
Director of Pharmacy Services
St. Francis Hospital and Medical
Center
Wilmington, Delaware

Judith A. Torpey, RN, MSN
Assistant Director
Visiting Nurse Association of Manchester
Manchester, Connecticut

Jennifer Trey
Senior Student
College of Nursing
University of Delware
Newark, Delaware

Marcus D. Wilkson, PharmD
Assistant Professor
Philadelphia College of Pharmacy
Philadelphia, Pennsylvania
Clinical Pharmacy Coordinator
HMO of Delaware
Wilmington, Delaware

Roni Zarge
Senior Student
College of Nursing
University of Delaware
Newark, Delaware

PREFACE

Welcome to a unique pharmacology pocket companion for nurses. This book was designed for both nurses in clinical practice and student nurses to provide complex information on prototype drugs complete with the nursing process and extensive drug tables. The easy-to-read format allows valuable information to be readily available to the reader.

More than 90 prototype drugs are illustrated in a unique graphic format that includes drug name (generic and brand); drug and pregnancy categories; drug forms, routes, and dosages; contraindications; drug, food, and laboratory interactions; pharmacokinetics and pharmacodynamics; therapeutic effects and uses and mode of action; and side effects and adverse reactions.

The nursing process—assessment, nursing diagnosis, planning, nursing interventions, client and family teaching, and evaluation—is integrated throughout the pocket reference. Two potential nursing diagnoses apply to each drug, including knowledge deficit and noncompliance. The most common nursing diagnoses related to the specific drug therapy are identified. The challenges of client and family teaching are described, and helpful teaching tips are offered. Client teaching focuses on general information, skills, diet, and side effects related to the drugs.

More than 1,000 drugs are described in approximately 100 drug tables that include generic and brand names, common dosages, pregnancy category, drug interactions, protein-binding capacity, half-life, and onset, peak, and duration of action. Refer to the prototype for a description of the side effects and adverse reactions.

The tables present essential information in a quick, easy-to-read format that enables the reader to not only pay attention to a single drug but also to compare and contrast aspects of the drug with those of related agents.

Complete abbreviation and laboratory test keys and a description of the drug pregnancy categories are given inside the front cover. Additional references are grouped at the beginning of the book, including sample dosage calculations, nomogram for body surface area, guide for calculation of intravenous flow rates, drugs that affect the color of urine and stool, therapeutic drug monitoring, table of metric and apothecary conversion, and additional prototype forms to be developed as needed.

Canadian drugs are listed in the Appendix according to US generic drug names with corresponding Canadian brand drug names (A), and Canadian brand drug names with corresponding US generic drug names (B).

Nurses in clinical practice and student nurses have an ongoing need for such a reference because of their responsibility for the administration of medications and evaluation of client response. This pocket reference details valuable information in a quick, easy-to-read format for clinical application.

ACKNOWLEDGMENTS

Sincere appreciation is given to the many professionals who assisted in the development of this reference. The perspectives of the reviewers were most helpful, and we gratefully thank them for their insightful suggestions: Michele Bockrath-Welch, RNC, MSN; Betty B. Laliberte, RN, MSN; Anne E. Lara, RN, MS, OCN, CS; Linda Laskowski-Jones, RN, MS, CCRN, CEN; Lois W. Lowry, PhD, RN; Nancy G.M. Miner, RNC, MSN; Donna Obra, PharmD; Joseph Peoples, RPh; Lisa Plowfield, PhD, RN; Nancy Sharts-Hopko, PhD, RN; Robert Thornton, RPh, BSc; Judith A. Torpey, RN, MSN; and Marcus D. Wilson, PharmD. We extend special thanks also to senior students Jennifer Trey and Roni Zarge.

We extend appreciation to Patricia Beauchesne, Katherine Dougherty, and Sandy Grim for their ongoing computer expertise.

Thanks are also due to the staff at W.B. Saunders Company, especially Daniel T. Ruth, Editor, Nursing Books, and Susan Bielitsky, Administrative Assistant.

We extend our appreciation and love to our families for their ongoing support.

NOTICE

Pharmacology is an ever-changing field. Standard safety precautions must be followed, but as new research and clinical experience broaden our knowledge, changes in treatment and drug therapy become necessary or appropriate. The editors of this work have carefully checked the generic and brand names and verified drug dosages to ensure that the dosage information in this work is accurate and in accord with the standards accepted at the time of publication. Readers are advised, however, to check the product information currently provided by the manufacturer of each drug to be administered to be certain that changes have not been made in the recommended dose or in the contraindications for administration. This is of particular importance in regard to new or infrequently used drugs. It is the responsibility of the treating physician or health care provider, relying on experience and knowledge of the patient, to determine dosages and the best treatment for their patient. The editors cannot be responsible for misuse or misapplication of the information in this work.

CONTENTS

ORIENTATION

INTRODUCTION TO USING THE DRUG PROTOTYPE

Comprehensive information is provided for each of the prototype drugs, including generic and brand names; dosage; forms available; pregnancy category; contraindication and cautions for use; drug, food, and laboratory interactions; pharmacokinetics; pharmacodynamics; therapeutic effects and mode of action; side effects; and adverse reactions.

Drug, food, and laboratory interactions are important and can be complex. For example, the interactions for hydrochlorothiazide are that the drug will:

> *Increase* digitalis toxicity with digitalis and hypokalemia; *increase* potassium loss with steroids; *decrease* antihypoglycemic effect; *decrease* thiazide effect with cholestyramine and colestipol
>
> *Lab: Decrease* serum potassium, sodium, and magnesium levels; *increase* serum calcium, glucose, and uric acid levels

Thus, it is evident that hydrochlorothiazide affects the action of other drugs and is affected by other drug actions.

The nursing process relates to the prototype drug as well as to other drugs within the category. In addition, comprehensive drug tables detail essential data about the most commonly prescribed drugs in that category.

Drug Category

Drug Generic Name

Drug Generic Name
Drug Brand Name(s)

Pregnancy Category:
Drug Forms:

Dosage

Contraindications

Caution:

Drug-Lab-Food Interactions

Pharmacokinetics

Absorption:
Distribution:
Metabolism:
Excretion:

Pharmacodynamics

Onset:
Peak:
Duration:

Therapeutic Effects/Uses:

Mode of Action:

Side Effects

Adverse Reactions

Life-threatening:

KEY:

Metric and Apothecary Conversion

Metric		Apothecary
Gram (g)	Milligram (mg)	Grain (gr)
1	1000	15
0.5	500	7½
0.3	300 (325)	5
0.1	100	1½
0.06	60 (64)	1
0.03	30 (32)	½
0.015	15 (16)	¼
0.010	10	⅙
0.0006	0.6	1/100
0.0004	0.4	1/150
0.0003	0.3	1/200

Drug Calculations: Ratio and Proportion

$$H \quad : \quad V \quad :: \quad D \quad : \quad X$$
on hand   vehicle   desired   unknown

means

extremes

Example:
Order: Amoxicillin 100 mg PO q6h
Available: Amoxicillin 250 mg/5 mL

$$H \quad : \quad V \quad :: \quad D \quad : \quad X$$
250 mg : 5 mL :: 100 mg : X mL

$$250 X = 500$$
$$X = 2 \text{ mL amoxicillin}$$

Liquid Conversion

30 mL (cc) = 1 oz (fl ℥) = 2 tbsp (T)
            = 6 tsp (t)
15 mL (cc) = ½ oz = 1 T = 3 t
1000 mL (cc) = 1 quart (qt) = 1 liter (L)
500 mL (cc) = 1 pint (pt)
5 mL (cc) = 1 tsp (t)
4 mL (cc) = 1 fl dr (fl℥)
1 mL (cc) = 15 (16) minims (℔)
          = 15 (16) drops (gtt)

Body Weight (Kilograms)

To change pounds to kilograms, divide by 2.2.

Example:
Change 44 pounds to kilograms (kg)
$$44 \div 2.2 = 20 \text{ kg}$$

$$\text{Dosage/kg/d} = \text{dosage/d}$$
$$(\text{dosage} \times \text{kg} = \text{dose/d})$$

Example:
Order: Drug 6 mg/kg/d in four divided doses

$$6 \text{ mg} \times 20 \text{ kg} \times 1 \text{ d} = 120 \text{ mg/d}$$
$$120 \div 4 = 30 \text{ mg per dose}$$

Drug Calculations: Basic Formula

$$\frac{D \text{ (desired)}}{H \text{ (on hand)}} \times V \text{ (vehicle, drug form)}$$

Example:
Order: Amoxicillin 100 mg PO q6h
Available: Amoxicillin 250 mg/5 mL

$$\frac{D}{H} \times V = \frac{100 \text{ mg}}{250 \text{ mg}} \times 5 \text{ mL}$$

$$= \frac{500}{250} = 2 \text{ mL amoxicillin}$$

Dimensional Analysis (Factor Labeling)

$$= \frac{V \text{ (vehicle)} \times C(H) \times D \text{ (desired)}}{H \text{ (on hand)} \times C(D) \times 1}$$
(drug label) (conversion factor) (drug order)

Conversion factor: 1 g = 1000 mg
                   1 g = 15 gr
                   1 gr = 60 mg

Order: Amoxicillin 0.1 g, PO q6h
Available: Amoxicillin 250 mg/5 mL
How many mLs would you give?

$$\frac{5 \text{ mL} \times \overset{4}{\cancel{1000 \text{ mg}}} \times 0.1 \cancel{g}}{\underset{1}{\cancel{250 \text{ mg}}} \times 1 \cancel{g} \times 1} =$$

$$5 \text{ mL} \times 4 \times 0.1 = 2 \text{ mL of amoxicillin}$$

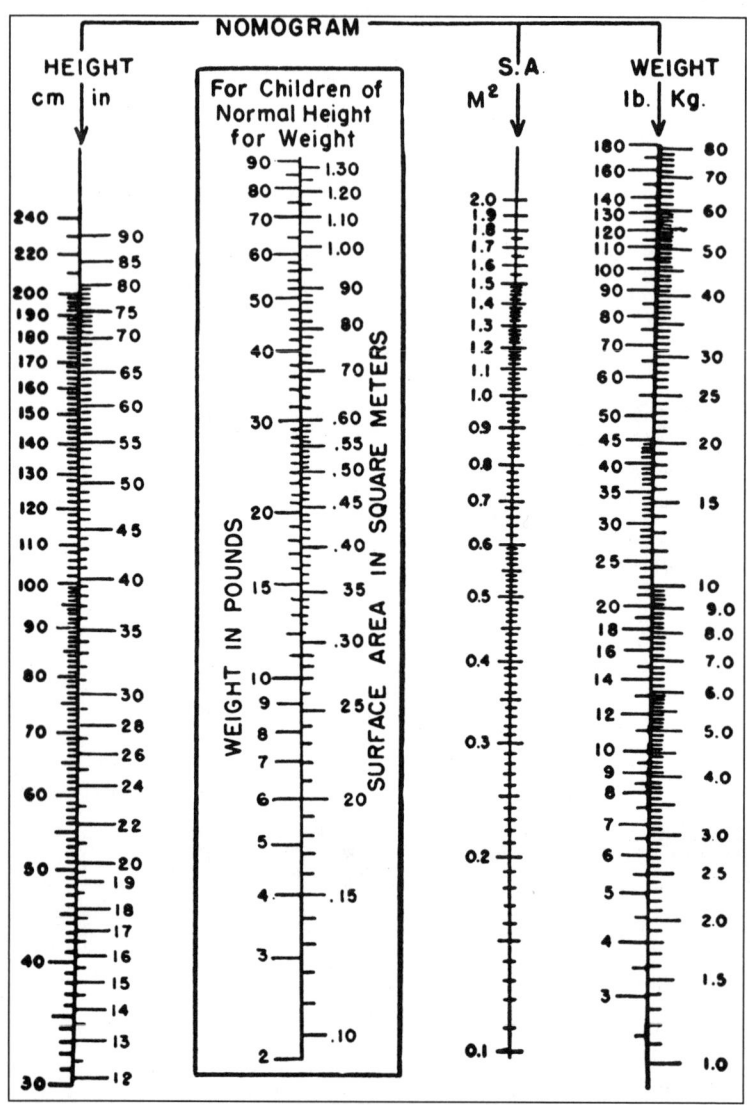

NOMOGRAM

West nomogram: for infants and children. *Directions*: (1) Find height. (2) Find weight. (3) Draw a straight line connecting the height and the weight, and where the line intersects on the SA column is the body surface area (m²). Modified from data of E. Boyd and C. D. West, in Behrman, R. E., and Vaughan, V. C.: *Nelson Textbook of Pediatrics*, (14th ed). Philadelphia, W.B. Saunders Co., 1992.

IV Flow Rate: Continuous

a. amount of fluid ÷ hours to administer
   = mL/h

b. $\dfrac{mL/h \times gtt/mL \text{ (IV set)}}{60 \text{ min/h}}$ = gtt/min

Example:
Order: 1,000 mL, $D_5/\frac{1}{2}$ NSS in 8 h.
IV set: Macrodrip: 10 gtt/mL.

a. 1,000 mL ÷ 8 h = 125 mL/h

b. $\dfrac{125 \text{ mL/h} \times \overset{1}{\cancel{10}} \text{ gtt/mL}}{\underset{6}{\cancel{60}} \text{ min/h}}$ = 21 gtt/min

IV Flow Rate: Intermittent Secondary Sets: Buretrol and Add-a-Line

$\dfrac{\text{Amount of solution} \times gtt/mL \text{ (set)}}{\text{Minutes to administer}}$ = gtt/min

Order: Administer 5 mL of drug solution in 50 mL of D_5W in 30 min
IV set: Buretrol (60 gtt/mL)

$\dfrac{55 \text{ mL} \times \overset{2}{\cancel{60}} \text{ gtt/mL}}{\underset{1}{\cancel{30}} \text{ min}}$ = 110 gtt/min

IV Flow Rate: Intermittent Volumetric Pump

Amount of solution ÷ $\dfrac{\text{minutes to administer}}{60 \text{ min/h}}$ = mL/h

Order: Administer 5 mL of drug solution in 100 mL of D_5W in 45 min

$105 \text{ mL} \div \dfrac{45 \text{ min}}{60 \text{ min/h}}$ (Invert divisor and multiply)

$= 105 \times \dfrac{\overset{4}{\cancel{60}}}{\underset{3}{\cancel{45}}} = 140 \text{ mL/h}$

Set volumetric pump at 140 mL/h to deliver 105 mL in 45 min.

Discoloration of Urine Due to Drugs

Black
Cascara
Ferrous salts
Iron dextran
Levodopa
Methocarbamol
Methyldopa
Naphthalene
Phenacetin
Phenols
Quinine
Sulfonamides

Blue
Anthraquinone
Indigo blue
Indigo carmine
Methocarbamol
Methylene blue
Nitrofurans
Triamterene

Blue-Green
Amitriptyline
Anthraquinone
Indigo blue
Indigo carmine
Methylene blue

Brown
Anthraquinone dyes
Cascara
Levodopa
Methocarbamol
Methyldopa
Metronidazole
Nitrofurans
Nitrofurantoin
Phenacetin
Primaquine
Quinine
Rifampin
Senna
Sodium diatrizoate
Sulfonamides

Brown-Black
Quinine

Yellow-Brown
Cascara
Chloroquine
Methylene blue
Metronidazole
Nitrofurantoin
Primaquine
Quinacrine
Senna
Sulfonamides

Dark
Cascara
Levodopa
Metronidazole
Nitrites
Primaquine
Quinine
Senna

Green
Anthraquinone
Indigo blue
Indigo carmine
Indomethacin
Methocarbamol
Methylene blue
Nitrofurans
Phenols

Green-Yellow
Methylene blue

Milky
Phosphates

Orange
Chlorzoxazone
Dihydroergotamine
  mesylate
Heparin sodium
Rifampin
Sulfasalazine
Warfarin

Orange-Red
Chlorzoxazone
Doxidan
Rifampin

Orange-Yellow
Fluorescein sodium
Rifampin
Sulfasalazine

Pink
Anthraquinone dyes
Danthron
Deferoxamine
Phenolphthalein
Phenothiazines
Phenytoin
Salicylates

Yellow-Pink
Cascara
Senna

Red
Anthraquinone
Cascara
Daunorubicin
Dimethylsulfoxide
DMSO
Doxorubicin
Heparin
Ibuprofen
Methyldopa
Oxyphenbutazone
Phenacetin
Phenolphthalein
Phenothiazines
Phenylbutazone
Phenytoin
Rifampin
Senna

Red-Brown
Cascara
Methyldopa
Oxyphenbutazone
Phenacetin
Phenolphthalein
Phenothiazines
Phenylbutazone
Phenytoin
Quinine

Red-Purple
Chlorzoxazone
Ibuprofen
Phenacetin
Senna

Rust
Cascara
Chloroquine
Metronidazole
Nitrofurantoin
Phenacetin
Riboflavin
Senna
Sulfonamides

Yellow
Nitrofurantoin
Phenacetin
Sulfasalazine

Adapted from *Drugdex®—Drug Consults, Micromedex, vol 62*. Denver, CO: Rocky Mountain Drug Consultation Center, November 1989. Published by Lexi-Comp Inc. for Medical Center of Delaware: *Formulary and Drug Therapy Guide, 1993–1994*. With permission.

Discoloration of Feces Due to Drugs

Black
Acetazolamide
Alcohols
Alkalies
Aminophylline
Amphetamine
Amphotericin
Antacids
Anticoagulants
Aspirin
Betamethasone
Charcoal
Chloramphenicol
Chlorpropamide
Clindamycin
Corticosteroids
Cortisone
Cyclophosphamide
Cytarabine
Dicumarol
Digitalis
Ethacrynic acid
Ferrous salts
Floxuridine
Fluorouracil
Halothane
Heparin
Hydralazine
Hydrocortisone
Ibuprofen
Indomethacin
Iodine drugs
Iron salts
Levarterenol
Levodopa
Manganese
Melphalan
Methylprednisolone
Methotrexate
Methylene blue
Oxyphenbutazone
Paraldehyde
Phenacetin
Phenolphthalein
Phenylbutazone
Phenylephrine
Phosphorus
Potassium salts
Prednisolone
Procarbazine
Reserpine
Salicylates
Sulfonamides
Tetracycline
Theophylline
Thiotepa
Triamcinolone
Warfarin

Blue
Chloramphenicol
Methylene blue

Dark Brown
Dexamethasone

Gray
Colchicine

Green
Indomethacin
Iron
Medroxyprogesterone

Green-Gray
Oral antibiotics
Oxyphenbutazone
Phenylbutazone

Light Brown
Anticoagulants

Orange-Red
Phenazopyridine
Rifampin

Pink
Anticoagulants
Aspirin
Heparin
Oxyphenbutazone
Phenylbutazone
Salicylates

Red
Anticoagulants
Aspirin
Heparin
Oxyphenbutazone
Phenolphthalein
Phenylbutazone
Salicylates
Tetracycline syrup

Red-Brown
Oxyphenbutazone
Phenylbutazone
Rifampin

Tarry
Ergot preparations
Ibuprofen
Salicylates
Warfarin

White/Speckling
Aluminum hydroxide
Antibiotics (oral)
Indocyanine green

Yellow
Senna

Yellow-Green
Senna

Adapted from *Drugdex®—Drug Consults, Micromedex, vol 62*. Denver, CO: Rocky Mountain Drug Consultation Center, November 1989. Published by Lexi-Comp Inc. for Medical Center of Delaware: *Formulary and Drug Therapy Guide, 1993–1994*. With permission.

THERAPEUTIC DRUG MONITORING (TDM)*

Selective drugs are monitored by serum and urine for the purpose of achieving and maintaining therapeutic drug effect and for preventing drug toxicity. Drugs with a wide therapeutic range (window), the difference between effective dose and toxic dose, are not usually monitored. Drug monitoring is important in maintaining a drug concentration-response relationship, especially when the serum drug range (window) is narrow, such as with digoxin and lithium. Therapeutic drug monitoring (TDM) is the process of following drug levels and adjusting drug doses to maintain a therapeutic level. Not all drugs can be dosed and/or monitored by their blood levels alone.

Drug levels are obtained at peak time and trough time after a steady state of the drug has occurred in the client. Steady state is reached after four or five half-lives of a drug and can be reached sooner if the drug has a short half-life. Once steady state is achieved, serum drug level is checked at the peak level (maximum drug concentration) and/or at trough/residual level (minimum drug concentration). If the trough or residual level is at the high therapeutic point, toxicity might occur. Careful assessment is needed by both physical and laboratory means.

TDM is required for drugs with a narrow therapeutic index or range (window); when other methods for monitoring drugs are noneffective, such as blood pressure (BP) monitoring; for determining when adequate blood concentrations are reached; for evaluating client's compliance to drug therapy; for determining whether other drugs have altered serum drug levels (increased or decreased) that could result in drug toxicity or lack of therapeutic effect; and for establishing new serum-drug level when dosage is changed.

Drug groups for TDM include analgesics, antibiotics, anticonvulsants, antineoplastics, bronchodilators, cardiac drugs, hypoglycemics, sedatives, and tranquilizers. To effectively conduct TDM, the laboratory must be provided with the following information: the drug name and daily dosage, time and amount of last dose, time blood was drawn, route of administration, and client's age. Without complete information, serum drug reporting might be incorrect.

*Revised by Ronald J. Lefever, RPh, Pharmacy Services, Medical College of Virginia, Richmond, VA.

Drug	Therapeutic Range	Peak Time	Toxic Level
Acetaminophen (Tylenol)	10–20 µg/mL	1–2.5 h	>50 µg/mL Hepatotoxicity: >200 µg/mL
Acetohexamide (Dymelor)	20–70 µg/mL (should be dosed according to blood glucose levels)	2–4 h	>75 µg/mL
Alcohol	Negative		Mild toxic: 150 mg/dL Marked toxic: >250 mg/L
Alprazolam (Xanax)	10–50 ng/mL	1–2 h	>75 ng/mL
Amikacin (Amikin)	Peak: 20–30 µg/mL Trough: ≤10 µg/mL	IV: ½ hour IM: 0.5–1.5 h	Peak: >35 µg/mL Trough: >10 µg/mL
Aminocaproic acid (Amicar)	100–400 µg/mL	1 h	>400 µg/mL
Aminophylline (see Theophylline)			
Amiodarone (Cordarone)	0.5–2.5 µg/mL	2–10 h	>2.5 µg/mL
Amitriptyline (Elavil)	125–200 ng/mL	2–12 h	>500 ng/mL
Amobarbital (Amytal)	1–5 µg/mL	2 h	>15 µg/mL Severe toxicity: >30 µg/mL
Amoxapine (Asendin)	200–400 ng/mL	1.5 h	>500 ng/mL
Amphetamine:			
Serum	20–30 ng/mL		0.2 µg/mL
Urine		Detectable in urine after 3 h; positive for 24–48 h	>30 µg/mL urine
Aspirin (see Salicylates)			
Atenolol (Tenormin)	200–500 ng/mL	2–4 h	>500 ng/mL
Bromide	20–80 mg/dL		>100 mg/dL
Butabarbital (Butisol)	1–2 µg/mL	3–4 h	>10 µg/mL
Caffeine	Adult: 3–15 µg/mL Infant: 8–20 µg/mL	0.5–1 h	>50 µg/mL
Carbamazepine (Tegretol)	4–12 µg/mL	6 h (Range 2–24 h)	>9–15 µg/mL
Chloral hydrate (Noctec)	2–12 µg/mL	1–2 h	>20 µg/mL

continued

Drug	Therapeutic Range	Peak Time	Toxic Level
Chloramphenicol (Chloromycetin)	10–20 mg/L		>25 mg/L
Chlordiazepoxide (Librium)	1–5 μg/mL	2–3 h	>5 μg/mL
Chlorpromazine (Thorazine)	50–300 ng/mL	2–4 h	>750 ng/mL
Chlorpropamide (Diabinese)	75–250 μg/mL	3–6 h	>250–750 μg/mL
Clonidine (Catapres)	0.2–2.0 ng/mL (hypotensive effect)	2–5 h	>2.0 ng/mL
Clorazepate (Tranxene)	0.12–1.0 μg/mL	1–2 h	>1.0 μg/mL
Cimetidine (Tagamet)	Trough: 0.5–1.2 μg/mL	1–1.5 h	Trough: >1.5 μg/mL
Clonazepam (Klonopin)	10–60 ng/mL	2 h	>80 ng/mL
Codeine	10–100 ng/mL	1–2 h	>200 ng/mL
Dantrolene (Dantrium)	1–3 μg/mL	5 h	>5 μg/mL
Desipramine (Norpramin)	125–300 ng/mL	4–6 h	>400 ng/mL
Diazepam (Valium)	0.5–2 mg/L 400–600 ng/mL Therapeutic	1–2 h	>3 mg/L >3000 ng/mL
Digitoxin (Rarely administered)	10–25 ng/mL	Noticeable: 2–4 h Peak: 12–24 h	>30 ng/mL
Digoxin	0.5–2 ng/mL	PO:6–8 h IV: 1.5–2 h	2–3 ng/mL
Dilantin (see Phenytoin)			
Diltiazem (Cardizem)	50–200 ng/mL	2–3 h	>200 ng/mL
Disopyramide (Norpace)	2–4 μg/mL	2 h	>4 μg/mL
Doxepin (Sinequan)	150–300 ng/mL	2–4 h	>500 ng/mL
Ethchlorvynol (Placidyl)	2–8 μg/mL	1–2 h	>20 μg/mL
Ethosuximide (Zarontin)	40–100 μg/mL	2–4 h	>150 μg/mL
Flecainide (Tambocor)	0.2–1.0 μg/mL	3 h	>1.0 μg/mL
Flurazepam (Dalmane)	20–110 ng/mL		>1500 ng/mL
Gentamicin (Garamycin)	Peak: 6–12 μg/mL Trough: <2 μg/mL	IV: 15–30 min	Peak: >12 μg/mL Trough: >2 μg/mL
Glutethimide (Doriden)	2–6 μg/mL	1–2 h	>20 μg/mL

continued

Drug	Therapeutic Range	Peak Time	Toxic Level
Haloperidol (Haldol)	5–15 ng/mL	2–6 h	>50 ng/mL
Hydromorphone (Dilaudid)	1–30 ng/mL	0.5–1.5 h	>100 ng/mL
Ibuprofen (Motrin, etc)	10–50 μg/mL	1–2 h	>100 μg/mL
Imipramine (Tofranil)	150–300 ng/mL	PO: 1–2 h IM: 0.5 h	>500 mg/mL
Isoniazid (INH, Nydrazid)	1–7 μg/mL (Dose usually adjusted based on liver function tests)	1–2 h	>20 μg/mL
Kanamycin (Kantrex)	Peak: 15–30 μg/mL Trough: 1–4 μg/mL	PO: 1–2 h IM: 0.5–1 h	Peak: >35 μg/mL Trough: >10 μg/mL
Lead	<20 μg/dL Urine: >80 μg/24 h		>80 μg/dL Urine: >125 μg/24 h
Lidocaine (Xylocaine)	1.5–5 μg/mL	IV: 10 min	>6 μg/mL
Lithium	0.8–1.2 mEq/L	0.5–4 h	1.5 mEq/L
Lorazepam (Ativan)	50–240 ng/mL	1–3 h	>300 ng/mL
Maprotiline (Ludiomil)	200–300 ng/mL	12 h	>500 ng/mL
Meperidine (Demerol)	0.4–0.7 μg/mL	2–4 h	>1.0 μg/mL
Mephenytoin (Mesantoin)	15–40 μg/mL	2–4 h	>50 μg/mL
Meprobamate (Equanil, Miltown)	15–25 μg/mL	2 h	>50 μg/mL
Methadone (Dolophine)	100–400 ng/mL	0.5–1 h	>2,000 ng/mL or >0.2 μg/mL
Methyldopa (Aldomet)	1–5 μg/mL	3–6 h	>7 μg/mL
Methyprylon (Noludar)	8–10 μg/mL	1–2 h	>50 μg/mL
Metoprolol (Lopressor)	75–200 ng/mL	2–4 h	>225 ng/mL
Mexiletine (Mexitil)	0.5–2 μg/mL	2–3 h	>2 μg/mL
Morphine	10–80 ng/mL	IV: Immediately IM: 0.5–1 h SC: 1–1.5 h	>200 ng/mL
Netilmicin (Netromycin)	Peak: 0.5–10 μg/mL Trough: <4 μg/mL	IV: 0.5 h	Peak: >16 μg/mL Trough: >4 μg/mL
Nifedipine (Procardia)	50–100 ng/mL	0.5–2 h	>100 ng/mL
Nortriptyline (Aventyl)	50–150 ng/mL	8 h	>200 ng/ml
Oxazepam (Serax)	0.2–1.4 μg/mL	1–2 h	—
Oxycodone (Percodan)	10–100 ng/mL	0.5–1 h	>200 ng/mL

Drug	Therapeutic Range	Peak Time	Toxic Level
Pentazocine (Talwin)	0.05–0.2 μg/mL	1–2 h	>1.0 μg/mL Urine: >30 μg/mL
Pentobarbital (Nembutal)	1–5 μg/mL	0.5–1 h	>10 μg/mL Severe toxicity: >30 μg/mL
Phenmetrazine (Preludin)	5–30 μg/mL (urine)	2 h	>50 μg/mL (urine)
Phenobarbital (Luminal)	15–40 μg/mL	6–18 h	>40 μg/mL Severe toxicity: >80 μg/mL
Phenytoin (Dilantin)	10–20 μg/mL	4–8 h	>20–30 μg/mL Severe toxicity: >40 μg/mL
Pindolol (Visken)	0.5–6.0 ng/mL	2–4 h	>10 ng/mL
Primidone (Mysoline)	5–12 μg/mL	2–4 h	>12–15 μg/mL
Procainamide (Pronestyl)	4–10 μg/mL	1 h	>10 μg/mL
Procaine (Novocain)	<11 μg/mL	10–30 min	>20 μg/mL
Prochlorperazine (Compazine)	50–300 ng/mL	2–4 h	>1,000 ng/mL
Propoxyphene (Darvon)	0.1–0.4 μg/mL	2–3 h	>0.5 μg/mL
Propranolol (Inderal)	>100 ng/mL	1–2 h	>150 ng/mL
Protriptyline (Vivactil)	50–150 ng/mL	8–12 h	>200 ng/mL
Quinidine	2–5 μg/mL	1–3 h	>6 μg/mL
Ranitidine (Zantac)	100 ng/mL	2–3 h	>100 ng/mL
Reserpine (Serpasil)	20 ng/mL	2–4 h	>20 ng/mL
Salicylates (Aspirin)	10–30 mg/dL	1–2 h	Tinnitis: >20–40 mg/mL Hyperventilation: >35 mg/dL Severe toxicity: >50 mg/dL
Secobarbital (Seconal)	2–5 μg/mL	1 h	>15 μg/mL Severe toxicity: >30 μg/mL
Theophylline (Thodur, Aminodur)	10–20 μg/mL	PO: 2–3 h IV: 15 min (Depends on smoking or nonsmoking)	>20 μg/mL
Thioridazine (Mellaril)	100–600 ng/mL 1.0–1.5 μg/mL	2–4 h	>2,000 ng/mL >10 μg/mL

Drug	Therapeutic Range	Peak Time	Toxic Level
Timolol (Blocadren)	3–55 ng/mL	1–2 h	>60 ng/mL
Tobramycin (Nebcin)	Peak: 5–10 µg/mL Trough: 1–1.5 µg/mL	IV: 15–30 min IM: 0.5–1.5 h	Peak: >12 µg/mL Trough: >2 µg/mL
Tocainide (Tonocard)	4–10 µg/mL	0.5–3 h	>12 µg/mL
Tolbutamide (Orinase)	80–240 µg/mL	3–5 h	>640 µg/mL
Trazodone (Desyrel)	500–2500 ng/mL	1–2 wk	>4,000 ng/mL
Trifluoperazine (Stelazine)	50–300 ng/mL	2–4 h	>1,000 ng/mL
Valproic acid (Depakene)	50–100 µg/mL	0.5–1.5 h	>100 µg/mL Severe toxicity: >150 µg/mL
Vancomycin (Vanocin)	Peak: 20–40 µg/mL Trough: 5–10 µg/mL	IV: Peak: 5 min IV: Trough: 12 h	Peak: >80 µg/mL
Verapamil (Calan)	100–300 ng/mL	PO: 1–2 h IV: 5 min	>500 ng/mL
Warfarin (Coumadin)	1–10 µg/mL (Dose usually adjusted by 1 to 2.5 × control)	1.5–3 d	>10 µg/mL

Source: Kee, J. L. (1995): *Laboratory and Diagnostic Tests With Nursing Implications* (4th ed). Norwalk, CT: Appleton and Lange. (Used with permission.)

PHARMACOLOGY

**Pocket
Companion
for Nurses**

VITAMINS, MINERALS, AND ELECTROLYTES

Vitamin A, Fat-Soluble

Antianemia, Mineral: Iron

Electrolyte:
  Potassium
  Calcium

Vitamin A, fat-soluble

Vitamin A	Dosage
Vitamin A (Acon, Aquasol A) Fat-soluble vitamin *Pregnancy Category:* A *Drug Forms:* Liquid (gtt) 5,000 U/0.1 mL Cap 50,000 U Inj 50,000 U/mL	A & C > 8 y: PO: 100,000–500,000 IU daily × 3 d; then 50,000 daily × 14 d *Maintenance:* 10,000–20,000 IU q.d. × 60 d C 1–8 y: IM: 17,000–35,000 IU daily × 10 d *Maintenance:* 4–8 y: 15,000 daily × 60 d 1–<4 y: 10,000 IU daily × 60 d

Contraindications	Drug-Lab-Food Interactions
Hypervitaminosis A, pregnancy (massive doses)	Decreased absorption of mineral oil, cholestyramine, oral contraceptives, corticosteroids

Pharmacokinetics	Pharmacodynamics

Absorption: PO: 1 h
Distribution: PB: UK
Metabolism: t 1/2: weeks–months
Excretion: Urine and feces
	PO: Onset: 1–2 h
	     Peak: 4–5 h
	     Duration: UK

Therapeutic Effects/Uses: To treat vitamin A deficiency, prevent night blindness, treat skin disorders, promote bone development

Mode of action: Essential for growth, bone and teeth development, vision, integrity of skin and mucous membrane, and reproduction

Side Effects	Adverse Reactions
Headache, fatigue, drowsiness, irritability, anorexia, vomiting, diarrhea, dry skin, visual changes	Evident only with toxicity: leukopenia, aplastic anemia, papilledema, increased intracranial pressure, hypervitaminosis A

KEY: For complete abbreviation key, see inside front cover.

■ **NURSING PROCESS: Vitamin A**

ASSESSMENT
- Assess the client for vitamin A deficiency before start of and regularly throughout therapy. Explore such areas as inadequate nutrient intake, debilitating disease, and GI disorders.
- Assess 24–48-h diet history for foods rich in vitamin A.

POTENTIAL NURSING DIAGNOSIS
- Altered nutrition; less than body requirements

PLANNING
- Client will eat a well-balanced diet that includes the foods and servings recommended in the food pyramid.
- Client with vitamin deficiency will take vitamin supplements as prescribed.

NURSING INTERVENTIONS
- Administer vitamin A with food to promote absorption.
- Store drug in light-resistant container.
- When administering drop form, use the supplied calibrated dropper for accurate dosage. Solution may be administered mixed with food or dropped into the mouth.
- Administer IM primarily for clients unable to take by PO route (e.g., GI malabsorption syndrome).
- Recognize need for vitamin E supplements for infants receiving vitamin A to avoid hemolytic anemia.

CLIENT TEACHING

General
- Instruct client to take the prescribed amount of drug.
- Discourage the client from taking megavitamins over a long period unless these are prescribed for a specific purpose by the health care provider. To discontinue long-term megavitamin therapy, a gradual decrease in vitamin intake is advised to avoid a vitamin deficiency. Megadoses of vitamin A can be toxic.
- Inform the client that missing vitamins for 1 or 2 d is not a cause for concern because deficiencies do not occur for some time.
- Advise the client to check the expiration dates on vitamin containers before purchasing and taking them. Potency of the vitamin is reduced after the expiration date.
- Instruct the client to avoid taking mineral oil with vitamin A on a regular basis because it interferes with the absorption of the vitamin. If needed, take mineral oil at bedtime.

Diet
- Advise the client to eat a well-balanced diet that includes the recommended amounts and types of food detailed in the food pyramid. Vitamin supplements are not necessary if the person is healthy and receives proper nutrition on a regular basis.
- Instruct the client about foods rich in vitamin A, including whole milk, butter, eggs, leafy green and yellow vegetables, fruits, and liver.

Side Effects
- Instruct the client that nausea, vomiting, headache, loss of hair, and cracked lips (symptoms of hypervitaminosis A) should be reported to health care provider.

EVALUATION
- Evaluate the effectiveness of the client's diet for the inclusion of the appropriate amounts and types of food from the food pyramid. Have client keep periodic diet chart for a complete week.
- Determine if the client with malnutrition is receiving appropriate vitamin therapy.

Vitamins: Functions, Suggested Food Sources, and Selected Deficiency Conditions

Vitamin (Adult RDA)	Function	Food Sources	Deficiency Conditions
A (800–1000 μg)	Required to develop and maintain healthy eyes, gums, teeth, skin, hair, and selected glands. Needed for fat metabolism.	Whole milk, butter, eggs, leafy green and yellow vegetables,* fruits, liver	Dry skin, poor tooth development, night blindness
B_1 (thiamine) (1.0–1.5 mg)	Promotes use of sugars (energy). Required for good function of nervous system and heart.	Enriched breads and cereals, yeast, liver, pork, fish, milk	Sensory disturbances, retarded growth, fatigue, anorexia
B_2 (riboflavin) (1.2–1.7 mg)	Promotes body's use of carbohydrates, proteins, and fats by releasing energy to cells. Required for tissue integrity.	Milk, enriched breads and cereals, liver, lean meat, eggs, leafy green vegetables†	Visual defects, such as blurred vision and photophobia; cheilosis; rash on nose; numbness of extremities
B_3 (pyridoxine) (1.6–2 mg)	Important in metabolism, synthesis of proteins, and formation of RBCs	Lean meat, leafy green vegetables, whole-grain cereals, yeast, bananas	Neuritis, convulsions, dermatitis, anemia, lymphopenia
B_{12} (cobalamin) (2.0 mg)	Functions as a building block of nucleic acids and to form RBCs. Facilitates functioning of nervous system.	Liver, kidney, fish, milk	Gastrointestinal disorders, poor growth, anemias
Biotin (no RDA)	Synthesis of fatty acids and energy production from glucose. Required by body chemical systems.	Eggs, milk, leafy green vegetables, liver, kidney.	Natural deficiency unknown in humans

Vitamin (RDA)	Function	Sources	Deficiency
C (ascorbic acid) (60 mg)	Helps tissue repair and growth. Required in formation of collagen.	Citrus fruits, tomatoes, leafy green vegetables, potatoes	Poor wound healing, bleeding gums, scurvy, predisposition to infection
D calciferol (5 μg)	Promotes use of phosphorus and calcium. Important for strong teeth and bones.	Vitamin D–fortified milk, egg yolk, tuna, salmon	Rickets, deficit of phosphorus and calcium in blood
E tocopherol (8–10 mg)	Protects fatty acids and promotes the formation and functioning of RBCs, muscle, and other tissues.	Whole-grain cereals, wheat germ, vegetable oils, lettuce	Breakdown of RBCs
Folic acid‡ (180–200 μg)	Helps in formation of genetic materials and proteins for the cell nucleus. Assists with intestinal functioning and prevents selected anemias.	Leafy green vegetables, yellow fruits and vegetables, yeast, meats	Decreased WBC count and clotting factors, anemias, intestinal disturbances, depression
K (60–80 μg)	Essential for blood clotting.	Leafy green vegetables, liver, cheese, egg yolk	Increased clotting time, leading to increased bleeding and hemorrhage
Niacin (13–19 mg)	In all body tissues. Necessary for energy-producing reactions. Assists nervous system.	Eggs, meat, liver, beans, peas, enriched bread, and cereals	Retarded growth, pellegra, headache, memory loss, anorexia, insomnia
Pantothenic acid (no RDA)	Promotes body's use of carbohydrates, fats, and proteins. Essential for formation of specific hormones and nerve-regulating substances.	Eggs, leafy green vegetables, nuts, liver, kidney, skimmed milk	Natural deficiency unknown in humans

RDAs are daily nutrient allowances recommended for healthy adults by the National Research Council, American Institute for Cancer Research.
*Yellow fruits and vegetables include apricots, cantaloupe, carrots, rutabaga, pumpkin, squash, and sweet potatoes.
†Leafy green vegetables include brussel spouts, chard, broccoli, kale, spinach, and turnip and mustard greens.
‡Women of childbearing age should consume 400 μg/d of folic acid.

Antianemia, Mineral: Iron

Iron

Ferrous sulfate (Feosol, Fer-Iron)
Ferrous gluconate (Fergon, Fetinic)
Ferrous fumarate (Feostat, Fumerin)
Mineral
Pregnancy Category: A
Drug Forms:
Sulfate
Tab 195, 300, 325 mg
Tab, enteric-coated 325 mg
Tab, extended-release 525 mg
Cap, time-release 525 mg

Dosage

A: PO: 300–325 mg q.i.d.: increase to
650 mg q.i.d. as needed and/or
tolerated
Pregnancy: PO: 300–600 mg/d
C ≥2 y: PO: 8 mg/kg q.d. in divided
doses

Contraindications

Hemolytic anemia, peptic ulcer,
ulcerative colitis

Drug-Lab-Food Interactions

Increased effect of iron with vitamin
C; *decreased* effect of tetracycline,
antacids, penicillamine

Pharmacokinetics

Absorption: PO: 5–30%
intestines
Distribution: PB: UK
Metabolism: t 1/2: UK
Excretion: Urine, feces, bile

Pharmacodynamics

PO: Onset: 4 d
Peak: 7–14 d
Duration: 3–4 mon

Therapeutic Effects/Uses: To prevent and treat iron deficiency anemia
Mode of Action: Enables RBC development and oxygen transport via hemoglobin

Side Effects:

Nausea, vomiting, diarrhea,
constipation, epigastric pain; elixir
may stain teeth

Adverse Reactions:

Pallor, drowsiness
Life-Threatening: Cardiovascular
collapse, metabolic acidosis

KEY: For complete abbreviation key, see inside front cover.

■ NURSING PROCESS: Antianemia, Mineral: Iron

ASSESSMENT

- Obtain a history of anemia or health problems that may lead to anemia.
- Assess the client for signs and symptoms of iron deficiency anemia, such as fatigue, malaise, pallor, shortness of breath, tachycardia, and cardiac dysrhythmia.
- Assess the client's RBC count, hemoglobin, hematocrit, iron level, and reticulocyte count before start of and throughout drug therapy.

POTENTIAL NURSING DIAGNOSIS

- Fatigue
- Altered nutrition; less than body requirements

PLANNING

- Client will consume foods rich in iron.
- Client with iron deficiency anemia or with low hemoglobin will take iron replacement as recommended by the health care provider, resulting in laboratory results within the desired range.

NURSING INTERVENTIONS

- Encourage the client to eat a nutritious diet to obtain sufficient iron. Iron supplements are not needed unless the person is malnourished or pregnant.
- Store drug in light-resistant container.
- Administer IM injection of iron by the Z-track method to avoid leakage of iron into the subcutaneous tissue and skin because it irritates and stains the skin.

CLIENT TEACHING

General

- Instruct the client to take the tablet or capsule between meals with at least 8 oz of juice or water to promote absorption. If gastric irritation occurs, instruct to take with food.
- Advise client to swallow whole the tablet or capsule.
- Instruct client to maintain sitting upright position for 30 min to prevent esophageal corrosion from reflux.
- Do not administer the drug within 1 h of ingesting antacid or milk.
- Advise client to increase fluids, activity, and dietary bulk to avoid or relieve constipation. Slow-release iron capsules decrease constipation and gastric irritation.
- Instruct adults not to leave iron tablets within reach of children. If a child swallows many tablets, induce vomiting and immediately call the local poison control center; the telephone number is in the front of most telephone books (include this number on emergency reference list).
- Instruct client to take prescribed amount of drug to avoid iron poisoning.
- Be alert that iron content varies among iron salts; therefore, do not substitute one for another.
- Advise client that drug treatment for anemia is generally less than 6 mon.

Diet

- Counsel the client to include iron-rich foods in diet, such as liver, lean meats, egg yolk, dried beans, green vegetables, and fruit.

Side Effects

- Instruct the client taking the liquid iron preparation to use a straw to prevent discoloration of teeth enamel.
- Alert the client that the drug turns stools a harmless black or dark green.
- Instruct client about signs and symptoms of toxicity, including nausea, vomiting, diarrhea, pallor, hematemesis, shock, and coma, and report occurrence to health care provider.

EVALUATION

- Evaluate the effectiveness of the drug therapy by determining that the client is not fatigued or short of breath and that the hemoglobin is within the desired range.

Electrolyte: Potassium

Potassium

Potassium chloride
   (Kaochlor, Kaon-Cl, Kay Ciel,
   Micro-K, K-Dur)
Potassium replacement
Pregnancy Category: A
Drug Forms:
Tablet, SR cap, elixir, liq mEq/5 mL
   Inj (mEq/mL): All in various doses

Dosage

A: *Hypokalemia (maintenance):*
PO: 20 mEq in 1–2 divided doses
Hypokalemia (correction):
PO: 40–80 mEq in 3–4 divided doses
IV: 20–40 mEq diluted in 1L of IV
   solution

Contraindications

Renal insufficiency or failure,
   Addison's disease, hyperkalemia,
   severe dehydration, acidosis,
   potassium-sparing diuretics
Caution:
Cardiac disorders, burns

Drug-Lab-Food Interactions

Increase serum potassium level with
   ACE inhibitors, potassium-sparing
   diuretics
Lab: May *increase* serum potassium
   level (>5.5 mEq/L)

Pharmacokinetics

Absorption: PO: rapidly absorbed,
   95% in body fluids
Distribution: PB: UK
Metabolism: t 1/2: UK
Excretion: 80–90% in urine; 10% in
   feces

Pharmacodynamics

PO: Onset: 30 min
       Peak: 1–2 h
       Duration: UK
IV: Onset: Rapid
       Peak: 1–1.5 h
       Duration: UK

Therapeutic Effects/Uses: To correct potassium deficit; strengthen cardiac and muscular activities

Mode of Action: Transmits and conducts nerve impulses; contracts skeletal, smooth,
and cardiac muscles

Side Effects:

Nausea, vomiting, diarrhea,
   abdominal cramps, irritability, rash
   (rare)

Adverse Reactions:

Oliguria, ECG changes (peaked T
   waves, widened QRS complex,
   prolonged PR interval), GI
   ulceration
Life-threatening: Cardiac
   dysrhythmias, respiratory distress,
   cardiac arrest

KEY: For complete abbreviation key, see inside front cover.

■ NURSING PROCESS: Electrolyte: Potassium

ASSESSMENT

• Assess for signs and symptoms of hypokalemia (decreased serum potassium) and hyperkalemia (elevated serum potassium). Symptoms of hypokalemia include nausea, vomiting, cardiac dysrhythmias, abdominal distension, and soft flabby muscles. Symptoms of hyperkalemia include oliguria, nausea, abdominal cramps, and tachycardia and, later, bradycardia, weakness, and numbness or tingling in the extremities.

• Assess serum potassium level; normal serum potassium level is 3.5–5.3 mEq/L. Report serum potassium deficit or excess to the physician or health care prescriber.

• Obtain baseline VS and ECG readings. Report abnormal findings. The VS and ECG results can be compared with future VS and ECG readings.

• Assess the client for signs and symptoms of digitalis toxicity when receiving a digitalis preparation (digoxin) and a potassium-wasting diuretic (chlorohydrothiazide, furosemide) or a cortisone preparation (prednisone). A decreased serum potassium level enhances the action of digitalis. Signs and symptoms of digitalis toxicity are nausea, vomiting, anorexia, bradycardia (pulse rate <60 or markedly decreased), cardiac dysrhythmias, and visual disturbances.

POTENTIAL NURSING DIAGNOSIS

• Altered nutrition, less than body requirements.
• Impaired tissue integrity.

PLANNING

• Client's serum potassium level will be within normal range in 2–4 d.
• Client with hypokalemia will eat foods rich in potassium, such as fruits, fruit juices, and vegetables. Client with hyperkalemia will avoid potassium-rich foods.

NURSING INTERVENTIONS

• Give oral potassium with a sufficient amount of water or juice (at least 6–8 oz) or at mealtime. Potassium is extremely irritating to the gastric mucosa.

• Dilute IV potassium chloride in the IV bag and invert the bag several times to promote thorough mixing of potassium with IV fluids. Potassium CANNOT be given IM. **Potassium should never be given as an IV bolus or push.** Giving IV potassium directly into the vein causes cardiac dysrhythmias and cardiac arrest.

• Monitor the amount of urine output. If the client is receiving potassium and the urine output is <25 mL/h or <600 mL/d, potassium accumulation occurs. Remember, 80–90% of potassium is excreted in the urine. Report results to the health care provider.

• Monitor the serum potassium level. Hypokalemia occurs if the serum potassium value is <3.5 mEq/L; hyperkalemia occurs when the serum potassium value is >5.3 mEq/L.

• Monitor the ECG. With hypokalemia, the T wave is flat or inverted, the ST segment is depressed, and the QT interval is prolonged. With hyperkalemia, the T wave is narrow and peaked, the QRS complex is spread, and the PR interval is prolonged.

• Check the IV site for infiltration if the client is receiving potassium in the IV fluids. Potassium can cause tissue necrosis if it infiltrates into the fatty

tissue (subcutaneous tissue). The IV fluid with potassium should be discontinued when infiltration occurs.
• Monitor clients receiving various medications for hyperkalemia, such as sodium bicarbonate, calcium gluconate, insulin and glucose, and Kayexalate and sorbitol, for signs and symptoms of continuing hyperkalemia or of developing hypokalemia.
• Prepare and administer Kayexalate orally or by retention enema. Prepare according to the drug circular. The client should have a cleansing enema before the retention enema.

CLIENT TEACHING

General

• Advise the client to have serum potassium level checked at regular intervals when taking drugs that are potassium supplements or that decrease potassium levels.
• Instruct the client to drink a full glass of water or juice when taking oral potassium supplements. Potassium preparations can be taken during or after a meal. Explain to the client that potassium is very irritating to the stomach.
• Instruct the client to comply with the prescribed potassium dose, regular laboratory tests, and medical follow-up related to the health problem and drug regimen.

Diet

• Instruct the client who is taking a potassium-wasting diuretic or a cortisone preparation to eat potassium-rich foods, including citrus fruit juice, fruits (bananas, plums, oranges, canteloupes, raisins), vegetables, and nuts.

Side Effects

• Instruct the client to report signs and symptoms of hypokalemia and hyperkalemia. See assessment for the list. When taking large amounts of potassium supplements, hyperkalemia could result.

EVALUATION

• Evaluate the client's serum potassium level and ECG. Report to the health care provider if the level remains abnormal. Potassium replacements and diet may need modification.

Electrolyte: Potassium

Selected Potassium Supplements

Preparation	Drug
PO liquid	Potassium chloride: 10% = 20 mEq/15 mL, 20% = 40 mEq/15 mL. Kaochlor 10% (potassium chloride) Kaon-Cl 20% (potassium chloride) Kay Ciel (potassium chloride) Potassium triplex (potassium acetate, bicarbonate, citrate). Rarely used.
PO tablet or capsule	Kaochlor (potassium chloride) Kaon (potassium gluconate) Kaon-Cl (potassium chloride) K-Dur (potassium chloride) K-Lyte (potassium bicarbonate, effervescent tablet) K-Lyte/Cl (potassium chloride) K-Tab (potassium chloride) Micro-K (potassium chloride) Potassium chloride (enteric-coated tablet) Slow-K (potassium chloride, 8 mEq) Ten-K (potassium chloride)
IV potassium	Potassium chloride in clear liquid in multidose vial or ampule (2 mEq/mL)

Electrolyte: Calcium

Calcium

Calcium chloride (IV)

Calcium carbonate
   (Os = cal, Tums, Caltrate, Mega-
   Cal)

Calcium gluconate (Kalcinate)

Calcium lactate

Calcium replacement

Pregnancy Category: C

Drug Forms: Tab, cap, liq, inj

Dosage

Antacid use:
A: PO: 0.5–1 g q4–6h (dose varies
   according to the calcium salt)
Osteoporosis:
A: PO: 1–2 g b.i.d.
   IV: 0.5–1 g q.d., q.o.d.
Tetany:
A: IV 4–16 mEq
C: IV: 0.5–0.7 mEq/kg t.i.d., q.i.d.
Hypocalcemia
C: PO: 500 mg/d in divided doses

Contraindications

Hypercalcemia, renal calculi, digitalis
   toxicity, ventricular fibrillation
Caution:
Renal or respiratory disorders, GI
   hypomotility

Drug-Lab-Food Interactions

Increase digitalis toxicity: digoxin;
   Decrease calcium effect: saline
   solution; *decrease* effect of calcium
   channel blockers, verapamil;
   decrease absorption of tetracycline;
   increase serum calcium level:
   thiazide diuretics

Pharmacokinetics

Absorption: PO: 35% absorbed,
   requires vitamin D
Distribution: PB: UK
Metabolism: t 1/2: UK
Excretion: 20% in urine; 70% in feces,
   some in saliva

Pharmacodynamics

PO: Onset: UK
    Peak: UK
    Duration: 2–4 h
IV: Onset: Rapid
    Peak: UK
    Duration: 2–3 h

Therapeutic Effects/Uses: To correct calcium deficit or tetany symptoms, prevent osteoporosis

Mode of Action: Transmits nerve impulses, contracts skeletal and cardiac muscles, maintains cellular permeability; promotes strong bone and teeth growth

Side Effects:

Nausea, vomiting, constipation, pain,
   drowsiness, headache, muscle
   weakness

Adverse Reactions:

Hypercalcemia, ECG changes
   (shortened QT interval), metabolic
   alkalosis, heart block, rebound
   hyperacidity
Life-threatening: Renal failure, cardiac
   dysrhythmias, cardiac arrest

KEY: For complete abbreviation key, see inside front cover.

■ NURSING PROCESS: Electrolyte: Calcium

ASSESSMENT

• Assess the client for signs and symptoms of hypocalcemia (decreased serum calcium), such as tetany (twitching of the mouth, tingling and numbness of the fingers, facial spasms, spasms of the larynx, and carpopedal spasm), muscle cramps, bleeding tendencies, and weak cardiac contractions.

• Check the serum calcium levels (normal, 4.5–5.5 mEq/L or 8.5–10.5 mg/dL) for hypocalcemia and hypercalcemia. Report abnormal test results. Serum ionized calcium (iCa) indicates free circulating calcium and is more accurate for determining calcium imbalance.

• Obtain VS and ECG readings. Report abnormal findings. VS and ECG results can be compared with future VS and ECG readings.

• Obtain a current drug history for the client. Calcium enhances the effect of digoxin. An elevated serum calcium level (due to excess calcium), when taken with digoxin, can cause digitalis toxicity. Signs and symptoms of digitalis toxicity include nausea, vomiting, anorexia, bradycardia (pulse rate <60 or markedly decreased), cardiac dysrhythmias, and visual disturbances. Thiazide diuretics can increase the serum calcium level. Drugs that decrease the effect of calcium are calcium channel blockers, tetracycline, and sodium chloride.

POTENTIAL NURSING DIAGNOSIS

• Altered nutrition, less than body requirements.
• Impaired tissue integrity.

PLANNING

• Client's serum calcium level will be within normal range by 3–7 d.
• Tetany symptoms will cease. Client will eat foods rich in calcium or take calcium supplements as ordered.
• Client with hypercalcemia will avoid foods rich in calcium, such as milk products.

NURSING INTERVENTIONS

• Monitor VS. Report abnormal findings. Compare with baseline VS. Monitor pulse rate if the client is taking digoxin. Bradycardia is a sign of digitalis toxicity.

• Administer IV fluids slowly with 10% calcium gluconate or chloride. Calcium should be administered with D_5W and not saline solution because sodium promotes calcium loss. Calcium should not be added to solutions containing bicarbonate because rapid precipitation occurs.

• Check IV site for infiltration if the client is receiving calcium in IV fluids. Calcium can cause tissue necrosis (sloughing of the tissue) if it infiltrates into the subcutaneous tissue. Calcium gluceptate is the only calcium preparation that can be given IM.

• Monitor the serum calcium and iCa levels. Hypocalcemia occurs if the serum calcium value is <4.5 mEq/L or <8.5 mg/dL or if iCa is <2.2 mEq/L. Hypercalcemia occurs if the serum calcium value is >5.5 mEq/L or > 10.5 mg/dL or if iCa is >2.5 mEq/L.

• Monitor ECGs. With hypocalcemia, the ST segment is lengthened and the QT interval is prolonged. With hypercalcemia, the ST segment is decreased and the QT interval is shortened.

CLIENT TEACHING

General

• Instruct the client to avoid overuse of antacids and to prevent the habit of chronic use of laxatives. Excessive use of certain antacids may cause alkalosis, decreasing calcium ionization. Chronic use of laxatives decreases calcium absorption from the GI tract. Suggest fruits and foods rich in fiber for improving bowel elimination.

• Instruct the client taking calcium supplements to check that the calcium tablet is absorbable. To do this, put 1 tablet into 1 oz of white vinegar. Stir every 3 min. The tablet should break up or dissolve within 30 min.

• Take oral calcium supplements with meals or after meals to increase absorption.

Diet

• Suggest that the client consume foods high in calcium, such as milk, milk products, and protein-rich foods. Protein and vitamin D are needed to enhance calcium absorption.

Side Effects

• Instruct the client to report symptoms related to calcium excess or hypercalcemia, including flabby muscles, pain over bony areas, ECG changes, and kidney (calcium form) stones.

EVALUATION

• Evaluate the client's serum calcium level. Report if calcium imbalance continues.

• Determine if side effects due to previous untreated hypocalcemia are absent.

CENTRAL NERVOUS SYSTEM STIMULANTS AND DEPRESSANTS

Central Nervous System Stimulants

Sedative-Hypnotics:
  Barbiturates
  Benzodiazepines

Analgesics:
  Aspirin
  Acetaminophen

Narcotics:
  Opiate: Morphine Sulfate
  Nonopiate: Meperidine
  Agonist-Antagonist: Pentazocine
    Lactate

Central Nervous System Stimulant

Methylphenidate HCl

Methylphenidate HCl
    (Ritalin, Ritalin SR)
Cerebral stimulant
CSS II
Pregnancy Category: C
Drug Forms:
Tab 5, 10, 20 mg
Tab SR 20 mg

Dosage

Attention deficit disorder:
C > 6 y: PO: 5 mg before breakfast
    and lunch; if necessary increase
    dosage weekly by 5–10 mg; max:
    60 mg/d
SR not recommended for initial
    treatment
Narcolepsy:
A: PO: 10 mg b.i.d./t.i.d. 30 min
    before meals

Contraindications

Hypersensitivity, hyperthyroidism,
    anxiety, history of seizures or
    Tourette syndrome
Caution: Hypertension, depression,
    pregnancy

Drug-Lab-Food Interactions

Hypertensive crises within 14 days of
    MAOIs
Decrease effects of decongestants,
    antihypertensives, barbiturates
Increase effects of oral anticoagulants,
    anticonvulsants, tricyclic
    antidepressants
Food: Caffeine (coffee, tea, colas,
    chocolate)

Pharmacokinetics

Absorption: PO: well absorbed; SR:
    delayed
Distribution: PB: UK
Metabolism: t 1/2: 1–3 h
Excretion: In urine 40% unchanged

Pharmacodynamics

PO: Onset: 0.5–1 h
    Peak: 1–3 h
    Duration: 4–6 h
PO: Onset: UK
    Peak: UK
    Duration: 4–8 h

Therapeutic Effects/Uses: Adjunct to treatment to correct hyperactivity caused by attention deficit disorder (ADD), to increase attention span, to treat fatigue, and to control narcolepsy.

Mode of Action: Respiratory and CNS stimulation; exact drug action unknown.

Side Effects

Anorexia, restlessness, nervousness,
    headache, dizziness, irritability,
    insomnia, vomiting, diarrhea,
    talkativeness

Adverse Reactions

Tachycardia, palpitations, transient
    loss of weight gain in children,
    growth suppression, increased
    hyperactivity
Life-threatening: Exfoliative
    dermatitis, uremia,
    thrombocytopenia

KEY: For complete abbreviation key, see inside front cover.

■ NURSING PROCESS: Central Nervous System Stimulant: Methylphenidate HCl (Ritalin)

ASSESSMENT

• Determine if there is a history of heart disease, hypertension, hyperthyroidism, or glaucoma; in such cases, drug is usually contraindicated.

Central Nervous System Stimulant

- Assess vital signs to be used for future comparisons. Pay close attention to clients with cardiac disease as drug may reverse effects of antihypertensives.
- Assess the client's mental status: e.g., mood, affect, aggressiveness.
- Assess height, growth, and weight of children.
- Assess CBC, differential WBCs, and platelets before and during therapy.

POTENTIAL NURSING DIAGNOSES
- Behavior disorders (impulsiveness, short attention span, and distractibility) that interfere with peer relationships, learning, and discipline.
- Potential for family crisis related to dysfunctional behavior.

PLANNING
- Client will be free of hyperactivity.
- Client will not experience side effects or adverse reactions to therapy. Child will increase attention span and ability to organize.

NURSING INTERVENTIONS
- Monitor vital signs. Report irregularities.
- Monitor height, weight, and growth of child.
- Monitor the client for withdrawal symptoms, e.g., nausea, vomiting, weakness, headache.
- Monitor the client for side effects, e.g., insomnia, restlessness, nervousness, tremors, irritability, tachycardia, or elevated blood pressure. Report findings.

CLIENT TEACHING
General
- Instruct the client to take drug before meals.
- Instruct the client to avoid alcohol consumption.
- Encourage the use of sugarless gum to relieve dry mouth.
- Instruct the client to monitor weight 2×/wk and to report weight loss.
- Instruct the client to avoid driving and using hazardous equipment when experiencing tremors, nervousness, or increased heart rate.
- Instruct the client not to abruptly discontinue the drug; the dose must be tapered off to avoid withdrawal symptoms. Consult the health care provider before modifying the dose.
- Encourage the client to read the labels on OTC products because many contain caffeine. A high caffeine plasma level could be fatal.
- Instruct the nursing mother to avoid taking all CNS stimulants. These drugs pass into the breast milk and can cause the infant to be "jittery."
- Encourage the family to seek counseling for children with attention deficit disorder. Drug therapy alone is not an appropriate therapy program. Notify school nurse of drug therapy regimen.
- Explain to client/family that long-term use may lead to drug abuse.
Diet
- Instruct the client to avoid caffeine-containing foods.
- Instruct parents to provide children with a good-quality breakfast because drug may have anorexic effects.
Side Effects
- Instruct the client about drug side effects and the need to report tachycardia and palpitations. Monitor children for onset of Tourette syndrome.

EVALUATION
- Evaluate the effectiveness of drug therapy. The client is not hyperactive and does not have adverse effects from drug.
- Monitor weight, sleep patterns, and mental status.

Amphetamines and Amphetaminelike Drug

Generic (Brand)	Route and Dosage	Preg Cat	Interaction	t 1/2	PB	Action		
						Onset	Peak	Duration
Amphetamines Amphetamine sulfate CSS II	A: PO: 5–20 mg q.d.–t.i.d. C > 6 y: PO: 2.5–5 mg daily for ADD; increase dose as needed	C	*Decrease* effects of tricyclic antidepressants, barbiturates; hypertensive crisis within 14 d of MAOIs	10–30 h	UK	30–45 min	1–3 h	4–20 h
Dextroamphetamine sulfate (Dexedrine) CSS II	Same as amphetamine sulfate	C	Similar to amphetamine sulfate	10–30 h	UK	30 min	1–3 h	4–20 h
Methamphetamine HCl (Desoxyn) CSS II	C: PO: 2.5–5 mg daily; increase to 20 mg as needed	C	Similar to amphetamine sulfate	UK	UK	UK	6–12 h	3–6 h
Amphetamine-like Drugs Methylphenidate (Ritalin) CSS II	See Prototype Drug Chart							
Pemoline (Cylert) CSS IV	C > 6 y: PO: 37.5 mg daily and increase weekly; average: 50–75 mg/d	B	*Increase* effects with other CNS stimulants	9–12 h	50%	ADD: days–weeks CNS stimulants: UK	2–3 wk	days
							2–4 h	8 h

Anorexiants

Drug	Dosage	Pregnancy Category	Drug Interactions	Half-Life	Onset	Peak	Duration	
Benzphetamine HCl (Didrex) CSS III	A: PO: 25–50 mg q.d.–t.i.d.	X	Hypertensive crisis may result if given within 14 d of MAOIs *Increase* effects with tricyclic antidepressants	6–12 h	UK	30 min	1–4 h	4–20 h
Dextroamphetamine sulfate (Dexedrine) CSS II	A: PO: 5–30 mg daily in divided doses 30–60 min ac of 5–10 mg	C	*Decrease* effects of tricyclic antidepressants, barbiturates; may have hypertensive crisis within 14 d of MAOIs	30–34 h	UK	30 min	1–3 h	4–20 h
Diethylpropion HCl (Dospan, Tenuate, Tepanil) CSS IV	A: PO: 25 mg t.i.d.; SR: 75 mg daily	B	Hypertensive crisis with MAOIs	2–3 h	UK	UK	UK	4 h SR: 12 h
Fenfluramine HCl (Pondimin) CSS IV	A: PO: 20 mg t.i.d.; max: 120 mg/d	C	Hypertensive crisis with MAOIs *Increase* effects with antacids, bicarbonates *Decrease* effects with tricyclic antidepressants	20 h	UK	1–3 min	2–4 h	4–6 h
Mazindol (Mazanor, Sanorex) CSS IV	A: PO: 1 mg t.i.d. ac or 2 mg daily	C	Similar to fenfluramine	2.5–9 h	UK	30–60 min	UK	10–15 h
Phendimetrazine tartrate (Anorex, Adipost, Bacarate) CSS III	A: PO: 17.5–35 mg 1 h ac b.i.d.–t.i.d.; max: 70 mg t.i.d.	C	Similar to fenfluramine	2–10 h	UK	30 min	1–3 h	4–16 h

continued

Amphetamines and Amphetaminelike Drug— *Continued*

Generic (Brand)	Route and Dosage	Preg Cat	Interaction	t 1/2	PB	Onset	Peak	Duration
						Action		
Phenmetrazine HCl (Preludin) CSS II	A: PO: 25 mg b.i.d.–t.i.d.; SR: 75 mg daily; max: 75 mg daily	C	Similar to fenfluramine	UK	UK	UK	5–12	12 h
Phentermine HCl (Adipex-P, Fastin, Ionamin) CSS IV	A: PO: 8 mg t.i.d.; ac or 15–30 mg/d	C	Similar to fenfluramine; diabetics may require less insulin	20 h	UK	UK	UK	10–14 h
Phenylpropanolamine HCl (Acutrim, Control, Dexatrim, Prolamine)	A: PO: 25 mg ac t.i.d.; or SR: 75 mg/d in morning	C	*Increase* effects with beta blockers; hypertensive crisis with MAOIs *Decrease* effects of antihypertensives	4–7 h	UK	UK	1–2 h	3 h SR: 12 h
Analeptics: Methylxanthines Caffeine (Nō Dōz, Tirend, Vivarin)	*Neonatal apnea:* Infants and C: PO: IM-IV: 5–10 mg/kg on day 1; then 2.5–5 mg/d *Therapeutic range:* 5–20 mg/mL	C	*Increase* CNS stimulation with theophylline and beta-adrenergic agonists	Neonate: 40–144 h A: 3–5 h	25–35%	UK	15–45 min	UK

Drug	Route and Dosage	Category	Contraindications and Drug Interactions	$t\frac{1}{2}$	PB	Onset	Peak	Duration
Theophylline	Infants: NGT: 5 mg/kg on day 1; then 2 mg in divided doses	C	See Prototype Drug Chart					
CNS Stimulant for Migraine Sumatriptan succinate (Imitrex)	A: SC: 6 mg single dose; may repeat in 1 h; max: 12 mg/d	C	*Increase* effect of ergot-containing drugs	2 h	20%	10–30 min	UK	1–2 h
Respiratory Stimulant Doxapram HCl (Dopram)	A: IV: 0.5–1 mg/kg; inf: 1–2 mg/min; max: 3 g/d *Neonatal apnea:* Initially: 0.5 mg/kg/h Maintenance: 0.5–2.5 mg/kg/h titrated to lowest effective rate	B	*Increase* pressor effect with MAOIs or sympathomimetic amines	A: 2.5–4 h Neonate: 7–10 h	UK	20–40 sec	1–2 min	6–12 min

KEY: For complete abbreviation key, see inside front cover.

Sedative-Hypnotic: Barbiturate

Pentobarbital Sodium

Pentobarbital sodium
(Nembutal Sodium)
Short-acting barbiturate
CSS II
Pregnancy Category: D
Drug Forms:
Cap 50, 100 mg
Liq 18.2 mg/5 mL
Supp 30, 60, 120, 200 mg
Inj 50 mg/mL

Dosage

Sedative:
A: PO: 20–30 mg t.i.d.
C: PO: 2–6 mg/kg/d in 3 divided
    doses
Hypnotic:
A: PO: 100–200 mg h.s.
C: PO: 30–120 mg h.s.
Preoperative:
A: PO/IM/IV: 100 mg; repeat if
    needed

Contraindications

Respiratory depression, severe
    hepatic disease, pregnancy (fetal
    immaturity)

Drug-Lab-Food Interactions

Decrease respiration with alcohol,
    CNS depressants; incompatible in
    solution with numerous drugs
    such as codeine, insulin, penicillin
    G, hydrocortisone, phenytoin

Pharmacokinetics

Absorption: PO: 90% absorbed slowly
Distribution: PB: 35–45%
Metabolism: t 1/2: 4 h (first phase);
    30–50 h (second phase)
Excretion: In urine as metabolites

Pharmacodynamics

PO: Onset: 15–30 min
    Peak: 0.5–1 h
    Duration: 3–6 h
IM: Onset: 10–15 min
    Peak: 0.5–1 h
    Duration: 3–6 h
IV: Onset: Immediate
    Peak: 2–5 min
    Duration: 15–60 min

Therapeutic Effects/Uses: To treat insomnia; used for sedation, preoperative medication, barbiturate coma (for controlling increased intracranial pressure).

Mode of Action: Depression of the CNS, including the motor and sensory activities.

Side Effects

Nausea, vomiting, diarrhea, lethargy,
    drowsiness, hangover, dizziness,
    rash

Adverse Reactions

Drug dependence or tolerance,
    urticaria, hypotension (rapid IV)
Life-threatening: Respiratory distress,
    laryngospasm

KEY: For complete abbreviation key, see inside front cover.

■ NURSING PROCESS: Sedative-Hypnotic: Barbiturate

ASSESSMENT
- Obtain baseline vital signs for future comparison.
- Determine if there is a history of insomnia or sleep disorder.
- Assess renal function. Urine output should be >600 mL/d. Renal impairment could prolong drug action by increasing the half-life of the drug.
- Assess potential for fluid volume deficit, which would potentiate hypotensive effects.

POTENTIAL NURSING DIAGNOSIS
- Sleep pattern disturbance

PLANNING
- Client will receive adequate sleep without hangover when taking the hypnotic.

NURSING INTERVENTIONS
- Recognize that continuous use of a barbiturate might result in drug abuse.
- Monitor vital signs, especially respirations and blood pressure.
- Raise bedside rails of older adults and clients receiving a hypnotic for the first time. Confusion may occur, and injury may result.
- Observe the client, especially an older adult or a debilitated client, for adverse reactions to the pentobarbital; see prototype.
- Check the client's skin for rashes. Skin eruptions may occur in clients taking barbiturates.
- Observe the client for withdrawal symptoms when pentobarbital has been taken over a prolonged period of time and then discontinued.
- Administer IV pentobarbital at a rate of less than 50 mg/min. Do NOT mix pentobarbital with other medications. IM injection should be given deep in a large muscle such as the gluteus medius.

CLIENT TEACHING

General
- Instruct the client to use nonpharmacological ways to induce sleep, such as enjoying a warm bath, listening to music, drinking warm fluids, and avoiding drinks with caffeine after dinner.
- Instruct the client to avoid alcohol and antidepressant, antipsychotic, and narcotic drugs while taking the barbiturate. Respiratory distress may occur when these drugs are combined.
- Advise the client not to drive a motor vehicle or operate machinery. Caution is always encouraged.
- Instruct the client to take the hypnotic 30 min before bedtime. Short-acting hypnotics such as pentobarbital take effect within 15–30 min.
- Encourage the client to check with the health care provider about OTC sleeping aids. Drowsiness may result from taking these drugs, and therefore caution in driving is advised.

Side Effects
- Advise the client to report adverse reactions, such as hangover, to the health care provider. Drug selection or dosage might need to be changed.
- Instruct the client that hypnotics such as pentobarbital should be gradu-

ally withdrawn, especially if it has been taken for several weeks. Abrupt cessation of the hypnotic may result in withdrawal symptoms (tremors, muscle twitching).

EVALUATION

- Evaluate the effectiveness of pentobarbital. Usually, this drug is given before surgery.
- Evaluate respiratory status to ensure that respiratory distress has not occurred.

Sedative-Hypnotics: Barbiturates and Others

Generic (Brand)	Route and Dosage	Preg Cat	Interaction	t 1/2	PB	Action Onset	Action Peak	Action Duration
Barbiturates: Short Acting Pentobarbital sodium (Nembutal Sodium)	See Prototype Drug Chart							
Secobarbital sodium (Seconal Sodium) CSS II	*Preoperative sedative:* A: PO: 100–300 mg before surgery C: PO: 50–100 mg *Hypnotic:* A: PO/IM: 100–200 mg h.s. C: IM: 3–5 mg/kg; max: 100 mg *Status epilepticus:* A: IV: 5.5 mg/kg; repeat in 3–4 h *With spinal anesthesia:* A: IV: 50–100 mg; infuse over 30 s; max: 250 mg/dose	D	*Increase* CNS depression with alcohol, narcotics, other sedatives, MAOIs *Decrease* effect of anticoagulants, glucocorticoids, quinidine	15–30 h	UK	PO: 15–30 min IM: 10–15 min IV: 1–5 min	PO: 30 min IM: 20 min IV: 1–3 min	PO: 1–4 h IM: 1–4 h IV: 30–60 min

25

Sedative-Hypnotics: Barbiturates and Others

Generic (Brand)	Route and Dosage	Preg Cat	Interaction	t 1/2	PB	Onset	Action Peak	Duration
Barbiturates: Intermediate Acting Amobarbital sodium (Amytal Sodium)	*Sedative:* A: PO: 30–50 mg b.i.d.–t.i.d. C: PO: 2 mg/kg/d in 3–4 divided doses *Hypnotic:* A: PO/IM: 65–200 mg h.s. C: IM: 2–3 mg/kg A and C: IV: 65–200 mg	D	*Increase* CNS depression with alcohol, narcotics, other sedatives, antidepressants, some antihistamines *Decrease* effect of beta blockers, glucocorticoids, phenothiazines, oral contraceptives, anticoagulants, estrogen	20–30 h	50–60%	PO: 45 min–1 h IV: 5 min	PO: UK IV: UK	PO: 6–8 h IV: 3–6 h
Aprobarbital (Alurate)	*Sedative:* A: PO: 40 mg t.i.d. *Hypnotic* A: PO: 40–160 mg h.s.	D	Same as amobarbital	15–40 h	<50%	45 min–1 h	UK	3–5 h
Butabarbital sodium (Butisol Sodium) CSS III	*Sedative:* A: PO: 15–30 mg t.i.d. *Hypnotic* A: PO: 50–100 mg h.s.	D	Same as amobarbital	100 h	<50%	45 min–1 h	3–4 h	6–8 h

Sedative-Hypnotics: Barbiturates and Others

Generic (Brand)	Route and Dosage	Preg Cat	Interaction	t 1/2	PB	Onset	Peak	Duration
							Action	
Other Sedative-Hypnotics								
Chloral hydrate (Noctec) CSS IV	*Sedative:* A: PO: 250 mg t.i.d. pc; C: PO: 8 mg/kg t.i.d. pc; max: 1,000 mg/d *Hypnotic:* A: PO: 500 mg–1 g h.s. (15–30 min before sleep) C: PO: 50 mg/kg h.s.; max: 1,000 mg	C	*Increase* CNS depression with alcohol, barbiturates, paraldehyde, other CNS depressants; *Increase* effect of loop diuretics, oral anticoagulants	8–10 h	70–80%	30–60 min	1–3 h	4–8 h
Paraldehyde (Paral) CSS IV	*Sedative:* A: PO: 5–10 mL q4–6 h PRN in water or juice; max: 30 mL C: PO: 0.3 mL/kg *Hypnotic:* A: PO: 10–30 mL h.s.	C	Same as chloral hydrate; *increase* urine crystals with sulfonamides	7.5 h	UK	10–15 min	1–2 h	6–8 h

KEY: For complete abbreviation key, see inside front cover.

Sedative-Hypnotic: Benzodiazepine

Flurazepam HCl

Flurazepam HCl
  (Dalmane)
Benzodiazepine hypnotic
CSS IV
Pregnancy Category: X
Drug Forms:
Cap 15, 30 mg

Dosage

A: PO: 15–30 mg h.s.
Elderly: PO: 15 mg h.s.

Contraindications

Hypersensitivity to benzodiazepine,
  pregnancy, lactation, intermittent
  porphyria
Caution: Renal, liver, or mental
  disorders; elderly, debilitation

Drug-Lab-Food Interactions

May *increase* effect with cimetidine
Decrease effect with antacids
Decrease CNS function with alcohol,
  CNS depressants, anticonvulsants
Lab: Increase AST, ALT, ALP, bilirubin
False negatives: Clinistix, Diastix

Pharmacokinetics

Absorption: PO: well absorbed
Distribution: PB: 97%
Metabolism: t 1/2: 2–3 h; metabolites:
  45–100 h
Excretion: In urine as active
  metabolites

Pharmacodynamics

PO: Onset: 15–45 min
     Peak: 0.5–1 h
     Duration: 7–10 h

Therapeutic Effects/Uses: To treat insomnia.

Mode of Action: Depression of the CNS; neurotransmitter inhibition.

Side Effects

Drowsiness, lethargy, hangover
  (residual sedation), dizziness,
  lightheadedness, anxiety, nausea,
  vomiting, diarrhea, confusion,
  disorientation

Adverse Reactions

Tolerance, psychological and/or
  physical dependence, hypotension,
  mental depression
Life-threatening: Coma from overdose,
  leukopenia (rare)

KEY: For complete abbreviation key, see inside front cover.

■ NURSING PROCESS: Sedative-Hypnotic: Benzodiazepine

ASSESSMENT

- Obtain baseline vital signs and laboratory tests (AST, ALT, bilirubin) for future comparisons.
- Obtain drug history. Taking CNS depressants with benzodiazepine hypnotics can depress respirations. Flurazepam is highly protein-bound. Report if the client is taking other highly protein-bound drugs such as warfarin (Coumadin). Drug displacement can occur with two highly protein-bound drugs, causing an increase in circulating drug(s).
- Ascertain the client's problem with sleep disturbance.

POTENTIAL NURSING DIAGNOSIS

- Sleep pattern disturbance

PLANNING

- Client will remain asleep for 6–8 h.

NURSING INTERVENTIONS

- Monitor vital signs. Check for signs of respiratory distress, such as slow, irregular breathing patterns.
- Raise bedside rails of older adults or clients receiving flurazepam for the first time. Confusion may occur, and injury may result.
- Observe the client for side effects of flurazepam, such as hangover (residual sedation), lightheadedness, dizziness, or confusion. The metabolites of flurazepam have a long half-life, so cumulative effects of the drug can occur.

CLIENT TEACHING

General

- Instruct the client to use nonpharmacological ways to induce sleep, such as enjoying a warm bath, listening to music, drinking warm fluids such as milk, and avoiding drinks with caffeine after dinner.
- Instruct the client to avoid alcohol and antidepressant, antipsychotic, and narcotic drugs while taking sedative-hypnotics. Severe respiratory distress may occur when these drugs are combined.
- Advise the client to take flurazepam before bedtime. Flurazepam takes effect within 15–45 min.
- Suggest that the client urinate before taking flurazepam to prevent sleep disruption.
- Encourage the client to check with the health care provider about OTC sleeping aids. Drowsiness may result from taking these drugs; therefore, caution in driving is advised.

Side Effects

- Instruct the client to report adverse reactions, such as hangover, to the health care provider. Drug selection or dosage may need to be changed if hangover occurs.

EVALUATION

- Evaluate the effectiveness of flurazepam in promoting sleep.
- Determine if side effects such as hangover occur after several days of taking flurazepam. Another hypnotic may be prescribed if side effects remain.

Generic (Brand)	Route and Dosage	Preg Cat	Interaction	t1/2	PB	Action Onset	Action Peak	Action Duration
Benzodiazepines Estazolam (ProSom) CSS IV	A: PO: 1–2 mg h.s. Elderly: PO: 0.5 mg h.s.	X	*Increase* estazolam effect with cimetidine, INH, oral contraceptives; *increase* CNS depression with alcohol, narcotics, anticonvulsants *Decrease* estazolam effect with theophylline, rifampin, smoking	10–24 h	93%	15–45 min	1.5–2 h	7–8 h
Flurazepam HCl (Dalmane)	See Prototype Drug Chart							
Lorazepam (Ativan) CSS IV	*Hypnotic:* A: PO: 2–4 mg h.s.	D	Similar to temazepam; *decrease* effect with oral contraceptives, valproic acid	12–14 h	85%	20–30 min	2–3 h	12–24 h
Quazepam (Doral) CSS IV	A: PO: 7.5–15 mg h.s.	X	*Increase* CNS depression with alcohol, narcotics, anticonvulsants	39 h	>95%	0.5 h	2 h	7–8 h
Temazepam (Restoril) CSS IV	*Hypnotic:* A: PO: 15–30 mg h.s.	X	*Increase* CNS depression with alcohol, anticonvulsants, CNS depressants, narcotics, other sedative-hypnotics; may *increase* phenytoin level *Decrease* absorption with antacids; may *decrease* effect of levodopa	10–20 h	96%	30–60 min	2–3 h	6–12 h

Drug	Dose		Drug Interactions					
Triazolam (Halcion) CSS IV	*Hypnotic:* A: PO: 0.125–0.5 mg h.s. Elderly: PO: 0.125–0.25 mg h.s.	X	Same as temazepam	2–4 h	89%	15–30 min	1–2 h	6–8 h
Nonbenzodiazepines								
Methyprylon (Noludar) CSS III	*Hypnotic:* A: PO: 200–400 mg h.s. C: PO: 50 mg h.s; may increase to 200 mg	B	Similar to glutethimide	3–6 h	60%	45–60 min	1–2 h	5–8 h
Zolpidem tartrate (Ambien)	*Hypnotic:* A: PO: Initially 5 mg; maint: 5–15 mg h.s.; average: 10 mg h.s.; use for 7–10 d	B	*Increase* CNS depression with alcohol, narcotics, antipsychotics	1.5–4 h	79–92%	10–30 min	0.5–2 h	6–8 h
Piperidinediones								
Glutethimide (Doriden) CSS III	*Hypnotic:* A: PO: 250–500 mg h.s.; repeat in 4 h if necessary	C	*Increase* CNS depression with alcohol, CNS antidepressants, barbiturates; *increase* anticholinergic effect with tricyclic antidepressants. *Decrease* anticoagulant effect with oral anticoagulants	10–20 h	50%	30 min	1–2 h	4–8 h

KEY: For complete abbreviation key, see inside front cover.

31

Analgesic: Aspirin

Aspirin

Aspirin
  (A.S.A., Bayer, Astrin, Ecotrin,
  Alka Seltzer [in some], Empirin)
Salicylate
Pregnancy Category: D
Drug Forms:
Tab 65, 325, 500, 650 mg
Cap SR 325, 500 mg
Supp 60, 120, 200, 325, 650 mg

Dosage

Analgesic:
A: PO: 325–650 mg q4h PRN; max: 4
  g/d
C: PO: 40–65 mg/d in 4–6 divided
  doses; max: 3.5 g/d
TIA and thromboembolic condition:
A: PO: 325–650 mg/d or b.i.d.
Arthritis:
A: PO: 3.6–5.4 g/d in divided doses
TDM: 15–30 mg/dL; 150–300 μg/
  mL

Contraindications

Hypersensitivity to salicylates or
  NSAIDs, flu or virus symptoms in
  children, third trimester of
  pregnancy
Caution: Renal or hepatic disorders

Drug-Lab-Food Interactions

Increase risk of bleeding with
  anticoagulants; *increase* risk of
  hypoglycemia with oral
  hypoglycemic drugs; *increase*
  ulcerogenic effect with
  glucocorticoids
Lab: Decrease cholesterol and
  potassium, T_3, T_4 levels; *increase* PT,
  bleeding time, uric acid

Pharmacokinetics

Absorption: PO: 80–100%
Distribution: PB: UK; crosses placenta
Metabolism: t 1/2: 2–3 h (low dose;
  2–20 h (high dose)
Excretion: 50% in urine

Pharmacodynamics

PO: Onset: 15–30 min
         Peak: 1–2 h
         Duration: 4–6 h
Rectal: Onset: 1–2 h
         Peak: 3–5 h
         Duration: 4–7 h

Therapeutic Effects/Uses: To reduce pain and inflammatory symptoms; to decrease body temperature; to inhibit platelet aggregation.

Mode of Action: Inhibition of prostaglandin synthesis, inhibition of hypothalamic heat-regulator center.

Side Effects

Anorexia, nausea, vomiting,
  diarrhea, dizziness, confusion,
  hearing loss, heartburn, rash,
  stomach pains, drowsiness

Adverse Reactions

Tinnitus, urticaria, ulceration
Life-threatening: Agranulocytosis,
  hemolytic anemia, bronchospasm,
  anaphylaxis, thrombocytopenia,
  hepatotoxicity, leukopenia

KEY: For complete abbreviation key, see inside front cover.

■ NURSING PROCESS: Analgesic: Aspirin

ASSESSMENT

• Obtain a medical history. Determine if there is any history of gastric upset, gastric bleeding, or liver disease. Aspirin can cause gastric irritation. It prolongs bleeding time by inhibiting platelet aggregation.
• Obtain a drug history. Report if a drug-drug interaction is probable.

POTENTIAL NURSING DIAGNOSIS
- High risk for injury
- Pain

PLANNING
- Client will be free of mild pain in 12–24 hours. Aspirin may be ordered for mild to severe arthritic conditions, pain relief, anti-inflammatory effects, fever reduction, and inhibition of platelet aggregation.

NURSING INTERVENTIONS
- Monitor serum salicylate (aspirin) level when the client is taking high doses of aspirin for chronic conditions such as arthritis. The normal therapeutic range is 15–30 mg/dL. Mild toxicity occurs at serum level of >30 mg/dL, and severe toxicity occurs at >50 mg/dL.
- Observe the client for signs of bleeding, such as dark (tarry) stools, bleeding gums, petechiae (round red spots), ecchymosis (excessive bruising), and purpura (large red spots) when the client is taking high doses of aspirin.

CLIENT TEACHING
General
- Advise the client not to take aspirin with alcohol or drugs that are highly protein-bound, such as the anticoagulant warfarin (Coumadin). Aspirin displaces drugs like warfarin from the protein-binding site, causing more free anticoagulant.
- Suggest that the client inform the dentist before a dental visit if the client is taking high doses of aspirin.
- With the health care provider's approval, instruct the client to discontinue aspirin 3–7 d before surgery to reduce the risk of bleeding.
- Keep aspirin bottle out of reach of small children.
- Instruct the parent to call the poison control center immediately if a child has taken a large or unknown amount of aspirin (also acetaminophen).
- Instruct the client NOT to administer aspirin for virus or flu symptoms in children. Reye's syndrome (vomiting, lethargy, delirium, and coma) has been linked with aspirin and viral infections. Acetaminophen is usually prescribed for cold and flu symptoms.
- Inform the client that old aspirin tablets can cause GI distress; discard.
- Inform the client with dysmenorrhea to take acetaminophen instead of aspirin 2 d before and 2 d during the menstrual period.

Diet
- Instruct the client to take aspirin (also ibuprofen) with food, at mealtime, or with plenty of fluids. Enteric-coated aspirin avoids GI disturbance.

Side Effects
- Instruct the client to report side effects such as drowsiness, tinnitus (ringing in the ears), headaches, flushing, dizziness, GI symptoms (bleeding, heartburn), visual changes, and seizures.

EVALUATION
- Evaluate the effectiveness of aspirin in relieving pain. If pain persists, another analgesic such as an NSAID such as ibuprofen may be prescribed.
- Determine if the client is having any side effects to aspirin.

Analgesic: Acetaminophen

Acetaminophen

Acetaminophen
  (Tylenol, Tempra, Panadol, Datril)
Para-aminophenol analgesic
Pregnancy Category: B
Drug Forms:
Tab and cap 325, 500, 650 mg
Chewable tab 80 mg
Liq 160 mg/5 mL
Supp 120, 325, 650 mg

Dosage

A: PO: 325–650 mg q4–6h PRN;
  max: 4,000 mg/d; rectal supp:
  650 mg q.i.d.
C: 0–3 mo: PO: 40 mg 4–5×/d
  4 mo–1 y: PO: 80 mg 4–5×/d
  1–2 y: PO: 120 mg 4–5×/d
  2–3 y: PO: 160 mg 4–5×/d
  4–5 y: PO: 240 mg 4–5×/d
  6–8 y: PO: 320 mg 4–5×/d
  9–10 y: PO: 400 mg 4–5×/d
  >11 y: PO: 480 mg 4–5×/d
C: 2–5 y: Rectal: 120 mg 4–5×/d
  6–12 y: Rectal: 325 mg 4–5×/d

Contraindications

Severe hepatic or renal disease,
  alcoholism

Drug-Lab-Food Interactions

Increase effect with caffeine, diflunisal
Decrease effect with oral
  contraceptives, anticholinergics,
  cholestyramine

Pharmacokinetics

Absorption: PO: rapidly absorbed;
  rectal: erratic
Distribution: PB: 20–50%; crosses the
  placenta, in breast milk
Metabolism: t 1/2: 1–3.5 h
Excretion: In urine as metabolites

Pharmacodynamics

PO: Onset: 10–30 min
       Peak: 1–2 h
       Duration: 3–5 h
Rectal: Onset: UK
       Peak: UK
       Duration: 4–6 h

Therapeutic Effects/Uses: To decrease pain and fever.

Mode of Action: Inhibition of prostaglandin synthesis, inhibition of hypothalamic heat-regulator center.

Side Effects

Anorexia, nausea, vomiting, rash

Adverse Reactions

Severe hypoglycemia, oliguria,
  urticaria
Life-threatening: Hemorrhage,
  hepatotoxicity, hemolytic anemia,
  leukopenia, thrombocytopenia

KEY: For complete abbreviation key, see inside front cover.

■ NURSING PROCESS: Analgesic: Acetaminophen

ASSESSMENT

• Obtain a medical history of liver dysfunction. Overdosing or extremely high doses of acetaminophen can cause hepatotoxicity.
• Ascertain the severity of the pain. Nonnarcotic NSAIDs such as ibuprofen or a narcotic may be necessary for relieving pain.

POTENTIAL NURSING DIAGNOSIS

• High risk for injury.
• Pain.

PLANNING

• Client's pain will be relieved or controlled.

NURSING INTERVENTIONS

• Check levels of ALT, ALP, GGT, 5-NT, bilirubin for elevations, if the client is on long-term therapy.

CLIENT TEACHING

• Instruct the client to keep acetaminophen out of children's reach. Acetaminophen for children is available in flavored tablets and liquid. High doses can cause hepatotoxicity. Self-medication of acetaminophen should not be used longer than 10 d for adults and 5 d for children without the health care provider's approval.
• Instruct the parent to call the poison control center immediately if a child has taken a large or unknown amount of acetaminophen. Ipecac should be available in the home.
• Check acetaminophen dosage on package level. Do NOT exceed the recommended dosage.

Side Effects

• Instruct the client to report side effects. Overdosing can cause severe liver damage and death.
• Check the serum acetaminophen level when toxicity is suspected. The normal serum level is 5–20 mg/mL; the toxic level is >50 µg/mL, and levels of >200 µg/mL could indicate hepatotoxicity. The antidote for acetaminophen is acetylcysteine (Mucomyst). The dosage is based on the serum acetaminophen level.

EVALUATION

• Evaluate the effectiveness of acetaminophen in relieving pain. If pain persists, another analgesic may be needed.
• Determine if the client is taking the dose as recommended and no side effects are observed or reported.

Generic (Brand)	Route and Dosage	Preg Cat	Interaction	t 1/2	PB	Onset	Peak	Duration
							Action	
NSAIDs: Propionic Acid Ibuprofen (Motrin, Advil, Nuprin, Medipren)	*Pain:* A: PO: 200–800 mg q4–6h; max: 3,200 mg/d *Fever:* A: PO: 200–400 mg t.i.d.-q.i.d. C: 6 mo–12 y: PO: 5–10 mg/kg t.i.d.-q.i.d.	B	*Increase* bleeding with heparin, oral anticoagulants; *increase* effects of phenytoin, sulfonamides, warfarin *Lab:* may *increase* lithium levels	2–4 h	98%	1/2 h	1–2 h	4–6 h
Para-aminophenol Acetaminophen (Tylenol, Panadol, Tempra)	See Prototype Drug Chart							

		Pregnancy Category	Drug-Lab-Food Interactions	t½	PB	Onset	Peak	Duration
Salicylates Aspirin (Bayer, Ecotrin, Astrin)	See Prototype Drug Chart							
Diflunisal (Dolobid)	A: PO: Initially: 1,000 mg; maint: 500 mg q8–12h	C	May *increase* lithium levels; may *increase* bleeding with warfarin; *increase* effects of acetaminophen, anticoagulants. *Decrease* effect with antacids, steroids; may *decrease* effects of diuretics, antihypertensives. *Lab:* may *increase* AST, ALT; may *decrease* T_4	8–12 h	99%	1 h	2–3 h	8–12 h
Methotrimeprazine HCl (Levoprome)	*Sedative-analgesic:* A: C: >12 y: PO: 6–25 mg/d in divided doses with meals IM: 10–12 mg q4–6h PRN (deep IM) Elderly: IM: 5–10 mg q4–6h *Postanalgesia:* A and C: >12 y: IM: 2.5–7.5 mg q4–6h PRN	C	*Increase* hypotensive effect with antihypertensives, MAOIs. *Increase* CNS depression with alcohol, narcotics	20 h	UK	15–30 min	1–2 h	4 h

KEY: For complete abbreviation key, see inside front cover.

37

Narcotic: Morphine

Morphine Sulfate

Morphine sulfate
   (Duramorph, MS Contin, Roxanol
   SR)
Narcotic opiate
CSS II
Pregnancy Category: B
Drug Forms:
Tab 15, 30 mg
Liq 10, 20/5 mL
Inj 2, 4, 5, 8, 10, 15 mg/mL
Supp 5, 10, 20 mg

Dosage

A: PO: 10–30 mg q4h PRN
   IM/SC: 5–15 mg PRN
   IV: 4–10 mg q4h PRN; diluted;
   inject over 5 min
C: IM/SC: 0.1–0.2 mg/kg PRN;
   max: <15 mg/dose

Contraindications

Asthma with respiratory depression,
   increased intracranial pressure,
   shock
Caution: Respiratory, renal, or hepatic
   diseases; myocardial infarction;
   elderly; very young

Drug-Lab-Food Interactions

Increase effects of alcohol, sedatives-
   hypnotics, antipsychotic drugs,
   muscle relaxants
Lab: Increase AST, ALT

Pharmacokinetics

Absorption: PO: varies; IV: rapid
Distribution: PB: UK; crosses placenta,
   in breast milk
Metabolism: t 1/2: 2.5–3 h
Excretion: 90% in urine

Pharmacodynamics

PO: Onset: variable
         Peak: 1–2 h
         Duration: 4–5 h
SC/IM: Onset: 15–30 min
         Peak: SC: 50–90 min
              IM: 0.5–1 h
         Duration: 3–5 h
IV: Onset: rapid
         Peak: 20 min
         Duration: 3–5 h

Therapeutic Effects/Uses: To relieve severe pain.

Mode of Action: Depression of the CNS, depression of pain impulses by binding with the opiate receptor in the CNS.

Side Effects

Anorexia, nausea, vomiting,
   constipation, drowsiness,
   dizziness, sedation, confusion,
   urinary retention, rash, blurred
   vision, bradycardia, flushing
   euphoria, pruritus

Adverse Reactions

Hypotension, urticaria, seizures
Life-threatening: Respiratory
   depression, increased intracranial
   pressure

KEY: For complete abbreviation key, see inside front cover.

■ NURSING PROCESS: Narcotic Analgesic: Morphine Sulfate

ASSESSMENT

- Obtain a medical history. Contraindications to use of morphine include severe respiratory disorders, increased intracranial pressure (ICP), and severe renal disease. Morphine may increase ICP and seizures.
- Obtain a drug history. Report if a drug-drug interaction is probable. Morphine increases the effects of alcohol, sedatives or hypnotics, antipsychotic drugs, and muscle relaxants and might cause respiratory depression.
- Assess vital signs and urinary output. Note the depth and rate of respirations. Morphine can cause urinary retention.

POTENTIAL NURSING DIAGNOSIS

- Pain related to surgery, injury
- Ineffective breathing patterns related to excess morphine dosage

PLANNING

- Client will be free of pain, or the intensity of pain will be lessened.

NURSING INTERVENTIONS

- Administer the narcotic before pain reaches its peak to maximize the effectiveness of the drug.
- Monitor vital signs at frequent intervals to detect respiratory changes. Respirations of <10/min can indicate respiratory distress.
- Monitor the client's urine output; urine output should be at least 600 mL/d.
- Check bowel sounds for decreased peristalsis, a cause of constipation due to morphine. Mild laxative or dietary change might be needed.
- Check for pupil changes and reaction. Pinpoint pupils can indicate morphine overdose.
- Have naloxone (Narcan) available as an antidote if morphine overdose occurs.
- Check child's dose of morphine before its administration; dose is 0.1–0.2 mg/kg.

CLIENT TEACHING

General

- Instruct the client not to take alcohol or CNS depressants with any narcotic analgesics such as morphine. Respiratory depression can result.
- Suggest nonpharmacological measures to relieve pain as client is recuperating from surgery. If necessary, a nonnarcotic analgesic may be prescribed.

Side Effects

- Alert the client that with continuous use, narcotics such as morphine can become addicting. If addiction occurs, inform the client about methadone treatment programs and other resources in the area.
- Instruct the client to report dizziness or difficulty in breathing while taking morphine. Dizziness could be due to orthostatic hypotension. Advise the client to ambulate with caution or only with assistance.

EVALUATION

- Evaluate the effectiveness of morphine in lessening or alleviating the pain.
- Evaluate the stability of vital signs. Report any decrease in blood pressure.

Narcotic: Meperidine

Meperidine HCl

Meperidine HCl
  (Demerol HCl)
Synthetic narcotic
CSS II
Pregnancy Category: B
Drug Forms:
Tab 50, 100 mg
Liq 50 mg/5 mL
Inj 25, 50, 75, 100 mg/mL

Dosage

A: PO/SC/IM/IV: 50–150 mg q3–4h
  PRN
C: PO/IM/IV: 1 mg/kg q4–6h; max:
  <100 mg q4h

Contraindications

Alcoholism; head trauma; increased
  intracranial pressure; severe
  hepatic, renal, and pulmonary
  diseases

Drug-Lab-Food Interactions

Increase CNS depression with alcohol,
  sedative-hypnotics, and other CNS
  depressants
Lab: Increase serum amylase, AST,
  ALT, bilirubin

Pharmacokinetics

Absorption: PO: 50% absorbed; IM:
  well absorbed
Distribution: PB: 60–70%
Metabolism: t 1/2: 3–8 h
Excretion: In urine, mostly as
  metabolites

Pharmacodynamics

PO:	Onset: 15 min
	Peak: 1 h
	Duration: 4 h
IM/SC:	Onset: 10–15 min
	Peak: 0.5–1 h
	Duration: 2–4 h
IV:	Onset: 1–5 min
	Peak: 5–10 min
	Duration: 2 h

Therapeutic Effects/Uses: To relieve moderate to severe pain.

Mode of Action: Synthetic morphine-like substance, depression of pain impulses by
binding to the opiate receptor in the CNS.

Side Effects

Nausea, vomiting, constipation,
  headache, dizziness, drowsiness,
  hypotension, sedation, confusion,
  abdominal cramps, euphoria,
  blurred vision, rash, tinnitus

Adverse Reactions

Bradycardia, severe hypotension,
  convulsion, physical and/or
  psychologic dependence
Life-threatening: Respiratory
  depression, cardiovascular
  collapse, increased intracranial
  pressure

KEY: For complete abbreviation key, see inside front cover.

■ **NURSING PROCESS: Narcotic Analgesic: Meperidine (Demerol)**

ASSESSMENT
- Obtain drug history from the client of drugs he or she is currently taking. Report if a drug-drug interaction is probable. CNS depressants enhance the action of meperidine; thus, respiratory depression can occur.
- Obtain baseline vital signs for future comparisons. Meperidine tends to decrease systolic blood pressure.
- Assess type of pain, location, and duration before giving meperidine.

POTENTIAL NURSING DIAGNOSIS
- Pain related to surgery or injury

PLANNING
- Client's pain will be decreased or alleviated. Drug dosing may need to be repeated.

NURSING INTERVENTIONS
- Administer meperidine before the pain reaches its peak to maximize the effectiveness of the drug.
- Monitor vital signs to compare blood pressure with baseline pressure. Hypotension is a side effect of meperidine. Note if client is having any breathing dysfunction.
- Have available naloxone (Narcan), which can reverse respiratory depression due to narcotic overdose.
- Check urine output and bowel sounds. Urinary retention and constipation are side effects of meperidine.
- Check older adults for side effects of meperidine. Confusion may occur, so use of side rails and other precautions should be taken. Dosgae may need to be decreased.

CLIENT TEACHING

General
- Instruct the client not to take alcohol or CNS depressants with meperidine because of increased depression of the CNS and of respirations.
- Inform the client that drug dependence could occur with continual use of meperidine. If severe pain is still present, another narcotic analgesic or analgesic may be prescribed.

Side Effects
- Instruct the client to report side effects such as dizziness due to orthostatic hypotension, headaches, constipation, blurred vision, or decreased urine output. Report findings to the health care provider.

EVALUATION
- Evaluate the effectiveness of the narcotic analgesic in lessening or alleviating the pain. If pain persists after several days, the cause should be determined or the narcotic should be changed.
- Evaluate the stability of vital signs. Abnormal signs, such as decreased blood pressure, should be reported.

Narcotics: Opium and Synthetics

Generic (Brand)	Route and Dosage	Preg Cat	Interaction	t 1/2	PB	Onset	Peak	Duration
							Action	
						Onset	Peak	Duration
Codeine (sulfate, phosphate) CSS II	A: PO/SC/IM: 15–60 mg q4–6h PRN C: PO/SC/IM: 0.5 mg/kg/dose q4–6h	C	*Increase* CNS depression with alcohol, sedative-hypnotics, antipsychotics, muscle relaxants, tricyclic antidepressants	2.5–4 h	70%	15–30 min	1–1.5 h	4–6 h
Hydromorphone HCl (Dilaudid) CSS II	A: PO: 1–6 mg q4–6h PRN SC/IM/IV: 1–4 mg q4–6h PRN Rectal: 3 mg h.s., PRN	C	Same as codeine	1–3 h	62%	15–30 min	0.5–1.5 h	4–5 h
Levorphanol tartrate (Levo-Dromoran) CSS II	A: PO/SC/IV: Initially: 2 mg PO/SC/IV: 2–3 mg q6–8 h PRN	B	Same as oxycodone	10–16 h	50–60%	PO: 1–1.5 h SC: 30 min–1 h IV: 20 min	PO: 2 h SC: 1–2 h IV: UK	PO: 6–8 h SC: 6–8 h IV: 6–8 h
Meperidine (Demerol)	See Prototype Drug Chart							
Morphine sulfate	See Prototype Drug Chart							
Oxycodone HCl (Percocet) and terephthalate (Percodan) (Percocet with acetominophen; Percodan with aspirin) CSS II	A: PO: 5 mg q4–6h PRN or 5–10 mg q6h PRN C: 6–12 y: 1.25 mg q6h PRN 12–17 y: 2.5 mg q6h PRN	B	*Increase* CNS depression with alcohol, sedative-hypnotics, other narcotics, antipsychotics, tricyclic antidepressants, muscle relaxants	2–3 h	UK	10–15 min	0.5–1 h	4–5 h

Drug	Dosage	CSS	Interactions					
Propoxyphene HCl (Darvon) Propoxyphene napsylate (Darvon-N) CSS IV	A: PO: HCl: 65 mg q4h PRN A: PO: napsylate: 100 mg q4h PRN	C (short time use)	Same as oxycodone	12 h	>90%	30 min–1 h	2–3 h	4–6 h
Sufentanil citrate (Sufenta) CSS II	*Primary anesthetic:* A: IV: 8–30 µg/kg with 100% O_2 and muscle relaxant C: IV: 10–25 µg/kg with 100% O_2 and muscle relaxant *Adjunct to anesthesia:* IV: 1–8 µg/kg	C	*Increase* additive effect with alcohol, sedative-hypnotics, antipsychotics	1–3 h	93%	1.5–3 min	UK	40 min
For Narcotic Addiction: Levomethadyl acetate HCl (ORLAMM)	A: IM: Initially: 10–40 mg 3×/wk; maint: 60–90 mg 3×/wk; max: 140 mg 3×/wk (M, W, F regimen)	UK	*Increase* CNS depression with CNS depressants	UK	UK	UK	UK	UK

KEY: For complete abbreviation key, see inside front cover.

43

Narcotic: Agonist-Antagonist

Pentazocine lactate
  (Talwin)
Narcotic agonist-antagonist
CSS IV
Pregnancy Category: C
Drug Forms:
Tab 50 mg
Inj 30 mg/mL

Dosage

A: PO: 50–100 mg q3–4h PRN; max:
  600 mg/d
IM/IV: 30 mg q3–4h PRN

Contraindications

Alcoholism; head trauma; severe
  respiratory, renal, and/or hepatic
  disease
Caution: Severe heart disease

Drug-Lab-Food Interactions

Increase CNS depression with alcohol,
  sedative-hypnotics, antipsychotics,
  muscle relaxants

Pharmacokinetics

Absorption: PO: well absorbed
Distribution: PB: 60%
Metabolism: t 1/2: 2–3 h
Excretion: In urine (small amount
  excreted unchanged); in feces
  (small amount)

Pharmacodynamics

PO: Onset: 15–30 min
     Peak: 1–2 h
     Duration: 2–4 h
IM: Onset: 15–20 min
     Peak: 1 h
     Duration: 2–4 h
IV: Onset: minutes
     Peak: 15 min
     Duration: 1–2 h

Therapeutic Effects/Uses: To relieve moderate to severe pain.

Mode of Action: Inhibition of pain impulses transmitted in the CNS by binding with
the opiate receptor, pain threshold is increased.

Side Effects

Nausea, vomiting, constipation,
  dizziness, sedation, headaches,
  confusion, euphoria, rash, blurred
  vision, dysuria

Adverse Reactions

Hallucinations, urinary retention,
  urticaria, tachycardia
Life threatening: Respiratory
  depression, shock

KEY: For complete abbreviation key, see inside front cover.

Narcotic: Agonist-Antagonist

■ NURSING PROCESS: Narcotic Analgesic: Pentazocine (Talwin)

ASSESSMENT
● Obtain a drug history from the client. Report if a drug-drug interaction is probable. When taken with pentazocine, CNS depressants can cause respiratory depression.
● Obtain baseline vital signs for future comparison.
● Assess the type of pain, duration, and location before giving the drug.

POTENTIAL NURSING DIAGNOSIS
● Pain related to surgery or trauma

PLANNING
● Client will be free of pain, or the intensity of pain will be lessened.

NURSING INTERVENTIONS
● Monitor vital signs. Note any changes in respirations.
● Check bowel sounds. Decreased peristalsis may result in constipation. A mild laxative may be necessary.
● Check urine output. Report if urine output is <30 mL/h or <600 mL/d.
● Administer IV pentazocine diluted in sterile water or undiluted. Do not mix with barbiturates.

CLIENT TEACHING
General
● Instruct the client not to consume alcohol or CNS depressants while taking pentazocine. Respiratory depression can occur.
● Suggest nonpharmacological methods for lessening pain, such as changing position or ambulation.

Side Effects
● Instruct the client to report side effects to pentazocine such as dizziness, headaches, constipation, dysuria, rash, or blurred vision. Hallucinations, tachycardia, and respiratory depression are adverse reactions that might occur.

EVALUATION
● Evaluate the effectiveness of pentazocine in relieving pain. If ineffective, another narcotic analgesic may be ordered.
● Evaluate the stability of the vital signs. Note if there is a change in respirations, pulse rate, or blood pressure. Report abnormal findings.

Narcotics: Agonist-Antagonists and Narcotic Antagonist

Generic (Brand)	Route and Dosage	Preg Cat	t 1/2	PB	Action Onset	Action Peak	Action Duration	Interaction
Buprenorphine HCl (Buprenex) CSS V	A: IM/IV: Initially: 0.3 mg q6h; may increase to 0.6 mg q6h PRN	C	2–3 h	96%	IM: 15–30 min IV: 1–2 min	IM: 1 h IV: 1 h	IM: 3–5 h IV: 2–6 h	Same as butorphanol
Butorphanol tartrate (Stadol)	A: IM: 1–4 mg q3–4h PRN IV: 0.5–2 mg q3–4h PRN	C	2.5–4 h	>90%	IM: 10–30 min IV: 1–2 min	IM: 0.5–1 h IV: 4–5 min	IM: 3–4 h IV: 2–4 h	*Increase* butorphanol effect with narcotics, sedative-hypnotics, antipsychotics, muscle relaxants
Nalbuphine HCl (Nubain) CSS II	A: SC/IM/IV: 10–20 mg q3–4h PRN; max: 160 mg/d	B	5 h	UK	IM: 15 min IV: 2–3 min	IM: UK IV: 30 min	IM: 3–6 h IV: 3–6 h	Same as butorphanol
Pentazocine lactate (Talwin)	See Prototype Drug Chart							
Narcotic Agonist-Antagonists Dezocine (Dalgan)	A: IM: 5–20 mg q3–6h PRN; max: 120 mg/d IV: 2.5–10 mg q3–6 h PRN	C	IM: 2.2 h IV: 2.6 h	UK	IM: 30 min IV: 10 min	IM: 1–1.5 h IV: 0.5 h	IM/IV: 2–4 h	*Increase* depressive effects with alcohol, sedative-hypnotics, antipsychotics, tranquilizers, general anesthesia *Lab: May increase* ALP, AST

Fentanyl (Duragesic, Sublimaze) CSS II	*Preoperative* A: IM/IV: 50–100 µg q1–2h PRN (0.05–0.1 mg) C: 2–12 y: 1.7–3.3 µg/kg A: Transdermal patch: 72-h effect	C	Similar to dezocine	UK	80–89%	IM:10–15 min IV: 1–2 min	IM: 20–30 min IV: 3–5 h	IM: 1–2 h IV: 0.5–1 h
Narcotic Antagonist Naloxone HCl (Narcan)	*Narcotic-induced respiratory distress:* A: IV: 0.4–2 mg; may repeat q2–3min; max: 10 mg C: IV: 0.1 mg/kg; may repeat q2–3min; max: 10 mg *Postoperative RD:* A: IV: 0.1–0.2 mg; may repeat q2–3min PRN C: IV/IM: 0.01 mg/kg; may repeat q2–3min PRN	B	None significant	1–1.5 h	UK	IV: 1–2 min	IV: 5–15 min	IV: 45 min–1 h

KEY: For complete abbreviation key, see inside front cover.

ANTICONVULSANTS

Barbiturates

Benzodiazepines

Hydantoins

Iminostilbenes

Oxazolidones

Succinimides

Valproate

Miscellaneous

Anticonvulsants

Phenytoin

Phenytoin
  (Dilantin)
Anticonvulsant, hydantoin
Pregnancy Category: D
Drug Forms:
Susp: 30, 125 mg/5 mL
Tab chewable 50 mg
Cap ext 30, 100 mg
Cap prompt 30, 100 mg
Inj 50 mg/mL

Dosage

A: PO: 100 mg t.i.d.
  IV: LD: 10–15 mg/kg; infusion
  <50 mg/min; max: 300 mg/d
C: 4–8 mg/kg/d in divided doses
Therapeutic range: 10–20 μg/mL

Contraindications

Hypersensitivity, heart block, psychiatric disorders, pregnancy

Drug-Lab-Food Interactions

Increase effects with cimetidine,
  isoniazid, chloramphenicol;
  decrease effects with cisplatin, folic
  acid, and vinblastine
Decrease effects of anticoagulants,
  oral contraceptives, antihistamines,
  corticosteroids, theophylline,
  cyclosporin, quinidine, dopamine,
  rifampin
Foods: Those rich in folic acid

Pharmacokinetics

Absorption: PO: slowly absorbed; IM:
  erratic rate of absorption
Distribution: PB: 85–95%
Metabolism: t 1/2: 6–45 h; averge: 22 h
Excretion: In urine, small amount; in
  bile and feces, moderate amount

Pharmacodynamics

PO: Onset: 0.5–2 h
  Peak: 1.5–3 h
  Duration: 6–12 h
IV: Onset: minutes–1 h
  Peak: 2 h
  Duration: >12 h

Therapeutic Effects/Uses: To prevent grand mal and complex partial seizures.
Mode of Action: Reduces motor cortex activity by altering transport of ions.

Side Effects

Headache, diplopia, confusion,
  dizziness, sluggishness, decreased
  coordination, ataxia, slurred
  speech, rash, anorexia, nausea,
  vomiting, hypotension (IV), pink-
  red/brown discoloration of urine

Adverse Reactions

Leukopenia, hepatitis, depression,
  gingival hyperplasia, gingivitis,
  nystagmus, hirsutism
Life-threatening: Aplastic anemia,
  thrombocytopenia,
  agranulocytosis, Stevens-Johnson
  syndrome, hypotension,
  ventricular fibrillation

KEY: For complete abbreviation key, see inside front cover.

■ NURSING PROCESS: Phenytoin

ASSESSMENT

• Obtain a medication history from the client, including current drugs. Report if a drug-drug interaction is probable.

Anticonvulsants

- Check urinary output to determine if adequate (>600 mL/d).
- Check laboratory values related to renal and liver function. If both BUN and creatinine levels are elevated, a renal disorder should be suspected. Elevated serum liver enzymes, such as ALP, ALT, or SGPT, γ-glutamyl transferase (GGT), and/or 5′-nucleotidase indicate a hepatic disorder.

POTENTIAL NURSING DIAGNOSIS
- High risk for injury
- Altered oral mucous membranes

PLANNING
- Client will be free of seizures and will adhere to anticonvulsant therapy.
- Side effects of phenytoin will be minimal and closely monitored.

NURSING INTERVENTIONS
- Monitor serum drug levels of anticonvulsant to determine overdosing or underdosing of drug; compliance to regimen.
- Protect the client from hazards in the environment, such as sharp objects and table corners, during a seizure.
- Determine if the client is receiving adequate nutrients. Phenytoin may cause anorexia, nausea, and vomiting.
- Women taking oral contraceptives and anticonvulsants may need to use an addtional contraceptive method.

CLIENT TEACHING

General
- Instruct the client to shake well the suspension form before pouring.
- Instruct the client not to drive or perform other hazardous activity when beginning anticonvulsant therapy.
- Instruct the client to inform the health care provider of adverse reactions such as gingivitis, nystagmus, slurred speech, and rash.
- Alert female clients contemplating pregnancy to consult with the health care provider as phenytoin may have a teratogenic effect on the fetus.
- Inform the client that alcohol and other CNS depressants can cause an added depressive effect on the body and should be avoided.
- Advise the client to obtain an alert ID card and medic alert bracelet or tag that indicate the health problem and the drug taken.
- Instruct the client not to abruptly stop the drug therapy but rather to withdraw the prescribed drug gradually under medical supervision to prevent seizure rebound (reoccurrence of seizures).
- Instruct the client of the need for preventative dental check-ups.

Side Effects
- Advise the client that urine may be a harmless pinkish-red or reddish-brown.
- Instruct the client to maintain good oral hygiene; use a soft toothbrush to prevent gum irritation and bleeding.

EVALUATION
- Evaluate the effectiveness of the drug in controlling seizures.
- Continue to monitor phenytoin serum levels to determine if they are within the desired range. High serum levels of phenytoin are frequently indicators of phenytoin toxicity.

Generic (Brand)	Route and Dosage	Preg Cat	Interaction	t 1/2	PB	Action Onset	Action Peak	Action Duration
Barbiturates Amobarbital (Amytal) CSS II	*Status epilepticus* A: IM/IV: 75–500 mg; max: IM: 500 mg; IV: 1,000 mg Therapeutic range: 1–5 µg/mL	D	*Increase* effect with antidepressants, CNS depressants *Decrease* effect of tricyclic antidepressants, cimetidine	*Biphasic:* 1–40 min; 2–20 h	50–60%	<5 min	UK	3–6 h
Mephobarbital (Mebaral) CSS II	A: PO: 400–600 mg/d C: PO: 6–12 mg/kg/d in divided doses or C >5 y: 32–64 mg t.i.d./q.i.d. C <5 y: 16–32 mg t.i.d./q.i.d. Therapeutic range: 15–40 µg/mL	D	*Decrease* effects of oral anticoagulants	34 h	UK	20–60 min	UK	6–8 h
Phenobarbital (Luminal) CSS IV	*Status epilepticus* Neonate: IV: LD: 15–20 mg/kg single or divided dose A&C: IV: 15–18 mg/kg; max: 30 mg/kg *Maintenance:* Neonate: PO/IV: 3–4 mg/kg/d in 1–2 divided doses Infant: 5–6 mg/kg/d in 1–2 divided doses	D	*Increase* effects of other CNS depressants *Decrease* effects of oral contraceptives, oral anticoagulants, theophylline, phenothiazines	A: 50–140 h C: 35–75 h Neonate: 50–500 h	20–40%	PO: 30–60 min IV: <5 min	UK 30 min	6–10 h 4–10 h

Drug	Route and Dosage	Pregnancy Category	Drug Interactions	Half-life	Protein Binding	Onset	Peak	Duration
Primidone (Mysoline)	C: 1–5 y: 6–8 mg/kg/d in 1–2 divided doses; 6–12 y: 4–6 mg/kg/d in 1–2 divided doses; A: Therapeutic range: 1–3 mg/kg/d 15–40 µg/mL; A: PO: 125–250 mg b.i.d./q.i.d.; C <8 y: PO: 1/2 of adult dose	D	Same as phenobarbital	10–24 h	99%	4–7 d	7–10 d	8–12 h
Benzodiazepines (anxiolytics)								
Clonazepam (Klonopin)	A: PO: 0.5–1 mg t.i.d.; gradually increase dose q3d until seizures are controlled; C: PO: 0.01–0.03 mg/kg/d; gradually increase	C	*Increase* effects with CNS depressants, phenytoin	A: 20–50 h; C: 24–36 h	85%	15–60 min	1–2 h	6–8 h
Clorazepate (Tranxene) CSS IV	Therapeutic range: 20–80 ng/mL; A: PO: 7.5 mg t.i.d.; C: PO: 7.5 mg b.i.d.	D	*Increase* effect of drug with CNS depressants, oral contraceptives, alcohol; *Decrease* effects with rifampin, barbiturates, valproic acid	48 h	97%	1–2 h	1–2 h	24 h

continued

Generic (Brand)	Route and Dosage	Preg Cat	Interaction	t 1/2	PB	Action Onset	Action Peak	Action Duration
Lorazepam (Ativan) CSS IV	*Status epilepticus:* Neonate: IV: 0.05 mg/kg over 2–5 min; Infants & C: 0.1 mg/kg over 2–5 min; max: 4 mg/single dose A: IV: 4 mg over 2–5 min; max: 8 mg; may repeat in 10–15 min for all ages Therapeutic range: 50–240 ng/mL	D	*Increase* effect with morphine *Decrease* effect with oral contraceptives, smoking; toxicity with MAOIs, CNS depressants, alcohol	10–16 h	85%	IV: 1–5 min	UK	UK
Diazepam (Valium)	See Prototype Drug Chart for Anxiolytics							
Hydantoins Ethotoin (Peganone)	A: PO: 1–3 g/d in divided doses C: PO: 0.5–1 g/d Therapeutic range: 15–50 µg/mL	D	Same as mephenytoin	3–9 h	UK	UK	UK	UK
Mephenytoin (Mesantoin)	A: PO: Initially: 50–100 mg; 100–200 mg t.i.d. C: PO: Initially: 50–100 mg; 100–400 mg/d in divided doses Therapeutic range: 25–40 µg/mL	C	*Increase* effects of oral contraceptives, oral anticoagulants, phenothiazines *Decrease* effects of antineoplastics	7 h Metabolite: 100–144 h	UK	30 min	1–4 h	24–48 h
Phenytoin (Dilantin)	See Prototype Drug Chart							

Iminostilbene Carbamazepine (Tegretol)	A: PO: 200 mg b.i.d.; increasing doses as needed C: PO: 10–20 mg/kg/d in divided doses Therapeutic range: 5–12 µg/mL	C	*Increase* effects of drug with verapamil, isoniazid, cimetidine, erythromycin	15–30 h	75–90%	2–4 d	2–12 h	UK
Oxazolidones Paramethadione (Paradione)	A: PO: 300–600 mg t.i.d./q.i.d. C: PO: 13 mg/kg t.i.d. or 335 mg/m² t.i.d. or 300–900 mg/d in divided doses	D	None significant	1–4 h	UK	15–30 min	1–2 h	4–6 h
Trimethadione (Tridione)	Same as paramethadione	D	None significant	6–12 d	<10%	UK	1/2–2 h	UK
Succinimides Ethosuximide (Zarontin)	A: PO: 250 mg b.i.d.; increase dose gradually C: 3–6 y: PO: 250 mg/d Therapeutic range: 40–100 µg/mL	C	MAOIs and antidepressants lower seizure threshold; *increase* effects with CNS depressants	A: 50–60 h C: 25–30 h	UK	UK	>4 h	12–60 h
Methsuximide (Celontin)	A&C: PO: Initially: 300 mg/d for 1 wk; may increase at intervals	C	*Decrease* effects of oral contraceptives	2–4 h	UK	15–30 min	1–3 h	4–6 h
Phensuximide (Milontin)	A&C: PO: 0.5–1 g b.i.d./t.i.d.	C	Similar to ethosuximide	5–12 h	UK	UK	1–4 h	UK

continued

55

Anticonvulsants—Continued

Generic (Brand)	Route and Dosage	Preg Cat	Interaction	t 1/2	PB	Onset	Peak	Duration
							Action	
Valproate								
Valproic acid (Depakene)	A&C: PO: 15 mg/kg; max: 60 mg/kg/d in divided doses Therapeutic range: 40–100 µg/mL	D	*Increase* effects of drug with CNS depressants, barbiturates	6–16 h	90%	15–30 min	1–4 h	4–6 h
Miscellaneous								
Acetazolamide (Diamox)	Commonly used with other anticonvulsants: A: PO/IM/IV: 375 mg daily; max: 250 mg q.i.d. or PO SR: 250–500 mg daily or b.i.d. C: PO: 8–30 mg/kg in divided doses; max: 1.5 g/d	C	*Increase* effects of tricyclic antidepressants, ephedrine, procainamide, amphetamines; toxicity with salicylates	2.5–6 h	90%	PO: 1h SR: 2 h IV: 2 min	2–4 h 8–18 h <1 min	8–12 h 18–24 h 4–5 h
Gabapentin (Neurontin)	*Adjunctive therapy for partial seizures:* PO: 900–1,800 mg/d in 3 divided doses; max time between doses: 12 h	C	*Decrease* effects with antacids	5–7 h	<3%	UK	UK	UK

| Magnesium sulfate | *Preeclampsia or eclampsia:*
A: IV: Initially: 4 g in 250 mL D_5W; then 4 g IM; follow with 4 g IM q4h PRN or Inf: 1–4 g/h
Hypomagnesemic seizures:
A: IV: 1–2 g (19% sol) over 20 min; follow with 1 g IM q4–6h based on blood levels | B | Use cautiously with anesthesia and CNS depressants to avoid additive effect
Increase neuromuscular blockade of vecuronium tubocurarine | UK | UK | IV: Immediate
IM: 1 h | UK | IV: 30 min |

ANTIPSYCHOTICS, ANXIOLYTICS, AND ANTIDEPRESSANTS

Antipsychotics
  Phenothiazine
  Nonphenothiazine

Anxiolytics

Antidepressants

Antimanic

Antipsychotic

Chlorpromazine
  (Thorazine)
Antipsychotic neuroleptic, antiemetic
  (phenothiazine)
Pregnancy Category: C
Drug Forms:
Tab 10, 25, 50, 100, 200 mg
Cap SR 30, 75, 150, 200, 300 mg
Syrup 10 mg/5 mL
Conc 30, 100 mg/mL
Supp 25, 100 mg
Inj IM/IV 25 mg/mL

Dosage

Psychoses
A: PO: 10–25 mg b.i.d./q.i.d.;
  increase by 20–50 mg/d q3–4d to
  max 800 mg/d in 4 divided doses
  (usual dose is 200 mg/d)
IM: Initially: 25–50 mg; may repeat
  in 1 h; increase to max of 400 mg
  q4–6h
C: PO: 0.55 mg/kg q4–6h
C: > 6 mon: IM: 0.55 mg/kg or 15
  mg/m^2 q6–8h; max: 6 mon–5 y:
  40 mg/d; 5–12 y: 75 mg/d
Consult other references for dosages
  for nausea, vomiting, preoperative
  sedation, and intractable hiccups.

Contraindications

Coma; hepatic, renal, or coronary
  disease; cerebral insufficiency;
  severe hypotension; bone marrow
  depression; blood dyscrasias; CNS
  depression

Drug-Lab-Food Interactions

Increase CNS depression with alcohol,
  CNS depressants, narcotics,
  sedative-hypnotics; tricyclic
  antidepressants *increase*
  hypotensive and anticholinergic
  effects

Decrease absorption with antacids,
  antidiarrheals

Lab: Increase AST, ALT, and alkaline
  phosphatase; false pregnancy test

Decrease hematocrit, hemoglobin
  leukocytes, platelets

Pharmacokinetics

Absorption: PO: Varies
Distribution: PB: 95%
Metabolism: t 1/2: 8–30 h
Excretion: In urine

Pharmacodynamics

PO:	Onset: 30–60 min
	Peak: 2–4 h
	Duration: 4–6 h
PO SR:	Onset: 30–60 min
	Peak: 2–4 h
	Duration: <10–12 h
Rectal:	Onset: 1–2 h
	Peak: 3 h
	Duration: 3–4 h
IM:	Onset: 15–30 min
	Peak: 30 min
	Duration: 4–8 h
IV:	Onset: 15 min
	Peak: 10 min
	Duration: UK

Therapeutic Effects/Uses: To treat psychosis (mania, schizophrenia), anxiety, agitation, intractable hiccups, nausea, vomiting, preoperative sedation, behavioral problems in children

Mode of Action: Alteration in dopamine effect on CNS, depression of limbic system and cerebral cortex that controls aggression, mechanism for antipsychotic effects unknown

Antipsychotics

Side Effects	Adverse Reactions
Sedation, hypotension, dizziness, extrapyramidal symptoms (EPS), constipation, headache, dry mouth and eyes, nausea, vomiting, diarrhea, urinary retention	Anemia, tachycardia, leukopenia, tardive dyskinesia *Life-threatening:* Agranulocytosis, seizures, laryngospasm, respiratory depression, circulatory failure

KEY: For complete abbreviation key, see inside front cover.

■ NURSING PROCESS: Chlorpromazine

ASSESSMENT
- Obtain baseline vital signs for use in future comparison.
- Obtain a history from the client of present drug therapy. If client is taking an anticonvulsant, drug dose might need to be increased as antipsychotics tend to lower seizure threshold.
- Assess mental status before start of drug therapy and continue daily.

POTENTIAL NURSING DIAGNOSES
Altered thought processes
Activity intolerance
Sensory-perceptual alteration

PLANNING
- Client's psychotic behavior will be controlled by drug(s) and psychotherapy.

NURSING INTERVENTIONS
- Monitor vital signs. Orthostatic hypotension is likely to occur.
- Remain with client while he or she takes the medication. Some clients hide drugs.
- Avoid skin contact with liquid concentrates to prevent contact dermatitis. Liquid must be protected from light and should be diluted with fruit juice.
- Administer oral doses with food or milk to decrease gastric irritation.
- Administer IM phenothiazines deep into the muscle because the drug is irritating to the fatty tissue. Do NOT inject into subcutaneous tissue. Check blood pressure for marked decrease 30 min after IM phenothiazine is injected.
- Do not mix in same syringe with heparin, pentobarbital, cimetidine, or dimenhydrinate.
- Chill suppository in the refrigerator for 30 min before removing foil wrapper.
- Observe the client for extrapyramidal syndrome (EPS): acute dystonia (spasms of the tongue, face, neck, and back), akathisia (restlessness, inability to sit still, foot tapping), pseudoparkinsonism (muscle tremors, rigidity, shuffling gait), and tardive dyskinesia (lip smacking, protruding and darting tongue, and constant chewing movement). Report these promptly to the health care provider.
- Monitor for symptoms of neuroleptic malignant syndrome (NMS): increased fever, pulse, and blood pressure; muscle rigidity; increased creatine phos-

phokinase and WBC; altered mental status; acute renal failure; varying levels of consciousness; pallor; diaphoresis, tachycardia; and dysrhythmias.
- Monitor urine output. Urinary retention may result.
- Monitor serum glucose level.

CLIENT TEACHING

General

- Instruct the client to take the drug exactly as ordered. In schizophrenia and other psychotic disorders, antipsychotics do not cure the mental illness but do prevent symptoms. Many clients on medication can function outside the institution setting.
- Advise the client that medication may take 6 wk or longer to achieve full clinical effect.
- Instruct the client not to consume alcohol or other CNS depressants such as narcotics; these drugs intensify the depressant effect on the body.
- Instruct the client not to abruptly discontinue the drug. Seek advice from the health care provider before making any changes in dosage.
- Encourage the client to read labels on OTC preparations. Some are contraindicated when taking antipsychotics.
- Advise client to consult the health care provider if dry mouth persists for more than 2 wk.
- Encourage the client to talk with the health care provider regarding family planning. The effect of antipsychotics on the fetus is not fully known; however, there may be teratogenic effects on the fetus.
- Instruct the client on the importance of routine follow-up examinations.
- Encourage the client to obtain laboratory tests on schedule. WBCs are monitored for 3 mon, especially during the start of drug therapy. Leukopenia, or decreased WBCs, may occur. Be alert to symptoms of malaise, fever, and sore throat, which may be an indication of agranulocytosis, a serious blood dyscrasia. Report this promptly to the health care provider.
- Encourage the client to wear an ID bracelet indicating the medication taken.

Side Effects

- Inform the client about EPS; instruct the client to promptly report symptoms to the health care provider.
- Photosensitivity may occur; instruct the client to avoid direct sunlight or to use a sun block and protective clothing. Sunbathing can cause a skin rash.
- Advise the client of orthostatic hypotension and possible dizziness.
- Advise the client that urine might be pink or red-brown; this discoloration is harmless.
- Inform the client that changes may occur related to sexual functioning and menstruating. Women could have irregular menstrual periods or amenorrhea, and men might experience impotence and gynecomastia (enlargement of breast tissue).

EVALUATION

- Evaluate the effectiveness of the drug; the client is free of psychotic symptoms.
- The client can cope with everyday living situation.
- Identify any side effects of or adverse reactions to the drug.

NOTES:

_____

_____

_____

_____

_____

_____

_____

_____

_____

_____

Antipsychotics

Generic (Brand)	Route and Dosage	Preg Cat	Interaction	t 1/2	PB	Onset	Peak	Duration
Phenothiazines:								
Aliphatics								
Chlorpromazine HCl (Thorazine)	See Prototype Drug Chart							
Promazine HCl (Sparine)	A: PO: 10–200 mg q4–6h IM: 50–150 mg; may repeat ×1 C > 12 y: PO: 10–25 mg q4–6h	C	*Increase* effect with CNS depressants, epinephrine, anticholinergics *Lab: Increase* cholesterol, glucose	≥24 h	≥90%	PO: 30–60 min IM: 15–30 min	2–4 h 1 h	4–6 h 4–6 h
Triflupromazine (Vesprin)	A: PO: 10–50 mg b.i.d./ t.i.d. IM: 60–150 mg/d C > 2 y: PO: 0.5–2 mg/ kg/d in 3 divided doses	C	Similar to promazine	≥24 h	≥90%	PO: Erratic IM: 15–30 min	2–4 h 1 h	4–6 h 12 h
Piperazines								
Fluphenazine HCl (Prolixin)	A: PO: 1–5 mg t.i.d./q.i.d. Elderly: 1–2.5 mg/d; also long-acting weekly/ biweekly dosages Therapeutic range: 5–20 ng/mL	C	*Increase* effect of narcotics *Decrease* effect of barbiturates, lithium, levodopa *Lab: Increase* cholesterol, glucose	5–15 h	≥90%	PO/IM: 1 h	0.5–2 h	6–8 h
Perphenazine (Trilafon)	See Prototype Drug Chart							
Prochlorperazine maleate (Compazine)	A: PO: 5–10 mg t.i.d./ q.i.d.; max: 40 mg/d (can be higher for psychotic behavior)	C	*Increase* effect of anticonvulsants, CNS depressants, epinephrine	23 h	≥90%	PO: 30–40 min IM: 10–20 min	2–4 h 15–30 min	3–4 h 2–12 h

(header "Action" spans Onset, Peak, Duration columns)

64

Drug	Pregnancy category	Dosage	Drug interactions	t½	Protein binding	Onset	Peak	Duration
Thiothixene HCl (Navane)	C	A: PO: 2 mg t.i.d.; max: 60 mg/d; IM: 4 mg b.i.d/q.i.d.; Max: 30 mg/d	*Increase* effect of CNS depressants, hypotensive agents; *Decrease* effects of levodopa; *Lab: Increase* cholesterol, glucose	24–34 h	≥90%	PO: 2–7 d; IM: 15–30 min	2–8 h; 1–6 h	12–24 h; Up to 12 h
Trifluoperazine HCl (Stelazine)	C	A: PO: 1–5 mg b.i.d.; max: 40 mg/d; C: PO: 1 mg daily/b.i.d.	*Increase* effect with CNS depressants, propranolol; *Decrease* effects with anticoagulants, anticonvulsants	≥24 h	≥90%	PO: 30–40 min; IM: 10–20 min	2–4 h; 15–30 min	4–6 h; 12 h
Piperidine Mesoridazine besylate (Serentil)	C	A: PO: 50 mg t.i.d.; gradually increase; Elderly: 1/3–1/2 adult dose	*Increase* toxicity with CNS depressants; *Decrease* effects with anticholinergics, anticonvulsants	24–48 h	92–99%	PO: Erratic; IM: 15–30 min	2 h; 20 min	4–6 h; 6–8 h
Thioridazine HCl (Mellaril)	C	A: PO: 50–100 mg t.i.d.; max: 800 mg/d; Elderly: 1/3–1/2 adult dose	*Increase* effect with CNS depressants, epinephrine; *Decrease* effects with anticholinergics	24–30 h	≥90%	PO: 30–60 min	2–4 h	4–6 h

KEY: For complete abbreviation key, see inside front cover.

65

Antipsychotic: Nonphenothiazine

Haloperidol

Haloperidol
  (Haldol)
Antipsychotic, neuroleptic
  (nonphenothiazine)
Pregnancy Category: C

Drug Forms:
Tab 0.5, 1, 2, 5, 10, 20 mg
Conc 2 mg/mL
Inj 5 mg/mL
Depot 50, 100 mg/mL

Dosage

A: PO: 0.5–5 mg b.i.d./t.i.d.
C: PO: 0.15 mg/kg/d in divided
  doses (not for child <3 y)
Elderly: Decreased doses than for
  younger adult
Depot: 50–100 mg q4wk

Contraindications

Narrow-angle glaucoma; severe
  hepatic, renal, and cardiovascular
  diseases; bone marrow depression;
  Parkinson's disease; blood
  dyscrasias; CNS depression;
  subcortical brain damage

Drug-Lab-Food Interactions

Increase sedation with alcohol, CNS
  depressants
Increase toxicity with anticholinergics,
  CNS depressants, lithium
Decrease effects with phenobarbital,
  carbamazepine

Pharmacokinetics

Absorption: PO: 60% absorbed
Distribution: PB: 80–90%
Metabolism: t 1/2: 15–35 h
Excretion: In urine and feces

Pharmacodynamics

PO:	Onset: 2 h
	Peak: 2–6 h
	Duration: 24–72 h
IM:	Onset: 15–30 min
	Peak: 30–45 min
	Duration: 4–8 h
IM: Decanoate:	Onset: UK
	Peak: 6–7 d
	Duration: 3–4 wk

Therapeutic Effects/Uses: To treat acute and chronic psychoses, for children with severe behavior problems who are combative, to suppress narcotic withdrawal symptoms, to treat schizophrenia resistant to other drugs, to treat Tourette's syndrome.

Mode of Action: Alteration of the effect of dopamine on CNS; mechanism for antipsychotic effects are unknown.

Side Effects

Sedation, extrapyramidal symptoms,
  orthostatic hypotension,
  photosensitivity, dry mouth and
  eyes, blurred vision

Adverse Reactions

Tachycardia, seizures, urinary
  retention
Life-threatening: Laryngospasm,
  respiratory depression, cardiac
  dysrhythmias

KEY: For complete abbreviation key, see inside front cover.

■ NURSING PROCESS: Nonphenothiazine Antipsychotic

ASSESSMENT

- Obtain baseline vital signs for future comparison.
- Obtain a history from the client of present drug therapy. If client is taking an anticonvulsant, drug dose might need to be increased as antipsychotics tend to lower seizure threshold.
- Assess mental status before the start of drug therapy.

POTENTIAL NURSING DIAGNOSES

Altered thought processes; potential for violence

PLANNING

- Client's psychotic behavior will be controlled by drug and psychotherapy.

NURSING INTERVENTIONS

- Monitor vital signs. Orthostatic hypotension is likely to occur.
- Remain with client while he or she takes the medication. Some clients hide drugs. If necessary, do mouth checks or give concentrate.
- Administer by IM route deep into the muscle because the drug is irritating to the fatty tissue. Do NOT inject into subcutaneous tissue. Check blood pressure for marked decrease 30 min after drug is injected.
- Do not mix in same syringe with heparin, pentobarbital, cimetidine, or dimenhydrinate.
- Administer oral doses with food or 8 oz of water or milk to decrease gastric irritation.
- Observe the client for extrapyramidal syndrome (EPS): acute dystonia (spasms of the tongue, face, neck, and back), akathisia (restlessness, inability to sit still, foot tapping), pseudoparkinsonism (muscle tremors, rigidity, drooling, shuffling gait), and tardive dyskinesia (lip smacking, protruding and darting tongue, constant chewing movement, difficulty swallowing). Report these promptly to the health care provider.
- Monitor urine output. Urinary retention may result.
- Monitor serum glucose level.

CLIENT TEACHING

General

- Instruct the client to take the drug exactly as ordered. In schizophrenia and other psychotic disorders, antipsychotics do not cure the mental illness but do prevent symptoms. Many clients on medication can function outside the institution.
- Instruct the client not to consume alcohol or other CNS depressants such as narcotics; these drugs intensify the depressant effect on the body.
- Instruct the client not to abruptly discontinue the drug. Seek advice from the health care provider before making any changes in dosage.
- Encourage the client to read labels on OTC preparations. Some are contraindicated when taking antipsychotics.
- Instruct the client on the importance of routine follow-up examination.
- Encourage the client to talk with the health care provider regarding family planning. The effect of antipsychotics on the fetus is not fully known; however, there may be teratogenic effects on the fetus.
- Encourage the client to wear an ID bracelet indicating the medication taken.

Antipsychotic: Nonphenothiazine

Side Effects

● Instruct the client to avoid potentially dangerous situations, such as driving, until drug dosing has been stabilized.

● Advise the client to change position slowly to decrease orthostatic hypotension.

● Inform clients about EPS symptoms; promptly report these to the health care provider.

● Advise the client to consult health care provider if dry mouth persists for more than 2 wk.

● Instruct the client to have daily fluid intake of eight 8-oz glasses.

● Photosensitivity may occur; instruct the client to avoid direct sunlight or to use a sun block and protective clothing. Sunbathing can cause a skin rash.

● Advise the client to avoid extremes in temperatures and increased exercise.

● Inform the client that changes related to sexual functioning and menstruation may occur. Women could have irregular menstrual periods or amenorrhea, and men might experience impotence and gynecomastia (enlargement of breast tissue).

● Encourge the client to obtain laboratory tests on schedule. Weekly blood work is a must for clozapine. WBCs are monitored for 3 mon, especially during the start of drug therapy. Leukopenia, or decreased WBCs, may occur. Be alert to symptoms of malaise, fever, and sore throat, which may be an indication of agranulocytosis, a serious blood dyscrasia. Report this promptly to the health care provider, especially with clozapine.

EVALUATION

● Evaluate the effectiveness of the drug; the client is free of psychotic symptoms at the *lowest* dose possible.

● The client can cope with everyday living situation and attend to activities of daily living.

● Determine if any side effects of or adverse reactions to the drug have occurred.

NOTES:

_____

_____

_____

_____

_____

_____

_____

_____

_____

_____

Antipsychotics

Generic (Brand)	Route and Dosage	Preg Cat	Interaction	t 1/2	PB	Action Onset	Action Peak	Action Duration
Butyrophenone Droperidol (Inapsine)	A: IM/IV: 2.5–10 mg 30–60 min before anesthesia C: IM/IV: 0.088–0.165 mg/kg	C	*Increase* CNS depression with other CNS depressants, alcohol *Decrease* effect of guanethidine	2 h	UK	5–10 min	30 min	2–12 h
Haloperidol (Haldol)	See Prototype Drug Chart							
Dibenzoxazepine Loxapine (Loxitane)	A: PO: Initially: 10 mg b.i.d.; then may increase to 50–100 mg/d Elderly: 1/3–1/2 regular adult dose	C	Similar to droperidol	5 h	95%	20–30 min	1–3 h	12 h
Thioxanthenes Clorprothixene HCl (Taractan)	A: PO: 25–50 mg t.i.d.; gradually increase to 500–600 mg/d	C	*Increase* CNS depression with CNS depressants, alcohol *Decrease* effect of guanethidine	Initial phase: 3 h Late phase: 34 h	UK	30–60 min	2–4 h	4–6 h

Thiothixene HCl (Navane)	A: PO: Initially: 2 mg t.i.d.; gradually increase to 10–25 mg/d	C	Similar to droperidol	34 h	UK	2–7 d	2–8 h	12–24 h
Others								
Clozapine (Clozaril)	A: PO/IM: Initially: <50 mg/d; if tolerated, gradually increase to 300–450 mg/d in divided doses	B	*Increase* CNS depression with antihistamines, sedative-hypnotics, narcotics	8–12 h	95%	UK	2–4 wk	4–12 h
Molindone HCl (Moban)	A: PO: 5–50 mg t.i.d./q.i.d. Elderly: 1/3–1/2 adult dose	C	*Increase* toxicity with antihypertensives, anticonvulsants, CNS depressants	1.5 h	UK	UK	1/2 h	24–30 h
Risperidone (Risperdal)	A: PO: 1–3 mg b.i.d. Elderly: 1/3–1/2 adult dose	C	*Increase* effects with CNS depressants, alcohol *Increase* toxicity with warfarin, quinidine *Lab*: must monitor for agranulocytosis with WBCs weekly	24 h	90%	UK	1–2 h	UK

KEY: For complete abbreviation key, see inside front cover.

Anxiolytics

Diazepam

Diazepam
  (Valium)
Benzodiazepine
  CSS IV
Pregnancy Category: D
Drug Forms:
Tab 2, 5, 10 mg
Cap SR 15 mg
Oral solution 5 mg/5 mL, 5 mg/mL
Inj 5 mg/5 mL (1, 2, and 10 mL)

Dosage

Anxiety:
A: PO/IM/IV: 2–10 mg b.i.d./q.i.d.
Elderly: 2.5 mg b.i.d.
C >6 mon: 1–2.5 mg t.i.d./q.i.d.
Musculoskeletal spasm:
A: PO: 2–10 mg b.i.d./q.i.d.
  IM: 5–10 mg q3–4h
Preoperative sedation:
A: IV: 5–15 mg 15 min before event
Status epilepticus:
A: IV: 5–10 mg q10–20 min; max:
  30 mg
C <6 y: 0.2–0.5 mg/kg q15–30 min;
  max: 5 mg total dose
C >6 y: 0.2–0.5 mg/kg q15–30 min;
  max: 10 mg total dose
IV: max: 5 mg/3 min

Contraindications

Hypersensitivity, CNS depression,
  shock, coma, narrow-angle
  glaucoma, pregnancy, lactation
Caution: Hepatic or renal
  dysfunction; epilepsy, elderly and
  infants; history of drug abuse;
  depression, addiction-prone, or
  suicidal tendency

Drug-Lab-Food Interactions

Increase effects of diazepam with
  alcohol, oral contraceptives, CNS
  depressants, cimetidine,
  disulfiram, fluoxetine, isoniazid,
  ketoconazole, levodopa,
  phenytoin, metoprolol,
  propoxyphene, propranolol,
  valproic acid; toxic effects with
  MAOIs; *Decrease* effects with
  rifampin, caffeine, cigarettes
Do not mix or dilute with other drugs
  in syringe
Lab: Increase bilirubin

Pharmacokinetics

Absorption: Rapid from GI tract;
  erratic from IM administration;
  most rapid and complete from
  deltoid muscle
Distribution: Widely PB: 98%
Metabolism: t 1/2: 25–50 h
Excretion: In urine

Pharmacodynamics

PO: Onset: 30–60 min
    Peak: 1–2 h
    Duration: 2–3 h (varies)
IM: Onset: 15–30 min
    Peak: 1–2 h
    Duration: 1–1 1/2 h (varies)
IV: Onset: 1–5 min
    Peak: 15–30 min
    Duration: 15–60 min

Therapeutic Effects/Uses: To control anxiety, preoperative sedation, skeletal muscle
relaxant, to treat status epilepticus, alcohol withdrawal, convulsive disorders, an-
terograde amnesia.

Mode of Action: Depression of limbic and subcortical CNS and skeletal muscle relaxation, shortens stage 4 and REM sleep.

Side Effects	Adverse Reactions
Drowsiness, dizziness, syncope, orthostatic hypotension, blurred vision, nausea, vomiting, fatigue, confusion	ECG changes, tachycardia, psychological and physical dependence with long-term use *Life-threatening:* Laryngospasm

KEY: For complete abbreviation key, see inside front cover.

■ NURSING PROCESS: Anxiolytics: Diazepam

ASSESSMENT
- Assess for suicidal ideation.
- Obtain a history of the client's anxiety reaction.
- Determine the client's support system (family, friends, groups), if any.
- Obtain the client's drug history. Report possible drug-drug interaction.

POTENTIAL NURSING DIAGNOSES
Anxiety
Mobility, impaired physical

PLANNING
- Client's anxiety and stress will be reduced through nonpharmacological methods, anxiolytic drugs, or support/group therapy.

NURSING INTERVENTIONS
- Administer by IM route in large muscle mass, and inject drug slowly.
- Observe the client for side effects of anxiolytics. Recognize that drug tolerance and physical and psychological dependency can result with most anxiolytics.
- Recognize that anxiolytic drug dosages should be less for older adults and debilitated persons than for young and middle-aged adults.
- Monitor vital signs, especially blood pressure and pulse; orthostatic hypotension may occur.
- Encourage the family to be supportive of the client.

CLIENT TEACHING
General
- Advise the client not to drive a motor vehicle or operate dangerous equipment when taking anxiolytics since sedation is a common side effect.
- Instruct the client not to consume alcohol or CNS depressants such as narcotics while taking an anxiolytic.
- Instruct the client on ways to control excess stress and anxiety, such as relaxation techniques.
- Inform the client that effective response may take 1 to 2 wk.
- Encourage the client to follow drug regimen and not to abruptly stop taking the drug after prolonged use because withdrawal symptoms can occur.

Side Effects
- Instruct the client to arise slowly from the sitting to standing position to avoid dizziness from orthostatic hypotension.

EVALUATION
- Evaluate the effectiveness of drug therapy by determining if the client is less anxious and more able to cope with stresses and anxieties.
- Determine if the client is taking anxiolytic drug as prescribed and is adhering to client teaching instructions.

Anxiolytics

Generic (Brand)	Route and Dosage	Preg Cat	Interaction	t 1/2	PB	Action Onset	Action Peak	Action Duration
Antihistamines Hydroxyzine HCl (Atarax, Vistaril)	A: PO: 50–100 mg t.i.d./q.i.d. IM: 25–100 mg C <6 y: 25 mg b.i.d. C >6 y: 25 mg b.i.d./q.i.d.	C	*Increase* effect with anticholinergic, CNS depressants *Decrease* effect with epinephrine	3–7 h	UK	PO/IM: 15–30 min	2–4 h	4–6 h
Benzodiazepines Alprazolam (Xanax) CSS IV	A: PO: 0.25–0.5 mg t.i.d. Elderly: 0.25 mg b.i.d./t.i.d.; max: 4 mg/d	D	*Increase* effects of drug with CNS depressants	12–15 h	80%	1–2 h	1–2 h	12–24 h
Chlordiazepoxide HCl (Librium) CSS IV	*Anxiety disorders:* A: PO: 5–25 mg t.i.d./q.i.d. C: PO: 5 mg b.i.d./q.i.d. *Acute alcohol withdrawal:* A: PO/IM/IV: 50–100 mg; max: 300 mg/d	D	*Increase* effect of drug with CNS depressants, oral contraceptives, alcohol, barbiturates, valproic acid *Decrease* effects of drug with rifampin	6–30 h	90–98%	PO: 15–30 min	15–30 min	2–4 h
Clorazepate dipotassium (Tranxene) CSS IV	A: PO: 15–60 mg/d in divided doses Elderly: 7.5 mg b.i.d.	D	Similar to chlordiazepoxide	48 h	80–90%	30–60 min	1–2 h	24 h
Diazepam (Valium)	See Prototype Drug Chart							

Drug	Route and Dosage	Pregnancy Category	Drug Interactions	t½	PB	Onset	Peak	Duration
Halazepam (Paxipam)	A: PO: 20–40 mg t.i.d./q.i.d. Elderly: 20 mg daily/b.i.d.	D	Same as chlordiazepoxide	14 h	97%	30–60 min	1–3 h	UK
Lorazepam (Ativan) CSS IV	A: PO: 2–6 mg/d in divided doses A: IM/IV: 2–4 mg	D	*Increase* effects with probenecid, CNS depressants *Decrease* effect with smoking	10–20 h	90%	15–45 min	1–6 h	36–48 h
Oxazepam (Serax)	A: PO: 10–30 mg t.i.d./q.i.d.	D	Similar to chlordiazepoxide	3.5–21 h	85–95%	45–90 min	1–2 h	6–12 h
Prazepam (Centrax) CSS IV	A: PO: 10 mg t.i.d./q.i.d. Elderly: 10–15 mg/d in divided doses	D	Same as chlordiazepoxide	30–200 h	97%	UK	7–14 d	2–3 d
Propanediols Meprobamate (Equanil, Miltown) CSS IV	A: PO: 400 mg t.i.d./q.i.d. C: PO: 100–200 mg b.i.d./t.i.d.	D	*Increase* effects with CNS depressants, sedative-hypnotics	6–16 h	UK	1 h	1–3 h	6–12 h
Others Buspirone HCl (BuSpar)	A: PO: 15–30 mg/d in divided doses; max: 60 mg/d	B	*Increase* effect with cimetidine; hypertensive crises may result with MAOIs; avoid alcohol *Increase* toxicity of digoxin *Lab:* *Increase* AST, ALT	2–3 h	95%	7–14 d	3–4 wk	UK

KEY: For complete abbreviation key, see inside front cover.

Antidepressants

Amoxapine

Amoxapine
  (Asendin)
Antidepressant: Second-generation
  tricyclic
Pregnancy Category: C
Drug Forms:
Tab 25, 50, 100, 150 mg

Dosage

A: PO: 50 mg b.i.d./t.i.d.; increase
  dose gradually to <300 mg/d or
  give as single dose at h.s.; max:
  inpatient: 600 mg/d; max:
  outpatient: 400 g/d; generally not
  recommended for children <16 y

Contraindications

Severe depression with suicidal
  tendency, severe liver disease,
  seizures, narrow-angle glaucoma,
  within 14 d of receiving MAOIs,
  myocardial infarction recovery
  phase, urinary retention

Drug-Lab-Food Interactions

Increase effect of CNS depressants,
  alcohol, adrenergic agents,
  anticholinergics; *increase* effects
  with phenothiazines, haloperidol,
  smoking
Hypertensive crisis and death may
  occur with MAOIs
Decrease effect of clonidine;
  guanethidine

Pharmacokinetics

Absorption: PO: well absorbed
Distribution: PB: 90%
Metabolism: t 1/2: 8 h
Excretion: 80% in urine; 20% in feces

Pharmacodynamics

Antidepressant effect:
PO: Onset: 2–4 wk
       Peak: 90 min
       Duration: weeks

Therapeutic Effects/Uses: To treat depression with melancholia or psychotic symptoms, depressive phase of bipolar disorder, depression associated with organic disease, alcoholism, psychoneurotic anxiety or mixed symptoms of anxiety and depression.

Mode of Action: Serotonin and norepinephrine increased in nerve cells due to blockage from nerve fibers.

Side Effects

Sedation, drowsiness, hypotension,
  dry mouth and eyes, blurred
  vision, urinary retention,
  constipation, extrapyramidal
  syndrome, diarrhea, rash, weight
  gain

Adverse Reactions

Life-threatening: Cardiac
  dysrhythmias, agranulocytosis,
  thrombocytopenia, leukopenia,
  paralytic ileus, hepatitis,
  hypertension, neuroleptic
  malignant syndrome
  (hyperpyrexia, muscle rigidity,
  tachycardia, cardiac dysrhythmias)

KEY: For complete abbreviation key, see inside front cover.

■ NURSING PROCESS: Second-Generation Antidepressant

ASSESSMENT
- Assess the client's baseline vital signs and weight for future comparison.
- Check the client's liver and renal function by assessing urine output (> 600 mL/d), BUN, and serum creatinine and liver enzyme levels.
- Obtain a history of episodes of depression or manic-depressive behavior; assess mental status.
- Obtain the client's drug history. CNS depressants can cause an additive effect. Antidepressants cause anticholinergic-like symptoms and are contraindicated if the client has glaucoma.
- Assess for tardive dyskinesia and neuroleptic malignant syndrome (NMS), including hyperpyrexia, muscle rigidity, tachycardia, cardiac dysrhythmias.

POTENTIAL NURSING DIAGNOSES
Potential for violence and injury
Anxiety
Social isolation

PLANNING
- Client's depression or manic-depressive behavior will be decreased.

NURSING INTERVENTIONS
- Observe the client for signs and symptoms of depression: mood changes, insomnia, apathy, or lack of interest in activities.
- Check the client's vital signs. Orthostatic hypotension is common. Check for anticholinergic-like symptoms: dry mouth, increased heart rate, urinary retention, or constipation. Weight check two to three times per week.
- Monitor the client for suicidal tendencies when marked depression is present.
- If the client is taking anticonvulsant, observe the client for seizures; antidepressants lower the seizure threshold.
- Provide the client with a list of foods to avoid, especially with MAOIs.

CLIENT TEACHING
General
- Instruct the client to take the medication as prescribed.
- Inform the client that the effectiveness of the drug may not be evident until 1–2 wk after the start of therapy.
- Encourage the client to keep medical appointments.
- Instruct the client not to consume alcohol or any CNS depressants.
- Instruct the client not to drive or be involved in potentially dangerous mechanical activity until stabilization of drug dose has been established.
- Instruct the client not to abruptly stop taking drug.
- Encourage the client who is planning pregnancy to consult with the health care provider about possible teratogenic effects of the drug on the fetus.
Side Effects
- Advise the client that antidepressants may be taken at bedtime to decrease the dangers from the sedative effect.

EVALUATION
- Evaluate the effectiveness of the drug therapy.

Antidepressants

Generic (Brand)	Route and Dosage	Preg Cat	Interaction	t 1/2	PB	Action: Onset	Action: Peak	Action: Duration
Tricyclics Amitriptyline HCl (Elavil, Endep, Enovil)	A: PO: 25 mg t.i.d.; increase to 150 mg/d; dose may be given as single h.s. dose *Therapeutic range:* 100–200 ng/mL	D	*Increase* effects of CNS depressants, anticholinergics, warfarin, adrenergics; *increase* toxicity with MAOIs, clonidine *Decrease* effect of guanethidine *Lab:* Increase glucose	10–50 h	95%	7–21 d	2–6 wk	UK
Clomipramine HCl (Anafranil)	A: 25–100 mg/d in divided doses; max: 250 mg/d; after titration; entire dose may be given h.s.	C	*Decrease* effects of phenytoin, barbiturates *Increase* effects of CNS depressants, anticholinergics, alcohol Toxicity MAOIs *Lab:* Increase glucose	20–30 h	96–97%	1–6 wk	UK	UK
Desipramine HCl (Norpramin, Pertofrane)	A: PO: 25 mg t.i.d. or 75 mg h.s.; increase to 200 mg/d Elderly: 25–50 mg/d in divided doses *Therapeutic range:* 150–250 ng/mL	D	Similar to amitriptyline	15–90 h	90–95%	2–3 wk	6 wk	UK

Drug							
Doxepin HCl (Sinequan) A: PO: 75–100 mg/d h.s. or in divided doses; max: 300 mg/d *Therapeutic range:* 30–50 ng/mL	C	Similar to amitriptyline	6–8 h	80–85%	2–3 wk	4–6 wk	UK
Imipramine HCl (Tofranil) A: PO: 75 mg/d (h.s. or 25 mg t.i.d.); max: 300 mg/d IM: Initially: max: 100 mg/d in divided doses *Therapeutic range:* 150–250 ng/mL	D	Similar to amitriptyline	8–15 h	89–95%	1 h	2–4 wk	≥1 wk
Nortriptyline HCl (Aventyl) A: PO: 25 mg t.i.d./q.i.d.; max: 100 mg/d Elderly: 30–50 mg/d in divided doses *Therapeutic range:* 50–150 ng/mL	D	*Increase* effects of CNS depressants, alcohol, epinephrine, benzodiazepines, MAOIs *Lab:* May increase PT of patients on warfarin; increase glucose	18–28 h	90–95%	2–3 wk	6 wk	UK
Protriptyline HCl (Vivactil) A: PO: 15–40 mg/d in divided doses; increase gradually; max: 60 mg/d *Therapeutic range:* 70–250 ng/mL	C	Similar to amitriptyline	60–98 h	92%	15–30 min	UK	4–6 h
Trimipramine maleate (Surmontil) A: PO: 75–150 mg/d in divided doses or all h.s.; max: 200 mg/d Elderly: max: 100 mg/d	C	Similar to amitriptyline	20–26 h	95%	UK	6 h	UK

continued

Antidepressants

Generic (Brand)	Route and Dosage	Preg Cat	Interaction	t 1/2	PB	Action Onset	Action Peak	Action Duration
Second Generation								
Amoxapine (Asendin)	See Prototype Drug Chart							
Bupropion HCl (Wellbutrin)	A: PO: Initially: 200 mg/d as b.i.d.; increase gradually to 300 mg/d in divided doses; max: 150 mg	B	*Increase* toxicity with anticonvulsants, cimetidine, MAOIs, levodopa	50 h	>80%	3–4 wk	1–3 h	UK
Fluoxetine HCl (Prozac)	A: PO: 20 mg in a.m.; max: 80 mg/d in divided doses	B	*Increase* toxicity with MAOIs, L-tryptophan, highly protein-bound drugs (e.g., warfarin)	7–9 d (active metabolite)	95%	Steady state: 2–4 wk	4 wk	2 wk
Maprotiline HCl (Ludiomil)	A: PO: 75 mg h.s. or in divided doses	B	*Increase* effects of norepinephrine, MAOIs, CNS depressants *Decrease* effects with phenytoin, barbiturates	21–25 h	88%	3–7 d	2–3 wk	UK
Paroxetine HCl (Paxil)	A: PO: 20 mg/d in a.m.; max: 50 mg/d Elderly: PO: Initially: 10 mg/d; max: 40 mg/d	B	Avoid use with highly protein-bound drugs, cimetidine, MAOIs, phenobarbital, phenytoin, alcohol, digoxin	21 h Elderly: 68 h	90–95%	Steady state: 10 d	5–8 h	UK

Drug	Dosage		Drug Interactions and Considerations					
Sertraline HCl (Zoloft)	A: PO: 50 mg daily; max: 200 mg/d	B	Avoid use with highly protein-bound drugs, within 14 days of MAOIs; alcohol; caution with CNS depressants	26 h	98%	Steady state: 7 d	2–4 wk	UK
Trazodone HCl (Desyrel)	A: PO: 75 mg h.s. or 50 mg t.i.d./q.i.d.; max: 600 mg/d	C	*Increase* effects of CNS depressants, phenytoin, digitalis	5–10 h	85–95%	2 wk	2–4 wk	UK
Venlafaxine (Effexor)	A: PO: 225–375 mg/d in 3 divided doses	C	Do not give with MAOIs to avoid serotonin syndrome	3–5 h	25–30%	UK	UK	UK
Monoamine Oxidase Inhibitors								
Isocarboxazid (Marplan)	A: PO: 10–20 mg/d; max: 30 mg/d	C	*Increase* pressor effects of amphetamines, meperidine, vasoconstrictors, levodopa, tricyclic antidepressants, ephedrine, imipramine; foods with tyramine may cause hypertensive crisis	UK	UK	1–4 wk	3–4 wk	2 wk
Phenelzine sulfate (Nardil)	A: PO: 15 mg t.i.d.; 1 mg/kg in divided doses	C	Similar to isocarboxazid	UK	UK	1–4 wk	2–5 wk	2 wk
Tranylcypromine sulfate (Parnate)	A: PO: 10 mg b.i.d.; max: 30 mg	C	Similar to isocarboxazid	UK	UK	3–5 d	2–3 wk	3–5 d
Antimanic								
Lithium carbonate; lithium citrate	See Prototype Drug Chart							

KEY: For complete abbreviation key, see inside front cover.

Antimanic: Lithium

Lithium carbonate

Lithium carbonate
  (Eskalith, Lithane, Lithonate,
  Lithobid)
Antimanic
Pregnancy Category: D
Drug Forms:
Cap 150, 300 mg
  Tab 300 mg
  Tab ER 300, 450 mg
Oral solution 8 mEq/5 mL
  (300 mg/5 mL)

Dosage

A: PO: 600–1,200 mg/d in divided
  doses; individualized to maintain
  blood level at 0.5–1.5 mEq/L
Therapeutic range: 0.5–1.5 mEq/L

Contraindications

Liver and renal disease, pregnancy,
  lactation, severe cardiovascular
  disease, severe dehydration, brain
  tumor or damage, sodium
  depletion, children <12 y
Caution: Thyroid disease

Drug-Lab-Food Interactions

May *increase* lithium level with
  thiazide diuretics, methyldopa,
  haloperidol, NSAIDs,
  antidepressants, carbamazepine,
  theophylline, aminophylline,
  sodium bicarbonate,
  phenothiazines
Food: Increase sodium intake; lithium
  may cause sodium depletion
Lab: Increase urine and blood glucose,
  protein

Pharmacokinetics

Absorption: PO: well absorbed
Distribution: PB: UK
Metabolism: t 1/2: 21–30 h; >36 h
  with renal impairment or elderly
Excretion: 98% in urine, mostly
  unchanged

Pharmacodynamics

Antimanic effects:
PO: Onset: 5–7 d
       Peak: 10–21 d
       Duration: days
PO SR: Peak: 5–7 d

Therapeutic Effects/Uses: To treat bipolar manic-depressive psychosis, manic episodes.

Mode of Action: Alteration of ion transport in muscle and nerve cells; increased receptor sensitivity to serotonin.

Side Effects

Headache, lethargy, drowsiness,
  dizziness, tremors, slurred speech,
  dry mouth, anorexia, vomiting,
  diarrhea, polyuria, hypotension,
  abdominal pain, muscle weakness,
  restlessness

Adverse Reactions

Urinary incontinence, clonic
  movements, stupor, azotemia,
  leukocytosis
Life-threatening: Cardiac
  dysrhythmias, circulatory collapse

KEY: For complete abbreviation key, see inside front cover.

■ NURSING PROCESS: Lithium

ASSESSMENT

- Assess for suicidal ideation.
- Assess the client's baseline vital signs for future comparison.
- Assess client's neurological status, including gait, level of consciousness, reflexes, and tremors.
- Check the client's hepatic and renal function by assessing urine output (>600 mL/d), whether BUN, serum creatinine and liver enzyme levels are within normal range. Assess for toxicity. Draw weekly blood levels initially and then every 1–2 mon. Therapeutic serum levels for acute mania are 1.0–1.5 mEq/L; for maintenance, levels are 0.6–1.2 mEq/L. Signs and symptoms of toxicity at serum levels of 1.5–2.0 mEq/L are persistent nausea and vomiting, severe diarrhea, ataxia, blurred vision, and tinnitus; at 2.0–3.5 mEq/L, signs and symptoms are excessive output of dilute urine, increasing tremors, muscular irritability, psychomotor retardation, mental confusion, and giddiness; and at >3.5 mEq/L, levels are life threatening and may result in impaired consciousness, nystagmus, seizures, coma, oliguria/anuria, cardiac dysrhythmias, myocardial infarction, and cardiovascular collapse. Withhold medications and notify health care provider immediately if any of these occur.
- Obtain a history of episodes of depression or manic-depressive behavior.
- Obtain the client's drug history. CNS depressants can cause an additive effect. Antidepressants cause anticholinergic-like symptoms and are contraindicated if the client has glaucoma. Renal or liver disorders may result in drug accumulation.

POTENTIAL NURSING DIAGNOSES

Potential for injury or violence related to excessive hyperactivity
Ineffective individual coping
Noncompliance

PLANNING

- Client's depression or manic-depressive behavior will be decreased.

NURSING INTERVENTIONS

- Observe the client for signs and symptoms of depression: mood changes, insomnia, apathy, or lack of interest in activities.
- Check the client's vital signs. Orthostatic hypotension is common. Check for anticholinergic-like symptoms: dry mouth, increased heart rate, urinary retention, or constipation.
- When drawing blood to check for lithium levels, draw samples immediately before the next dose (8–12 h after the previous dose). Monitor for signs of lithium toxicity.
- Monitor client for suicidal tendencies when marked depression is present.
- If the client is taking an anticonvulsant, observe the client for seizures; antidepressants lower the seizure threshold. The anticonvulsant dosage might need to be increased.
- Provide the client with a list of foods and drugs to avoid.

CLIENT TEACHING

General

• Instruct the client to take lithium as prescribed. Emphasize the importance of adherence to the therapy and laboratory tests. If lithium is stopped, manic symptoms will reappear.

• Instruct the client to contact the health care provider if signs of toxicity occur: diarrhea, vomiting, unsteady gait, tremor, or muscle weakness.

• Encourage the client to keep medical appointments. Have client check with the health care provider before taking OTC preparations.

• Instruct the client not to drive a motor vehicle or be involved in potentially dangerous mechanical activity until stable lithium level is established.

• Advise the client to maintain adequate fluid intake: 2–3 L/d initially and 1–2 L/d maintenance.

• Instruct the client to take the lithium with meals to decrease gastric irritation.

• Inform the client that the effectiveness of the drug may not be evident until 1–2 wk after the start of therapy.

• Encourage the client who is planning pregnancy to consult with the health care provider about possible teratogenic effects of the drug on the fetus.

• Encourage the client to wear or carry an ID tag or bracelet indicating the drug taken.

Diet

• Advise the client to avoid caffeine products because they can aggravate the manic phase of the bipolar disorder.

• Instruct the client to maintain adequate sodium intake and to avoid crash diets that affect physical and mental health.

EVALUATION

• Evaluate the effectiveness of the drug therapy. The client is free of manic-depressive behavior.

• Client verbalizes understanding of symptoms of toxicity.

• Client demonstrates a subsiding or resolution of the symptoms.

NEUROLOGIC AND NEUROMUSCULAR AGENTS

Adrenergic Agonist

Adrenergic Blocker

Cholinergic

Anticholinergic

Antiparkinsonism:
   Anticholinergic
   Dopaminergic

Myasthenia Gravis

Muscle Relaxant

Adrenergic Agonist

Epinephrine
   (Adrenalin)
Sympathomimetic
Pregnancy Category: C
Drug Forms:
Aerosol spray 0.16, 0.2, 0.25 mg
Inj 1:1000 (1 mg/mL), 1:200
   (5 mg/mL)

Dosage

Asthma anaphylaxis:
A: SC: 0.1–0.5 mL of 1:1000 PRN
   IV: 0.1–0.25 mL of 1:1000
C: SC: 0.01 mL/kg of 1:1000
   IV: 0.01 mL/kg of 1:1000

Contraindications

Cardiac dysrhythmias, cerebral
   arteriosclerosis, pregnancy,
   narrow-angle glaucoma,
   cardiogenic shock
Caution: Hypertension, prostatic
   hypertrophy, hyperthyroidism,
   pregnancy

Drug-Lab-Food Interactions

Decrease epinephrine effect with
   methyldopa, beta blockers
Lab: Increase blood glucose, serum
   lactic acid

Pharmacokinetics

Absorption: SC/IM/IV: Rapidly
Distribution: PB: UK; in breast milk
Metabolism: t 1/2: UK
Excretion: In urine unchanged

Pharmacodynamics

SC/IM: Onset: 3–10 min
        Peak: 20 min
        Duration: 20–30 min
IV: Onset: Immediate
        Peak: 2–5 min
        Duration: 5–10 min
Inhal: Onset: 1 min
        Peak: 3–5 min
        Duration: 1–3 h

Therapeutic Effects/Uses: To treat allergic reaction, anaphylaxis, bronchospasm, cardiac arrest.

Mode of Action: Action on one or more adrenergic sites; promotion of CNS and cardiac stimulation, and bronchodilation.

Side Effects

Anorexia, nausea, vomiting,
   nervousness, tremors, agitation,
   headache, pallor, insomnia,
   syncope, dizziness

Adverse Reactions

Palpitations, tachycardia, dyspnea
Life threatening: Ventricular
   fibrillation, pulmonary edema

KEY: For complete abbreviation key, see inside front cover.

■ NURSING PROCESS: ADRENERGIC AGONIST: Epinephrine

ASSESSMENT

• Obtain VS for future comparison. Epinephrine stimulates the alpha$_1$ (increases blood pressure), beta$_1$ (increase heart rate), and beta$_2$ (dilates bronchial tubes) receptors. Isoproterenol (Isuprel) stimulates the beta$_1$ and beta$_2$ receptors. Albuterol (Proventil) stimulates the beta$_2$ receptor.

Adrenergic Agonist

- Assess the drugs the client is taking and report possible drug–drug interaction. Beta blockers decrease the effect of epinephrine.
- Assess the medical history. Most adrenergic drugs are contraindicated if the client has cardiac dysrhythmias, narrow-angle glaucoma, or cardiogenic shock.
- Assess the results of laboratory values and compare with future laboratory findings.

POTENTIAL NURSING DIAGNOSES
High risk for impaired tissue integrity
Decreased cardiac output

PLANNING
- Client's VS will be closely monitored and will be within normal or acceptable ranges.

NURSING INTERVENTIONS
- Monitor the client's VS. Report signs of increasing blood pressure and increasing pulse rate. If the client is receiving an alpha-adrenergic drug IV for shock, the blood pressure should be checked every 3–5 min or as indicated to avoid severe hypertension.
- Report side effects of adrenergic drugs, such as tachycardia, palpitations, tremors, dizziness, and increased blood pressure.
- Check the client's urinary output and assess for bladder distention. Urinary retention can result from high drug dose or continuous use of adrenergic drugs.
- For cardiac resuscitation, administer epinephrine 1:1000 IV (1 mg/mL), which may be diluted in 10 mL of saline solution (as prescribed).
- Check IV site frequently when administering norepinephrine bitartrate (Levarternol) or dopamine (Intropin) because infiltration of these drugs causes tissue necrosis. These drugs should be diluted sufficiently in IV fluids. An antidote for norepinephrine (Levophed) and dopamine is phentolamine mesylate (Regitine) 5–10 mg, diluted in 10–15 mL of saline infiltrated into the area.
- Offer food when giving adrenergic drugs to avoid nausea and vomiting.
- Monitor laboratory test results. Blood glucose levels may be increased.

CLIENT TEACHING

General
- Instruct the client to read labels on all OTC drugs for cold symptoms and diet pills. Many of these have properties of sympathetic (adrenergic, sympathomimetics) drugs and should not be taken if the client is hypertensive or has diabetes mellitus, cardiac dysrhythmias, or coronary artery disease.
- Instruct mothers not to take drugs containing sympathetic drugs while nursing infants. These drugs pass into the breast milk.
- Explain to the client that continuous use of nasal sprays or drops that contain adrenergics may result in nasal congestion rebound (inflamed and congested nasal tissue).

Skill
- Instruct the client and family how to administer cold medications by spray or drops in the nostrils. Spray should be used with head in upright position. The use of nasal spray lying down can cause systemic absorption. Coloration of nasal spray or drops might indicate deterioration.

Adrenergic Agonist

- Instruct the client not to use bronchodilator sprays in excess. If the client is using a nonselective adrenergic drug that affects $beta_1$ and $beta_2$ receptors, tachycardia may occur.

Side Effects

- Instruct the client to report side effects to health care provider, i.e., rapid heart rate, palpitations, or dizziness.

EVALUATION

- Evaluate the client's response to the adrenergic drug. Continue monitoring the client's VS and report abnormal findings.

Adrenergic Drugs (Alpha, Beta₁, and Beta₂)

Generic (Brand)	Route and Dosage	Preg Cat	Interaction	t 1/2	PB	Onset	Peak	Duration
							Action	
Albuterol (Proventil, Ventolin) Beta₂	A: PO: 2–4 mg t.i.d./q.i.d. PO/SR: 4–8 mg q12h Inhal: 1–2 puffs q4–6h PRN C: 2–6 y: PO: 0.1 mg t.i.d. 6–12 y: PO: 2 mg t.i.d./q.i.d. C: 6–12 y: Inhal: Same as A	C	Similar to norepinephrine	PO: 2.5–5 h Inhal: 2–3 h	UK	PO: 30 min Inhal: 5–15 min	PO: 2.5 h Inhal: 0.5–2 h	PO: 4–6 h SR: 8–12 h Inhal: 3–5 h
Dobutamine HCl (Dobutrex) Beta₁	A or C: IV: 2.5–10 µg/kg/min initially; increase dose gradually; max: 40 µg/kg/min	C	Decrease dobutamine effect with beta blockers; others: similar to norepinephrine	2 min	UK	1–2 min	10–20 min	UK
Dopamine HCl (Intropin) Beta₁	A: IV/Inf: 1–5 µg/kg/min initially; gradually increase 5–15 µg/kg/min; max: 50 µg/kg/min C: IV: usually the same	C	Similar to norepinephrine	2 min	UK	5 min	UK	<10 min

continued

Adrenergic Drugs (Alpha, Beta₁, and Beta₂)—Continued

Generic (Brand)	Route and Dosage	Preg Cat	Interaction	t 1/2	PB	Onset	Peak	Duration
							Action	
Ephedrine HCl (Efedron) Ephedrine sulfate (Efedrin) Alpha, beta₁, and beta₂	A: PO: 25–50 mg t.i.d./q.i.d. SC/IM: 25–50 mg IV: 10–25 mg PRN; max: 150 mg/24 h C >2 y: PO: 2–3 mg/kg/d or 25–100 mg/m²/d in 4–6 divided doses	C	Severely *increase* alpha-adrenergic effect with MAOIs, tricyclic antidepressants *Increase* cardiac dysrhythmic effect with digoxin, anesthetics *Decrease* effect with methyldopa, reserpine	3–6 h	UK	PO: 15–60 min IM: 10–20 min IV: 5 min	UK	PO: 2–4 h IV: 2 h
Epinephrine (Adrenaline) Alpha, beta₁, and beta₂	See Prototype Drug Chart							
Isoetharine HCl (Bronkosol) Beta₂	A: IPPB: 0.5–1.0 mL of 5% sol OR 0.5 mL of 1% sol diluted in 3 mL of NSS Inhal: 1–2 puffs	C	Similar to norepinephrine	UK	UK	Immediate	5–15 min	1–4 h
Isoproterenol HCl (Isuprel) Beta₁ and beta₂	A: SL: 10–20 mg t.i.d. Inhal: 1–2 puffs q4–6 h PRN IV: 2–20 μg/min via inf	C	Similar to norepinephrine	2.5–5 min	UK	SL: 15–30 min Inhal: Rapid IV: Rapid	UK	SL: 2 h Inhal: 1 h IV: 2–5 min

Metaproterenol sulfate (Alupent, Metaprel) Beta₁ and beta₂	C: SL: 5–10 mg t.i.d. Inhal: Same as adult IV: 2.5 µg/min OR 0.1–1.0 mg/kg/min via inf A&C: >9 y: PO: 10–20 mg t.i.d./q.i.d. C <2 y: PO: 0.4 mg/kg t.i.d./q.i.d. 2–6 y: PO: 1–2.6 mg/kg t.i.d./q.i.d. 6–9 y: PO: 10 mg t.i.d./q.i.d. A&C: >12 y: inhal: 2–3 puffs q3–4h; max: 12 puffs/d	C	Similar to norepinephrine	UK	UK	Inhal: <1 min PO: 15 min	Inhal/PO: 1 h	Inhal/PO: 1–5 h
Norepinephrine bitartrate (Levarterenol, Levophed) Alpha and beta₁	A: IV: 4 mg in 250–500 mL of D₅W or NSS infused initially 8–12 µg/min, then 4 µg/min; monitor blood pressure	D	Increase norepinephrine effect with MAOIs, tricyclic antidepressants, antihistamines Increase cardiac dysrhythmias with anesthetics Decrease norepinephrine effect with alpha-adrenergics	UK	UK	1 min	UK	2–4 min

continued

Adrenergic Drugs (Alpha, Beta₁, and Beta₂) — Continued

Generic (Brand)	Route and Dosage	Preg Cat	Interaction	t1/2	PB	Onset	Peak	Duration
							Action	
Phenylephrine HCl 12-hour spray (oxymetazoline HCl) (Neo-Synephrine) Alpha	*Nasal decongestant:* A: Instill: 2–3 sprays or gtt of 0.25%–0.5% sol C <6 y: Instill: 2–3 gtt of 0.125% sol C 6–12 y: Instill: 2–3 gtt of 0.25% sol Also available IM, IV	C	*Decrease* phenylephrine effect with alpha and beta blockers; others: similar to norepinephrine	2.5 h	UK	Rapid	UK	3–6 h
Phenylpropanolamine HCl *Decongestant:* Dimetapp, Dristan, Contac 12 Hour, Triaminicol, Triaminic *Anorexiant:* Dexatrim, Dietac, Control Alpha and beta₁	*Nasal decongestant:* A: PO: 25 mg q4h PRN PO/SR: 75 mg q12h PRN C 2–6 y: PO: 6.25 mg q4h PRN C 6–12 y: 12.5 mg q4h PRN *Appetite suppressant:* A: PO/SR: 75 mg q.d. (before breakfast) PO: 25 mg t.i.d. a.c.	C	*Decrease* antihypertensive effect with antihypertensives *Decrease* effects of phenothiazines, tricyclic antidepressants	3–4 h	UK	15–30 min	PO: 1–2 h SR: 4 h	PO: 3–4 h SR: 12 h
Pseudoephedrine HCl (Sudafed, Actifed, Co-Tylenol PediaCare) Alpha and beta₁	*Nasal decongestant:* A: PO: 60 mg q.i.d./q6h PO/SR: 120 mg q12h; max: 240 mg/d C 2–6 y: PO: 15 mg q6h; max: 60 mg/d C 6–12 y: PO: 30 mg q6h; max: 120 mg/d	C	Similar to ephedrine	9–16 h	UK	PO: 15–30 min	UK	PO: 4–6 h SR: 8–12 h

Drug	Dosage	Pregnancy Category	Drug-Lab-Food Interactions	Half-Life	% PB	Onset	Peak	Duration
Ritodrine HCl (Yutopar) Beta$_2$ and some beta$_1$	A: PO: Initially 10 mg q2h for first 24 h; maint: 10–12 mg q4–6h; max: 120 mg/d IV: 50–100 µg/min; dose may gradually increase to 300 µg/min	C	*Decrease* ritodrine effect with beta blockers; may cause pulmonary edema with corticosteroids	1.7–2.5 h Final: >10 h	32%	UK	PO: 30 min–1 h IV: 1 h	UK
Terbutaline sulfate (Brethine, Brethaire, Bricanyl) Beta$_2$	A: PO: 2.5–5 mg t.i.d. OR q8h Inhal: 2 puffs q4–6h IV: 10 µg/min, gradually increase; max: 80 µg/min C >12 y: PO: 2.5 mg t.i.d. OR q8h	B	Similar to norepinephrine	3–11 h	25%	PO: 30 min Inhal: 5–30 min UK	PO: 2–3 h Inhal: 1–2 h	PO: 4–8 h Inhal: 3–5 h UK

KEY: For complete abbreviation key, see inside front cover.

Adrenergic Blocker

Propranolol HCl

Propranolol HCl
  (Inderal)
Sympatholytic (beta$_1$ and beta$_2$
  blocker)
Pregnancy Category: C
Drug Forms:
Tab 10, 20, 40, 60, 80 mg
SR cap 80, 120, 160 mg
Liq 4, 8 mg/mL
Inj 1 mg/mL

Dosage

See Antihypertension, antianginal,
  and antidysrhythmics
A: PO: 10–40 mg b.i.d./t.i.d.
IV: 0.5–3 mg q4h PRN
C: PO: 1–4 mg/kg/d in 4 divided
  doses

Contraindications

Congestive heart failure, secondary
  heart block, cardiogenic shock,
  bronchial asthma, bronchospasm
Caution: Renal or hepatic dysfunction

Drug-Lab-Food Interactions

Increase atrioventricular block with
  digoxin, calcium channel blockers
Increase hypotensive effect with
  phenothiazines, diuretics,
  antihypertensives
Decrease absorption with antacids
Lab: Increase serum potassium, uric
  acid, AST (SGOT), ALT (SGPT),
  ALP; *decrease* blood sugar

Pharmacokinetics

Absorption: PO: Well absorbed
Distribution: PB: 93%
Metabolism: t 1/2: 2–4 h
Excretion: 90% excreted in urine as
  metabolites

Pharmacodynamics

PO: Onset: 30 min
     Peak: 1–1.5 h (SR: 6 h)
     Duration: 6 h
IV: Onset: Immediate
     Peak: 5 min
     Duration: UK

Therapeutic Effects/Uses: To treat cardiac dysrhythmias, hypertension, angina pectoris, myocardial infarction.

Mode of Action: Blocks beta$_1$-(cardiac) and beta$_2$-(pulmonary) adrenergic receptor sites

Side Effects

Bradycardia, confusion, drowsiness,
  fatigue, vertigo, pruritus, dry
  mouth, nasal stuffiness, brown
  discoloration of the tongue (rare)

Adverse Reactions

Visual hallucinations,
  thrombocytopenia
Life threatening: Laryngospasm,
  atrioventricular heart block,
  agranulocytosis

KEY: For complete abbreviation key, see inside front cover.

■ NURSING PROCESS: ADRENERGIC BLOCKER: Propranolol

Adrenergic alpha and beta blockers are also presented within the antihypertensive, antianginal, and antidysrhythmia sections.

ASSESSMENT

• Obtain baseline VS and ECG for future comparison. Bradycardia and decrease in blood pressure are common cardiac effects of adrenergic beta blockers. Adrenergic beta blockers are frequently referred to as beta blockers, blocking beta$_1$ and beta$_2$ (nonselective) or beta$_1$ (cardiac selective).

• Assess whether the client is having respiratory problems by listening for signs of wheezing or noting dyspnea (difficulty in breathing). If the beta blocker is nonselective, not only does the pulse rate decrease but also bronchoconstriction can result. Clients with asthma should take a beta$_1$ blocker, such as metoprolol (Lopressor), and avoid nonselective beta blockers.

• Assess the drugs the client is currently taking. Report if any are phenothiazines, digoxin, calcium channel blockers, or other antihypertensives.

• Assess the client's urine output and use for future comparison.

POTENTIAL NURSING DIAGNOSES

Decreased cardiac output
Impaired tissue integrity

PLANNING

• The client will comply with the drug regimen.
• The client's VS will be within desired range.

NURSING INTERVENTIONS

• Monitor the client's VS. Report marked changes.
• Administer IV propranolol undiluted or diluted in D$_5$W.
• Report any complaints of excessive dizziness or lightheadedness.
• Report any complaint of stuffy nose. Vasodilation results from use of alpha-adrenergic blockers, and nasal congestion can occur.
• Report if the client is a diabetic and receiving an adrenergic beta blocker; insulin dose or oral hypoglycemic may need to be adjusted.

CLIENT TEACHING

General

• Advise the client to avoid abruptly stopping a beta blocker; rebound hypertension, rebound tachycardia, or an angina attack could result.
• Instruct the client to comply with the drug regimen.
• Advise clients on insulin therapy that early warning signs of hypoglycemia may be masked by the beta blocker (i.e., tachycardia, nervousness).

Skill

• Instruct the client and family how to take pulse and blood pressure.

Side Effects

• Instruct the client to avoid orthostatic (postural) hypotension, such as by slowly rising from supine or sitting to standing positions.
• Inform the client and family of possible mood changes when taking beta blockers. Mood changes can include depression, nightmares, and suicidal tendencies.
• Advise the male client that certain beta blockers, such as propranolol, metoprolol, and pindolol, and alpha blockers, such as prazosin, may cause impotence. Usually the problem is dose related.

EVALUATION

• Evaluate the effectiveness of the adrenergic blocker. VS must be stable within desired range.

Adrenergic Blockers

Generic (Brand)	Route and Dosage	Preg Cat	Interaction	t 1/2	PB	Onset	Peak	Duration
							Action	
						Onset	Peak	Duration
Acebutolol HCl (Sectral) Beta$_1$	A: PO: 400–800 mg/d in 1–2 divided doses; max: 1200 mg/d	B	Same as nadolol	3–13 h	26%	1 h	3–4 h	21–24 h
Atenolol (Tenormin) Beta$_1$	A: PO: 25–100 mg/d	C	Same as nadolol; *Increase* absorption with anticholinergics; may *increase* lidocaine levels *Decrease* hypotensive effect with NSAIDs	6–7 h	6–16%	1 h	2–4 h	24 h
Metoprolol tartrate (Lopressor) Beta$_1$	*Hypertension:* A: PO: 50–100 mg/d in 1–2 divided doses; maint: 100–450 mg/d in divided doses; max: 450 mg/d in divided doses *Myocardial infarction:* A: IV: 5 mg q2min ×3 doses, then PO: 100 mg b.i.d.	C	Same as nadolol *Increase* bradycardia with digoxin	3–4 h	12%	PO: 15 min IV: Immediate	PO: 1.5 h IV: 20 min	PO: 10–19 h IV: 5–10 h
Nadolol (Corgard) Beta$_1$ and beta$_2$	A: PO: 40–80 mg/d; max: 320 mg/d	C	*Increase* hypotensive effect with diuretics, other antihypertensives	10–24 h	30%	1 h	2–4 h	18–24 h

Drug		Route and Dosage	Drug Interactions					
Phentolamine mesylate (Regitine) Alpha	C	A: IM/IV: 2.5–5 mg, repeat q5min until controlled, then q2–3h PRN; C: IM/IV: 0.05–0.1 mg/kg, repeat if needed	*Increase* hypotensive effect with antihypertensives	20 min	UK	UK	IM: 20 min IV: 2 min	IM: 3–4 h IV: 15 min
Pindolol (Visken) Beta$_1$ and beta$_2$	B	A: PO: 5 mg b.i.d./t.i.d.; maint: 10–30 mg in divided doses; max: 60 mg/d in divided doses	Same as nadolol	3–4 h	40%	3 h	UK	24 h
Prazosin HCl (Minipress) Alpha	C	A: PO: 1 mg b.i.d./t.i.d.; maint: 3–15 mg/d; max: 20 mg/d in divided doses	*Increase* hypotensive effect with alcohol, antihypertensives, nitrates	3 h	95%	0.5–2 h	2–4 h	10 h
Propranolol HCl (Inderal) Beta$_1$ and beta$_2$		See Prototype Drug Chart						
Timolol maleate (Blocadren) Beta$_1$ and beta$_2$	C	A: PO: Initially 10 mg b.i.d.; maint: 20–40 mg/d in 2 divided doses; max: 60 mg/d	Same as nadolol	3–4 h	<10%	1 h	2–4 h	12–24 h
Tolazoline (Priscoline HCl) Alpha	C	A: SC/IM/IV: 10–50 mg q.i.d. *Pulmonary hypertension:* NB: IV: 1–2 mg/kg infused over 10 min, followed by 1–2 mg/kg for 24–48 h	*Increase* tolazoline effect with alcohol, beta blockers, antihypertensives	3–10 h	UK	30 min	IM: 0.5–1 h	IM: 3–4 h

KEY: For complete abbreviation key, see inside front cover.

Cholinergic

Bethanechol Chloride

Bethanechol Chloride
  (Urecholine)
Parasympathomimetic
Pregnancy Category: C
Drug Forms:
Tab 5, 10, 25, 50 mg
Inj 5 mg/mL

Dosage

A: PO: 10–50 mg b.i.d./t.i.d./q.i.d.
SC: 2.5 mg

Contraindications

Severe bradycardia or hypotension,
  chronic obstructive pulmonary
  disease, asthma, peptic ulcer,
  parkinsonism, hyperthyroidism

Drug-Lab-Food Interactions

Decrease bethanechol effect with
  antidysrhythmics
Lab: Increase AST, bilirubin, amylase,
  lipase

Pharmacokinetics

Absorption: PO: Poorly absorbed
Distribution: PB: UK
Metabolism: t 1/2: UK
Excretion: In urine

Pharmacodynamics

PO: Onset: 0.5–1.5 h
     Peak: 1–2 h
     Duration: 4–6 h
SC: Onset: 5–15 min
     Peak: 0.5 h
     Duration: 2 h

Therapeutic Effects/Uses: To treat urinary retention, abdominal distention.

Mode of Action: Stimulation of the cholinergic (muscarinic) receptor. Promote contraction of the bladder; increase GI peristalsis, GI secretion, pupillary constriction, and bronchoconstriction.

Side Effects

Nausea, vomiting, diarrhea,
  salivation, sweating, flushing,
  frequent urination, rash, miosis,
  blurred vision

Adverse Reactions

Hypotension, bradycardia, muscle
  weakness
Life threatening: Acute asthmatic
  attack, heart block, circulatory
  collapse, cardiac arrest

KEY: For complete abbreviation key, see inside front cover.

■ NURSING PROCESS: CHOLINERGIC DIRECT ACTING: Bethanechol (Urecholine)

ASSESSMENT
- Obtain baseline VS for future comparison.
- Assess urine output that should be >600 mL/d. Report decrease in urine output.
- Obtain a history from the client of health problems, such as peptic ulcer, urinary obstruction, or asthma. Cholinergics can aggravate symptoms of these conditions.

POTENTIAL NURSING DIAGNOSES
Urinary retention
Anxiety

PLANNING
- Client will have increased bladder and GI tone after taking cholinergics.
- Client will have increased neuromuscular strength.

NURSING INTERVENTIONS

Direct Acting
- Monitor the client's VS. Pulse rate and blood pressure decrease when large doses of cholinergics are taken. Orthostatic hypotension is a side effect of a cholinergic such as bethanechol.
- Monitor fluid intake and output. Decreased urinary output should be reported for it may be related to urinary obstruction.
- Give cholinergics 1 h before or 2 h after meals. If the client complains of gastric pain, the drug may be given with meals.
- Check serum enzyme values for amylase and lipase, as well as AST (SGOT) and bilirubin levels. These laboratory values may increase slightly when taking cholinergics.
- Observe the client for side effects, such as gastric pain or cramping, diarrhea, increased salivary or bronchial secretions, bradycardia, and orthostatic hypotension.
- Auscultate for bowel sounds. Report decreased or hyperactive bowel sounds.
- Auscultate breath sounds for rales (cracking sounds from fluid congestion in lung tissue) or rhonchi (rough sounds due to mucus secretions in lung tissue). Cholinergic drugs can increase bronchial secretions.
- Have IV atropine sulfate (0.6 mg) available as an antidote for overdosing of cholinergics. Early signs of overdosing include salivation, sweating, abdominal cramps, and flushing.
- Note that diaphoresis (excessive perspiration) may occur; linens should be changed as needed.

Indirect Acting
- Beware of the possibility of cholinergic crisis (overdose); symptoms include muscular weakness and increased salivation.

CLIENT TEACHING

Direct Acting

General
• Instruct the client to take the cholinergic as prescribed. Compliance with the drug regimen is essential.

Side Effects
• Instruct the client to report severe side effects, such as profound dizziness or a drop in pulse rate below 60.
• Instruct the client to arise from a lying position slowly to avoid dizziness; this is most likely due to orthostatic hypotension.
• Encourage the client to maintain effective oral hygiene if excess salivation occurs.
• Advise the client to report any difficulty in breathing due to respiratory distress.

Indirect Acting: See Drugs for Myasthenia Gravis
• Instruct the client to take the drug on time to avoid respiratory muscle weakness.
• Instruct the client to assess changes in muscle strength. Cholinesterase inhibitors (anticholinesterases) increase muscle strength.

EVALUATION
• Evaluate the effectiveness of the cholinergic or anticholinesterase drug.
• Evaluate the stability of the client's VS, and note the presence of side effects or adverse reactions.

Generic (Brand)	Route and Dosage	Preg Cat	Interaction	t 1/2	PB	Onset	Peak	Duration
Direct Acting								
Bethanechol (Urecholine)	See Prototype Drug Chart							
Carbachol (Carcholin, Miostat)	Ophthalmic: 0.75–3%, 1 gt See Drugs for the Eye		See Drugs for the Eye					
Pilocarpine HCl (Pilocar)	Ophthalmic: 0.5–4%, 1 gt See Drugs for the Eye		See Drugs for the Eye					
Cholinesterase Inhibitor *For Alzheimer's Disease:*								
Tacrine HCl (Cognex)	A: PO: 40–160 mg/d pc	C	*Increase* effect of theophylline *Increase* effect with cimetidine	1.5–3.5 h	50%	0.5–1.5 h	2 h	24–36 h
Velnacrine (Mentane)	A: PO: 150–225 mg/d in divided doses		Investigational drug *Lab:* May *increase* liver enzymes	2–3 h	UK	UK	1 h	UK
Indirect Acting Irreversible Anticholinesterases								
Demecarium bromide (Humorsol)	0.125–0.25%, 1 gt q12–48h See Drugs for the Eye		See Drugs for the Eye					

continued

Generic (Brand)	Route and Dosage	Preg Cat	Interaction	t 1/2	PB	Onset	Peak	Duration
							Action	
Echothiophate iodide (Phospholine iodide)	0.03–0.06%, 1 gt q.d./b.i.d. See Drugs for the Eye		See Drugs for the Eye					
Isoflurophate (Floropryl)	0.25%, ointment q8–72h See Drugs for the Eye		See Drugs for the Eye					
Indirect Acting, Reversible Anticholinesterases								
Ambenonium Cl (Mytelease)	A: PO: 2.5–5.0 mg t.id./q.i.d.; dose may be increased; maint: 5–40 mg t.i.d./q.i.d.	C	Similar to neostigmine	UK	UK	30 min	UK	3–8 h
Edrophonium Cl (Tensilon)	A: IV: 2 mg; then 8 mg if no response IM: 10 mg; may repeat with 2 mg in 30 min C <34 kg: IV: 1 mg; repeat in 30–45 s if no response; max: 5 mg C >34 kg: IV: 2 mg; repeat with 1 mg if no response; max: 10 mg	C	*Increase* bradycardia with digoxin	1.2–2 h	UK	IV: 0.5–1 min IM: 2–10 min	IV/IM: UK	IV: 6–12 min IM: 5–30 min

Drug	Route and Dosage	Pregnancy Category	Uses and Considerations	t½	PB	Onset	Peak	Duration
Neostigmine bromide (Prostigmin) Neostigmine methysulfate (injectable form)	A: PO: Initially 15 mg t.i.d.; maint: 150 mg/d in divided doses; range: 15–375 mg/d IM/IV: 0.5–2.5 mg as needed C: PO: 2 mg/kg/d in 6 divided doses	C	*Increase* neostigmine effect with other cholinergics *Decrease* neostigmine effect with atropine, antidysrhythmics	1–1.5 h	15–25%	PO: 1–4 h IM: 15–30 min IV: 5–8 min	PO: UK IM: 20–30 min IV: UK	PO/IM: 2.5–4 h IV: 2–4 h
Physostigmine salicylate (Eserine salicylate)	0.25–0.5%, 1 gt q.d./q.i.d. See Drugs for the Eye		See Drugs for the Eye					
Pyridostigmine bromide (Mestinon)	A: PO: 60–120 mg t.i.d./q.i.d.; max: 2.5 g/d SR: 180–540 mg q.d./b.i.d. IM/IV: 2 mg q2–3h C: PO: 7 mg/kg/d in 5–6 divided doses	C	Same as neostigmine	3.5–4 h	<10%	PO: 30–45 min SR: 0.5–1 h IM: 15 min IV: 2–5 min	PO/SR/IM/IV: UK	PO: 3–6 h SR: 6–12 h IM: 2–4 h IV: 2–3 h

KEY: For complete abbreviation key, see inside front cover.

Anticholinergic

Atropine SO₄

Atropine SO$_4$
(Atropine)
Atropisol (Optic)
Parasympatholytic

Pregnancy Category: C

Drug Forms:
Tab 0.4 mg
Inj 0.1, 0.4, 1 mg/mL
Ophthalmic ointment and sol (1%)

Dosage

A: PO/IM/IV: 0.4–0.6 mg q4–6h
PRN
C: PO/IM/IV: 0.01 mg/kg/dose;
max: 0.4 mg/dose

Contraindications

Narrow-angle glaucoma, obstructive
GI disorders, paralytic ileus,
ulcerative colitis, tachycardia,
benign prostatic hypertrophy,
myasthenia gravis

Caution: Renal or hepatic disorders,
chronic obstructive pulmonary
disease, congestive heart failure

Drug-Lab-Food Interactions

Increase anticholinergic effect with
phenothiazines, antidepressants,
MAOIs

Pharmacokinetics

Absorption: PO/IM: Well absorbed
Distribution: PB: UK; crosses the
placenta
Metabolism: t 1/2: 2–3 h
Excretion: >75% excreted in urine

Pharmacodynamics

PO: Onset: 0.5–1 h
Peak: 1–2 h
Duration: 4 h
IM: Onset: 10–30 min
Peak: 0.5 h
Duration: 4 h
IV: Onset: Immediate
Peak: 5 min
Duration: UK
Instill: Onset: 20–30 min
Peak: 30–40 min
Duration: days

Therapeutic Effects/Uses: Preoperative medication to reduce salivation, increase
heart rate, dilate pupils of the eye.

Mode of Action: Inhibition of acetylcholine by occupying the receptors; increase
heart rate by blocking vagus stimulation; promote dilation of the pupil by blocking iris sphincter muscle.

Side Effects

Dry mouth, nausea, headache,
constipation, rash, dry skin,
flushing, blurred vision,
photophobia

Adverse Reactions

Tachycardia, hypotension, pupillary
dilatation, abdominal distention,
nasal congestion
Life threatening: Paralytic ileus, coma

KEY: For complete abbreviation key, see inside front cover.

■ NURSING PROCESS: ANTICHOLINERGIC DRUGS: Atropine

ASSESSMENT

- Obtain baseline VS for future comparison. Tachycardia is a side effect that occurs with large doses of anticholinergics such as atropine sulfate.
- Assess urine output. Urinary retention may occur.
- Check the client's medical history. Atropine and atropine-like drugs are contraindicated if the client has narrow-angle glaucoma, obstructive GI disorder, paralytic ileus, ulcerative colitis, benign prostatic hypertrophy (BPH), or myasthenia gravis.
- Obtain a history of the drugs the client is taking. Phenothiazines and antidepressants increase the effect of anticholinergics.

POTENTIAL NURSING DIAGNOSES

Urinary retention
Altered oral mucous membrane
Constipation

PLANNING

- The client's secretions will be decreased before surgery.
- Client will not have side effects that may become a health problem.

NURSING INTERVENTIONS

- Monitor the client's VS. Report if tachycardia occurs.
- Check intake and output. Encourage the client to void before taking the medication. Report decreased urine output. Anticholinergics can cause urinary retention. Maintain adequate fluid intake.
- Check bowel sounds. Absence of bowel sounds may indicate paralytic ileus due to decrease in GI motility (peristalsis).
- Check for constipation due to the decrease in GI motility. Encourage the client to ingest foods that are high in fiber, to drink adequate amounts of fluids, and to exercise if able.
- Raise bedside rails for clients who are confused, debilitated, or elderly. Atropine could cause CNS stimulation (excitement, confusion) or drowsiness.
- Administer mouth care. Atropine decreases oral secretions and can cause dryness of the mouth.
- Administer IV atropine undiluted or diluted in 10 mL of sterile water. Rate of administration is 0.6 mg/min.

CLIENT TEACHING

General

- Instruct the client with glaucoma to avoid atropine-like drugs. Anticholinergics cause mydriasis and increase the intraocular pressure. Clients should be alerted to check labels on OTC drugs to determine if they are contraindicated for glaucoma.
- Instruct the client not to drive a motor vehicle or participate in activities that require alertness. Drowsiness is common.
- Advise the client to avoid alcohol, cigarette smoking, caffeine, and aspirin at bedtime to decrease gastric acidity.
- Instruct the client with mydriasis from an eye examination to use sunglasses in bright light because of photophobia (intolerance of bright light).

Anticholinergic

• Instruct the client to avoid hot environments and excess physical exertion. Elevations in body temperature can result from diminished sweat gland activity.

Diet

• Suggest that the client's diet include foods high in fiber and increased water intake to prevent constipation.

Side Effects

• Advise the client of common side effects from long-term use of anticholinergics, such as dry mouth, decrease in urination, and constipation.
• Instruct the client to increase fluid intake to prevent constipation when taking anticholinergics for a prolonged period of time.
• Instruct the client to urinate before taking the anticholinergic. Urinary retention can be a problem. The client should report a marked decrease in urine output.
• Suggest that the client use hard candy, ice chips, or chewing gum and maintain effective oral hygiene if the client's mouth is dry. Anticholinergics decrease salivation.
• Encourage the client to use Artificial Tears (eye drops) for dry eyes due to decreased lacrimation (tearing).

EVALUATION

• Evaluate the client's response to the anticholinergic.
• Determine if constipation, urine retention, or increased pulse rate is or remains a problem.

Generic (Brand)	Route and Dosage	Preg Cat	Interaction	t 1/2	PB	Onset	Peak	Duration
							Action	
Eye								
Cyclopentolate HCl (Cyclogyl)	0.5–2% sol, 1–2 gtt See Drugs for the Eye		See Drugs for the Eye					
Homatropine (Isopto Homatropine)	2–5% sol, 1–2 gtt See Drugs for the Eye		See Drugs for the Eye					
Tropicamide (Mydriacyl Ophthalmic)	0.5–1% sol, 1–2 gtt See Drugs for the Eye		See Drugs for the Eye					
Gastrointestinal								
Atropine sulfate	See Prototype Drug Chart							
Dicyclomine HCl (Bentyl, Antispas, Di-Spaz)	A: PO: 10–20 mg t.i.d./q.i.d. IM: 20 mg q4–6h C >2 y: PO: 10 mg t.i.d./q.i.d.	B	*Increase* anticholinergic effect with MAOIs, tricyclic antidepressants, antihistamines (H₁)	9–10 h	UK	1–2 h	UK	3–4 h

continued

Anticholinergics—*Continued*

Generic (Brand)	Route and Dosage	Preg Cat	Interaction	t 1/2	PB	Action		
						Onset	*Peak*	*Duration*
Glycopyrrolate (Robinul)	*GI disorders:* A: PO: 1–2 mg b.i.d./t.i.d. IM/IV: 0.1–0.2 mg t.i.d./q.i.d. *Preoperative:* A: IM: 4.4 µg/kg 30 min–1 h before surgery	B	Same as dicyclomine *Decrease* levodopa effects; may *decrease* antipsychotic effects of phenothiazines	1–4.6 h	UK	PO: 1 h IM: 30 min IV: 1–10 min	PO: 1–2 h IM: 0.5–1 h IV: 10 min	PO: 8–12 h IM: 3–7 h IV: 3–4 h
Hyoscyamine SO₄ (Cystospaz, Anaspaz, Levisin)	A: PO/SL: 0.125–0.25 mg t.i.d./q.i.d. ac & h.s. SR: 0.375 mg q8h SC/IM/IV: 0.25–0.5 mg b.i.d./q.i.d. C 2–10 y: one-half of the adult dose	C	*Increase* hyoscyamine effect with antihistamines, tricyclic antidepressants, amantadine *Decrease* effect with antacids; *decrease* effects of phenothiazines, levodopa	3.5 h	50–60%	PO: 20–30 min IV: 2–3 min	PO: 0.5–1 h IV: 15–30 min	PO/IV: 4–6 h

Isopropamide iodide (Darbid)	A: PO: 5 mg b.i.d. or q12h; may increase to 10 mg b.i.d.	C	Similar to glycopyrrolate	UK	UK	UK	UK	10–12 h
Mepenzolate bromide (Cantil)	A: PO: 25–50 mg t.i.d. with meals and h.s.	C	Similar to glycopyrrolate	UK	UK	1 h	UK	3–4 h
Methscopolamine bromide (Pamine)	A: PO: 2.5–5 mg a.c., h.s. C: PO: 0.2 mg/kg q.i.d.	C	*Increase* additive effect with antihistamines, antiparkinsonism, disopyramide, phenothiazides, antihypertensives *Decrease* effect of phenothiazines, levodopa, ketoconazole	UK	UK	1 h	UK	4–8 h
Oxyphencyclimine HCl (Daricon)	A: PO: 5–10 mg b.i.d.	C	Same as methscopolamine	UK	UK	1–2 h	UK	>12 h
Propantheline bromide (Pro-Banthine)	A: PO: 15 mg a.c. t.i.d; 30 mg h.s.; max: 120 mg/d Elderly: 7.5 mg a.c. t.i.d.	C	Same as glycopyrrolate	9 h	UK	30–60 min	UK	4–6 h

continued

Anticholinergics—*Continued*

Generic (Brand)	Route and Dosage	Preg Cat	Interaction	t 1/2	PB	Onset	Peak	Duration
							Action	
						Onset	*Peak*	*Duration*
Scopolamine hydrobromide (also hyoscine hydrobromide)	*Preoperative:* A: PO: 0.5–1.0 mg SC/IM/IV: 0.3–0.6 mg C: SC: 0.006 mg/kg or 0.2 mg/m²; max: 0.3 mg *Motion sickness:* A: PO: 0.3–0.6 mg; transderm patch: 1 patch behind ear q72h	C	Same as glycopyrrolate	8 h	<30%	PO: 30 min IV: 10 min Transderm: 4 h	PO: 1 h IV: 1 h Transderm: UK	PO: 4–6 h IV: 2–4 h Transderm: 72 h
Neuromuscular (Atropine-like Agents: Antiparkinsonism Drugs) Benztropine mesylate (Cogentin) See Antiparkinsonism Drugs	*Parkinsonism:* A: PO: Initially 0.5–1.0 mg/d in 1–2 divided doses (larger dose at h.s.); maint: 0.5–6 mg/d in 1–2 divided doses	C	*Increase* anticholinergic effect with narcotics, antipsychotics, tricyclic antidepressants, antihistamines, some antidysrhythmics *Decrease* effect of levodopa	UK	UK	PO: 1 h	UK	PO: 6–24 h

Drug	Dosage	Pregnancy Category	Drug-Lab-Food Interactions	Onset			Peak	Duration
Biperiden lactate (Akineton) See Antiparkinsonism Drugs	Parkinsonism: A: PO: 2 mg t.i.d./q.i.d. IM/IV: 2 mg q30min for 4 doses	C	Same as benztropine	UK	UK	PO: 1 h	UK	PO: 6–24 h
Procyclidine HCl (Kemadrin) See Antiparkinsonism Drugs	Parkinsonism: A: PO: 2.5–5 mg pc t.i.d.	C	Same as benztropine	UK	UK	30–40 min	UK	4–6 h
Trihexyphenidyl HCl (Artane, Trihexy) See Antiparkinsonism Drugs	Parkinsonism: A: PO: Initially 1 mg/d, increase to 6–10 mg/d in divided doses	C	Same as benztropine *Decrease* trihexyphenidyl absorption with antacids	UK	UK	PO: 1 h SR: UK	PO: 2–3 h SR: UK	PO: 6–12 h SR: 12–24 h

KEY: For complete abbreviation key, see inside front cover.

Antiparkinsonism: Anticholinergic

Trihexyphenidyl HCl

Trihexyphenidyl HCl
(Artane, Aphen, Hexaphen,
Trihexane, Trihexy)
Anticholinergic
Pregnancy Category: C
Drug Forms:
Tab 2, 5 mg
SR cap 5 mg
Elix 2 mg/5 mL

Dosage

Parkinsonism:
A: PO: Initially 1 mg/d; increase to
6–10 mg/d in divided doses
*Extrapyramidal symptoms: Drug
induced:*
A: PO: 1 mg/d; increase to 5–15
mg/d in divided doses

Contraindications

Narrow-angle glaucoma, GI
obstruction, urinary retention,
severe angina pectoris, myasthenia
gravis
Caution: Tachycardia, benign
prostatic hypertrophy, children,
elderly, during lactation

Drug-Lab-Food Interactions

Increase anticholinergic effect with
phenothiazines, antihistamines,
tricyclic antidepressants,
quinidine
Decrease trihexyphenidyl absorption
with antacids

Pharmacokinetics

Absorption: PO: Well absorbed
Distribution: PB: UK
Metabolism: t 1/2: UK
Excretion: In urine

Pharmacodynamics

PO: Onset: 1 h
         Peak: 2–3 h
         Duration: 6–12 h
SR/PO: Onset: UK
         Peak: UK
         Duration: 12–24 h

Therapeutic Effects/Uses: To decrease involuntary symptoms of parkinsonism or drug-induced parkinsonism by inhibiting acetylcholine.

Mode of Action: Blocks cholinergic (muscarinic) receptors; thus decreases involuntary movements.

Side Effects

Nausea, vomiting, dry mouth,
constipation, anxiety, restlessness,
headache, dizziness, blurred
vision, photophobia, pupil
dilation, dysphagia

Adverse Reactions

Tachycardia, palpitations, urticaria,
postural hypotension, urinary
retention
Life threatening: Paralytic ileus

KEY: For complete abbreviation key, see inside front cover.

■ NURSING PROCESS: ANTIPARKINSONISM:
Anticholinergic: Trihexyphenidyl

ASSESSMENT
- Obtain a medical history. Report if the client has a history of glaucoma, GI dysfunction, urinary retention, angina pectoris, or myasthenia gravis. All anticholinergics are contraindicated if the client has glaucoma.
- Obtain a drug history. Report if a drug-drug interaction is probable. Phenothiazines, tricyclic antidepressants, and antihistamines increase the effect of trihexyphenidyl.
- Assess baseline VS for future comparisons. Pulse rate may increase.
- Assess urinary output for comparison. Urinary retention may occur with continuous use of anticholinergics.

POTENTIAL NURSING DIAGNOSES
Impaired physical mobility
High risk for activity intolerance

PLANNING
- Client will have decreased involuntary symptoms due to parkinsonism or drug-induced parkinsonism.

NURSING INTERVENTIONS
- Monitor VS, urine output, and bowel sounds. Increased pulse rate, urinary retention, and constipation are side effects of anticholinergics.

CLIENT TEACHING
General
- Advise the client to avoid alcohol, cigarette smoking, caffeine, and aspirin to decrease gastric acidity.

Diet
- Encourage the client to ingest foods that are high in fiber and to increase fluid intake to prevent constipation.

Side Effects
- Suggest that the client relieve dry mouth with hard candy, ice chips, or sugarless chewing gum. Anticholinergics decrease salivation.
- Suggest that the client use sunglasses in direct sun because of possible photophobia.
- Advise the client to void before taking the drug to minimize urinary retention. This is especially important if urine retention is present.
- Advise the client taking an anticholinergic to control symptoms of parkinsonism and to have routine eye examinations to determine the presence of increased intraocular pressure, which indicates glaucoma. Clients who have glaucoma should NOT take anticholinergics.

EVALUATION
- Evaluate the client's response to trihexyphenidyl to determine if parkinsonism symptoms are controlled.

Antiparkinsonism Drugs: Anticholinergics

Generic (Brand)	Route and Dosage	Preg Cat	Interaction	t 1/2	PB	Action			
						Onset	Peak	Duration	
Benztropine mesylate (Cogentin)	*Parkinsonism:* A: PO: Initially 0.5–1.0 mg/d in 1–2 divided doses (larger dose at h.s.); maint: 0.5–6 mg/d in 1–2 divided doses *Extrapyramidal syndrome:* A: PO: 1–4 mg/d in 1–2 divided doses IM/IV: 1–2 mg/d	C	*Increase* anticholinergic effect with narcotics, antipsychotics, tricyclic antidepressants, antihistamines, some antidysrhythmics *Decrease* effect of levodopa	UK	UK	PO: 1 h IM/IV: 15 min	UK	PO: 6–24 h IM/IV: 6–24 h	
Biperiden HCl (Akineton)	*Parkinsonism:* A: PO: 2 mg t.i.d./q.i.d. IM/IV: 2 mg every 30 min to 4 doses C: IM/IV: 0.04 mg/kg or 1.2 mg/m^2, repeat if necessary; max: 8 mg/d	C	Same as benztropine	UK	UK	PO: 1 h IM/IV: 15 min	UK	PO/IM/IV: 6–24 h	

Drug	Dose		Interactions					
Ethopropazine HCl (Parsidol)	*Parkinsonism:* A: PO: Initially 50 mg q.d./b.i.d.; maint: 100–400 mg/d in divided doses; max: 600 mg/d in divided doses	C	Similar to benztropine	UK	UK	0.5–1 h	UK	4 h
Orphenadrine HCl or citrate (Disipal, Norflex, Banflex)	A: PO: 50 mg t.i.d. or 100 mg b.i.d.	C	None significant	14 h	UK	1 h	2 h	4–6 h
Procyclidine HCl (Kemadrin)	*Parkinsonism:* A: PO: 2.5 mg p.c. t.i.d. *Extrapyramidal syndrome:* A: PO: Initially 2.5 mg p.c. t.i.d.; maint: 2.5–5 mg p.c. t.i.d.	C	Similar to benztropine	UK	UK	PO: 30–40 min	UK	4–6 h
Trihexyphenidyl HCl (Artane)	See Prototype Drug Chart							

KEY: For complete abbreviation key, see inside front cover.

Antiparkinsonism: Dopaminergic

Carbidopa-Levodopa	Dosage
Carbidopa-Levodopa (Sinemet) Dopaminergic *Pregnancy Category:* C *Drug Forms:* Tab 10/100, 25/250 mg (carbidopa/levodopa)	A: PO: 1:10 ratio; initially 10 carbidopa/100 levodopa t.i.d.; maint: 25/250 mg t.i.d.

Contraindications	Drug-Lab-Food Interactions
Narrow-angle glaucoma; severe cardiac, renal, or hepatic disease *Caution:* peptic ulcer, psychiatric disorders	*Increase* hypertensive crisis with MAOIs *Decrease* levodopa effect with other anticholinergics, phenytoin, tricyclic antidepressants, pyridoxine *Lab:* May *increase* BUN, AST, ALT, ALP, LDH *Food:* Avoid foods containing pyridoxine (vitamin B_6)

Pharmacokinetics	Pharmacodynamics
Absorption: PO: Well absorbed *Distribution:* PB: Carbidopa: 36%; levodopa: UK *Metabolism:* t 1/2: 1–2 h *Excretion:* In urine as metabolites	PO: Onset: 15 min Peak: 1–3 h Duration: 5–12 h

Therapeutic Effects/Uses: To treat parkinsonism, to relieve tremors and rigidity.

Mode of Action: Transmission of levodopa to brain cells for conversion to dopamine; carbidopa blocks the conversion of levodopa to dopamine in the periphery.

Side Effects	Adverse Reactions
Anorexia, nausea, vomiting, dysphagia, fatigue, dizziness, headache, dry mouth, bitter taste, twitching, blurred vision, insomnia	Involuntary choreiform movements, palpitations, orthostatic hypotension, urinary retention, psychosis, severe depression, hallucinations *Life threatening:* Agranulocytosis, hemolytic anemia, cardiac dysrhythmias, leukopenia

KEY: For complete abbreviation key, see inside front cover.

■ NURSING PROCESS: ANTIPARKINSONISM: Dopaminergic Agent: Carbidopa-Levodopa

ASSESSMENT

• Obtain the client's VS to use for future comparison.

116

Antiparkinsonism: Dopaminergic

- Assess the client for signs and symptoms of parkinsonism, including stooped, forward posture; shuffling gait; masked facies; and resting tremors.
- Obtain a history from the client of glaucoma, heart disease, peptic ulcers, kidney or liver disease, and psychosis.
- Report if drug–drug interaction is probable. Drugs that should be avoided or closely monitored are levodopa, bromocriptine, and anticholinergics.

POTENTIAL NURSING DIAGNOSES
Impaired physical mobility
High risk for activity intolerance

PLANNING
- Symptoms of parkinsonism will be decreased or absent after 1–4 wk of drug therapy.

NURSING INTERVENTIONS
- Monitor the client's VS and ECG. Orthostatic hypotension may occur during early use of levodopa and bromocriptine. Have the client rise slowly to avoid faintness.
- Check for weakness, dizziness, or faintness, which are symptoms of orthostatic hypotension.
- Administer carbidopa-levodopa (Sinemet) with low-protein foods. High-protein diets interfere with drug transport to the CNS.

CLIENT TEACHING
General
- Advise the client not to abruptly discontinue the medication. Rebound parkinsonism (increased symptoms of parkinsonism) can occur.
- Inform the client that urine may be discolored and will darken with exposure to air. Perspiration also may be dark. Explain that both are harmless but that clothes may be stained.
- Advise the diabetic client that the blood sugar should be checked with a OTC reagent strip (Hemastix or Chemstrip bG) and not done through urine testing. With Clinitest, a false-positive test result can occur; with Tes-Tape or Clinistix, a false-negative test result can occur.

Diet
- Suggest to the client that taking levodopa with food may decrease GI upset; however, food will slow the drug absorption rate.
- Advise the client to avoid vitamins that contain vitamin B_6 (pyridoxine) and foods rich in vitamin B_6, such as beans (lima, navy, kidney) and cereals that contain the vitamin.

Side Effects
- Instruct the client to report side effects and symptoms of dyskinesia. Explain to the client that it may take weeks or months before the symptoms are controlled.

EVALUATION
- Evaluate the effectiveness of the drug therapy in controlling the symptoms of parkinsonism.
- Determine that there is an absence of side effects.

Antiparkinsonism: Dopaminergics

Generic (Brand)	Route and Dosage	Preg Cat	Interaction	t 1/2	PB	Onset	Peak	Duration
Dopaminergics Carbidopa-Levodopa (Sinemet)	See Prototype Drug Chart							
Levodopa (or L-dopa) (Dopar, Larodopa)	A: PO: 0.5–1.0 g/d in 2–4 divided doses; increase dose gradually; average maint: 3–6 g/d with food, in divided doses; max: 8 g/d	C	*Increase* hypertensive crisis with MAOIs *Decrease* levodopa effect with anticholinergics, phenytoin, tricyclic antidepressants, pyridoxine, papaverine	1–3 h	UK	15–30 min	1–3 h	5–24 h
Dopamine Agonists Amantadine HCl; (Symmetrel)	*Parkinsonism:* A: PO: 100 mg b.i.d.; may increase dose; max: 400 mg/d	C	*Increase* anticholinergic effect with other anticholinergics	24 h; longer with poor renal function	60–70%	48 h	1–4 h	UK

Drug	Route and dosage	Pregnancy category	Drug interactions	Half-life	Protein-binding	Onset	Peak	Duration
Bromocriptine mesylate (Parlodel)	A: PO: Initially 1.25–2.5 mg/d; may gradually increase dose; maint: 30–60 mg/d in 3 divided doses; max: 100 mg/d	C	*Increase* hypotensive effect with antihypertensive drugs *Increase* CNS depression with alcohol, narcotics, sedative-hypnotics *Decrease* bromocriptine effect with phenothiazines, amitriptyline, haloperidol, methyldopa	6–8 h Terminal phase: 50 h	90–96%	30 min–1 h	1–2 h	4–8 h
Pergolide mesylate (Permax)	A: PO: Initially 0.05 mg/d ×2d; increase by 0.1–0.15 mg q3d ×12d; max: 5 mg/d	B	May *increase* highly protein-bound drugs May *decrease* effect with phenothiazines, thioxanthines, butyrophenones	UK	90%	UK	UK	UK
Selegiline HCl (Eldepryl)	A: PO: 10 mg/d in 2 divided doses	C	*Increase* toxicity with meperidine	2–20 h	UK	1 h	UK	UK

KEY: For complete abbreviation key, see inside front cover.

Myasthenia Gravis (Drugs for)

Pyridostigmine Bromide

Pyridostigmine Bromide
  (Mestinon)
Cholinesterase inhibitor
Pregnancy Category: C
Drug Forms:
Tab 60 mg
SR tab 180 mg
Liquid 60 mg/ 5 mL
Inj 5 mg/mL

Dosage

A: PO: 60–120 mg t.i.d./q.i.d.; max:
  1.5 g/d
  SR: 180–540 mg q.d. or b.i.d.
  IM/IV: 2 mg q2–3h
C: PO: 7 mg/kg/d in 5–6 divided
  doses

Contraindications

GI and GU obstruction, severe renal
  disease
Caution: Asthma, bradycardia, peptic
  ulcer, cardiac dysrhythmias,
  pregnancy

Drug-Lab-Food Interactions

Decrease pyridostigmine effect with
  atropine, muscle relaxants,
  antidysrhythmics, magnesium

Pharmacokinetics

Absorption: PO: Poorly absorbed; SR:
  50% absorbed
Distribution: PB: UK
Metabolism: t 1/2: PO: 3.5–4 h; IV: 2 h
Excretion: In urine and by liver

Pharmacodynamics

PO: Onset: 30–45 min
        Peak: UK
        Duration: 3–6 h
PO SR: Onset: 0.5–1 h
        Peak: UK
        Duration: 6–12 h
IM: Onset: 15 min
        Peak: UK
        Duration: 2–4 h
IV: Onset: 2–5 min
        Peak: UK
        Duration: 2–3 h

Therapeutic Effects/Uses: To control and treat myasthenia gravis.

Mode of Action: Transmission of neuromuscular impulses by preventing the destruction of acetylcholine.

Side Effects

Nausea, vomiting, diarrhea,
  headache, dizziness, abdominal
  cramps, sweating, rash, miosis

Adverse Reactions

Hypotension, urticaria
Life threatening: Respiratory
  depression, bronchospasm, cardiac
  dysrhythmias, seizures

KEY: For complete abbreviation key, see inside front cover.

■ NURSING PROCESS: MYASTHENIA GRAVIS (Drugs for): Pyridostigmine (Mestinon)

ASSESSMENT
- Obtain a drug history of drugs that the client is currently taking. Report if a drug-drug interaction is likely. Client should avoid atropine, atropine-like drugs, and muscle relaxants.
- Obtain baseline VS for future comparison.
- Assess the client for signs and symptoms of **myasthenia crisis**, such as muscle weakness with difficulty breathing and swallowing.

POTENTIAL NURSING DIAGNOSES
Inability to sustain spontaneous ventilation
High risk for activity intolerance
Anxiety related to possible recurrence of myasthenia crisis

PLANNING
- The client's symptoms of muscle weakness and difficulty breathing and swallowing due to myasthenia gravis will be eliminated or reduced in 2−3 d.

NURSING INTERVENTIONS
- Monitor the effectiveness of drug therapy (acetylcholinesterase [AChE] inhibitors). Muscle strength should be increased. Both depth and rate of respirations should be assessed and maintained within normal range.
- Administer IV pyridostigmine undiluted at rate of 0.5 mg/min. Do NOT add the drug to IV fluids.
- Observe the client for signs and symptoms of **cholinergic crisis** due to overdosing, including muscle weakness, increased salivation, sweating, tearing, and miosis.
- Have readily available an antidote for cholinergic crisis (atropine sulfate).

CLIENT TEACHING
General
- Instruct the client to take the drugs as prescribed to avoid recurrence of symptoms.
- Encourage the client to wear a medical ID bracelet or necklace, e.g., Medic Alert, indicating the health problem and the drug(s) taken.

Diet
- Instruct the client to take the drug before meals for best drug absorption. If gastric irritation occurs, take the drug with food.

Side Effects
- Advise the client to report to health care provider recurrence of symptoms of myasthenia gravis. Drug therapy may need to be modified.

EVALUATION
- Evaluate the effectiveness of the drug therapy. Muscle strength should be maintained.
- Determine the absence of respiratory distress.

Acetylcholinesterase Inhibitors: Myasthenia Gravis (Drugs for)

Generic (Brand)	Route and Dosage	Preg Cat	Interaction	t 1/2	PB	Onset	Peak	Duration
							Action	
Ambenonium (Mytelase)	A: PO: 2.5–5.0 mg t.i.d./q.i.d.; dose may be increased; maint: 5–40 mg t.i.d./q.i.d.	C	Similar to neostigmine	UK	UK	30 min	UK	3–8 h
Edrophonium Cl (Tensilon)	A: IV: 2 mg; then 8 mg if no response IM: 10 mg, may repeat with 2 mg in 30 min C <34 kg: IV: 1 mg, repeat in 30–45 s if no response; max: 5 mg C >34 kg: IV: 2 mg, repeat with 1 mg if no response; max: 10 mg	C	*Increase* bradycardia with digoxin	1.2–2 h	UK	IV: 30–60 s IM: 2–10 min	IV:UK IM: UK	IV: 6–12 min IM: 5–30 min

Neostigmine bromide (Prostigmin) Neostigmine methylsulfate (injectable form)	A: PO: 150 mg/d in divided doses; range: 15–375 mg/d IM/IV: 0.5–2.5 mg as needed C: PO: 2 mg/kg/d in divided doses or 10 mg/m² q4h	C	*Increase* neostigmine effect with other cholinergics *Decrease* neostigmine effect with atropine, antidysrhythmics	1–1.5 h	15–25%	PO: 1–4 h IM: 15–30 min IV: 5–8 min	PO: UK IM: 20–30 min IV: UK	PO: 2.5–4 h IM: 2.5–4 h IV: 2–4 h
Pyridostigmine (Mestinon)	See Prototype Drug Chart							

KEY: *For complete abbreviation key, see inside front cover.*

Muscle Relaxant

Carisoprodol	Dosage
Carisoprodol (Soma) Skeletal muscle relaxant *Pregnancy Category:* C *Drug Forms:* Tab 350 mg	A: PO: 350 mg q.i.d.

Contraindications	Drug-Lab-Food Interactions
Severe renal and hepatic disease	*Increase* CNS depression with alcohol, narcotics, sedative-hypnotics, antihistamines, tricyclic antidepressants

Pharmacokinetics	Pharmacodynamics
Absorption: PO: Well absorbed *Distribution:* PB: UK; in breast milk *Metabolism:* t 1/2: 8 h *Excretion:* In urine	PO: Onset: 30 min Peak: 3–4 h Duration: 4–6 h

Therapeutic Effects/Uses: To relax skeletal muscles.

Mode of Action: Depression of the CNS and, thus, relaxation of skeletal muscles.

Side Effects	Adverse Reactions
Nausea, vomiting, syncope, dizziness, drowsiness, weakness, insomnia, headache, depression, irritability, rash	Tachycardia, postural hypotension, diplopia *Life threatening:* Asthmatic attack, leukopenia, anaphylactic shock

KEY: For complete abbreviation key, see inside front cover.

■ NURSING PROCESS: MUSCLE RELAXANT: Carisoprodol

ASSESSMENT

- Obtain a medical history. Carisoprodol is contraindicated if the client has severe renal or liver disease.
- Obtain baseline VS for future comparison.
- Obtain the client's history to identify the cause of muscle spasm and to determine if it is acute or chronic.
- Obtain a drug history. Report if a drug-drug interaction is probable.
- Note if there is a history of narrow-angle glaucoma or myasthenia gravis. Cyclobenzaprine and orphenadrine are contraindicated with these health problems.

POTENTIAL NURSING DIAGNOSES

Impaired physical mobility
Activity intolerance

PLANNING

- Client will be free of muscular pain within 1 wk.

NURSING INTERVENTIONS

- Monitor serum liver enzyme levels of clients taking dantrolene and carisoprodol. Report elevated liver enzymes, such as ALP, ALT, and GGPT.
- Monitor VS. Report abnormal results.

CLIENT TEACHING

General

- Inform the client that the muscle relaxant should not be abruptly stopped. Drug should be tapered over 1 wk to avoid rebound spasms.
- Advise the client not to drive or operate dangerous machinery when taking muscle relaxants. These drugs have a sedative effect and can cause drowsiness.
- Inform the client that most of the centrally acting muscle relaxants for acute spasms are usually taken for no longer than 3 wk.
- Advise the client to avoid alcohol and CNS depressants. If muscle relaxants are taken with these drugs, CNS depression may be intensified.
- Inform the client that these drugs are contraindicated during pregnancy or by lactating mothers. Check with the health care provider.

Diet

- Advise the client to take muscle relaxants with food to decrease GI upset.

Side Effects

- Instruct the client to report side effects of the muscle relaxant, such as nausea, vomiting, dizziness, faintness, headache, and diplopia. Dizziness and faintness are most likely due to orthostatic (postural) hypotension.

EVALUATION

- Evaluate the effectiveness of the muscle relaxant to determine if the client's muscular pain has decreased or disappeared.

Muscle Relaxant (Skeletal)

Generic (Brand)	Route and Dosage	Preg Cat	Interaction	t 1/2	PB	Onset	Peak	Duration
							Action	
Anxiolytics Diazepam (Valium) CSS IV	A: PO: 2–10 mg b.i.d./q.i.d IM/IV: 5–10 mg; may repeat	D	*Increase* CNS depression with alcohol, narcotics, sedatives/hypnotics, anticonvulsants *Increase* phenytoin levels; increase diazepam effect with cimetidine, oral contraceptives *Decrease* diazepam effects with oral contraceptives, rifampin	20–50 h	98%	PO: 30–60 min IM: 15–30 min IV: 1–5 min	PO: 1–2 h IV: 10–15 min	PO: 3 h IV: 30–60 min
Meprobamate (Equanil, Miltown) CSS IV	A: PO: 400 mg–1.2 g/d in divided doses	D	Similar to diazepam	10–12 h	UK	1 h	1–3 h	6–12 h

Centrally Acting Muscle Relaxants	Route and Dosage		Drug Interactions					
Baclofen (Lioresal)	A: PO: Initially 5 mg t.i.d.; may increase dose; maint; 10–20 mg t.i.d./ q.i.d.; max: 80 mg/d	C	*Increase* CNS depression with alcohol, narcotics, sedative/ hypnotics, tricyclic antidepressants, MAOIs, some antihistamines *Lab:* may *increase* blood glucose levels	3–4 h	30%	UK	2–3 h	8 h
Carisoprodol (Soma)	See Prototype Drug Chart							
Chlorphenesin carbamate (Maolate)	A: PO: Initially 800 mg t.i.d.; maint: 400 mg q.i.d.	C	Same as baclofen	3–4 h	UK	1 h	1–2 h	4–6 h
Chlorzoxazone (Paraflex, Parafon Forte)	A: PO: 250–750 mg t.i.d./q.i.d; max: 3 g/d C: PO: 20 mg/kg/d or 600 mg/m²/d in 3–4 divided doses	C	Same as baclofen	1 h	UK	1 h	2–4 h	4–5 h
Cyclobenzaprine HCl (Flexeril)	A: PO: 10 mg t.i.d.; may increase dose; max: 60 mg/d	B	Same as baclofen; may cause hypertensive crisis with MAOIs	1–3 d	93%	1 h	3–8 h	12–24 h

continued

Muscle Relaxant (Skeletal)— *Continued*

Generic (Brand)	Route and Dosage	Preg Cat	Interaction	t1/2	PB	Onset	Peak	Duration
							Action	
						Onset	Peak	Duration
Methocarbamol (Robaxin, Delaxin, Marbaxin)	A: PO: Initially 1.5 g q.i.d.; maint: 1 g q.i.d. IM/IV: 0.5–1 g q8h; max: 3 g/d	C	Same as baclofen	1–2 h	UK	30 min	1–2 h	UK
Orphenadrine citrate (Norflex, Flexon)	A: PO: 100 mg b.i.d. IM/IV: 60 mg daily/b.i.d.	C	*Increase* CNS effects with other anticholinergics, oral contraceptives, propoxyphene	14 h	<20%	PO: 1 h IV: Immediate	PO: 2 h	PO: 4–6 h
Depolarizing Muscle Relaxants (adjunct to anesthesia)								

Drug								
Pancuronium bromide (Pavulon)	C	*Increase* neuromuscular blockade with local anesthetic, aminoglycosides, quinidine, narcotics, thiazides, lithium, bacitracin, lidocaine *Decrease* pancuronium effect with phenytoin	A: IV: 0.04–0.1 mg/kg; then 0.01 mg/kg every 30–60 min as needed C >10 y: same as for adult	2 h	<10%	30–45 s	2–3 min	45–60 min
Succinylcholine Cl (Anectine Cl, Quelicin, Sucostrin)	C	Same as pancuronium	A: IM: 2.5–4 mg/kg; max: 150 mg IV: 0.3–1.1 mg/kg; max: 150 mg C: IM/IV: 1–2 mg/kg; max: IM: 150 mg	UK	UK	IM: 2–3 min IV: 1 min	IM: UK IV: 2–3 min	IM: 10–30 min IV: 6–10 min
Vecuronium bromide (Norcuron)	C	Similar to pancuronium	A or C >9 y: IV: Initially 0.08–0.1 mg/kg/ dose; maint: 0.05–0.1 mg/kg/h as needed	1–1.5 h	60–80%	30–60 min	3–5 min	25–40 min

continued

Muscle Relaxant (Skeletal) — Continued

Generic (Brand)	Route and Dosage	Preg Cat	Interaction	t 1/2	PB	Onset	Peak	Duration
Muscle Relaxant Recuronium bromide (Flumadine)	*Anesthesia intubation:* A: IV: Initially: 0.45–0.6 mg/kg C: IV: 0.6 mg/kg *During surgery:* A: IV bolus: 0.9–1.2 mg/kg *Postoperative:* A: IV: 0.01–0.012 mg/kg/min	B	*Increase* effect with anesthetics	2–18 min	30%	2 min	4 min	UK
Peripherally Acting Muscle Relaxant Dantrolene sodium (Dantrium)	A: PO: Initially 25 mg/d; increase gradually; maint: 100 mg b.i.d.–q.i.d. C: PO: Initially 0.5 mg/kg b.i.d.; increase dose gradually by 0.5 mg/kg t.i.d./q.i.d.; max: 100 mg q.i.d.	C	*Increase* CNS depression with alcohol, narcotics, sedatives/ hypnotics, tricyclic antidepressants	8.7 h	95%	1 h	5 h	8 h

KEY: For complete abbreviation key, see inside front cover.

ANTI-INFLAMMATORY AGENTS

Nonsteroidal Anti-inflammatory Drugs

Gold Preparations

Antigout Drugs

Anti-inflammatory: Nonsteroidal Anti-inflammatory Drugs (NSAID)

Ibuprofen

Ibuprofen
  (Motrin, Advil, Nuprin, Medipren,
  Rufen)
NSAID: Propionic acid derivative
Pregnancy Category: B
Drug Forms:
Tab 200, 400, 600, 800 mg

Dosage

A: PO: 200–800 mg t.i.d./q.i.d.; max:
  <3.2 g/d (<3,200 mg/d)
C: PO: Average: 5–10 mg/kg/d;
  max: 40 mg/kg/d
1–4 y: 400 mg/d in divided doses
5–7 y: 600 mg/d in divided doses
>8 y: 800 mg/d in divided doses

Contraindications

Severe renal or hepatic disease,
  asthma, peptic ulcer
Caution: Bleeding disorders, early
  pregnancy, lactation, systemic
  lupus erythematosus (SLE)

Drug-Lab-Food Interactions

Increase bleeding time with oral
  anticoagulants; *increase* effects of
  phenytoin, sulfonamides, warfarin
Decrease effect with aspirin; may
  increase severe side effect of lithium

Pharmacokinetics

Absorption: PO: Well absorbed
Distribution: PB: 98%
Metabolism: t 1/2: 2–4 h
Excretion: In urine, mostly as inactive
  metabolites; some in bile

Pharmacodynamics

PO: Onset: 0.5 h
  Peak: 1–2 h
  Duration: 4–6 h

Therapeutic Effects/Uses: To reduce inflammatory process; to relieve pain; anti-inflammatory effect for arthritic conditions.

Mode of Action: Inhibition of prostaglandin synthesis, thus relieving pain and inflammation.

Side Effects

Anorexia, nausea, vomiting,
  diarrhea, edema, rash, purpura,
  tinnitus, fatigue, dizziness,
  lightheadedness, anxiety,
  confusion

Adverse Reactions

GI bleeding
Life-threatening: Blood dyscrasias,
  cardiac dysrhythmias,
  nephrotoxicity, anaphylaxis

KEY: For complete abbreviation key, see inside front cover.

■ NURSING PROCESS: ANTI-INFLAMMATORY: Nonsteroidal Anti-inflammatory Drug

ASSESSMENT

- Check the client's history of allergy to NSAIDs, including aspirin. If an allergy is present, notify the health care provider.
- Obtain a drug history and report any possible drug-drug interaction. NSAIDs can increase the effects of phenytoin (Dilantin), sulfonamides, and warfarin. Most NSAIDs are highly protein-bound and can displace other highly protein-bound drugs, like warfarin (Coumadin).
- Obtain a medical history. NSAIDs are contraindicated if the client has a severe renal or liver disease, peptic ulcer, or bleeding disorder.
- Assess the client for GI upset and peripheral edema, which are common side effects of NSAIDs.

POTENTIAL NURSING DIAGNOSES

Impaired tissue integrity
High risk for activity intolerance

PLANNING

- The inflammatory process will subside in 1−3 wk.

NURSING INTERVENTIONS

- Observe the client for bleeding gums, petechiae, ecchymoses, or black (tarry) stools. Bleeding time can be prolonged when taking NSAIDs, especially with a highly protein-bound drug such as warfarin (anticoagulant).
- Report if the client is having GI discomfort. Administer the NSAIDs at mealtime or with food to prevent GI upset.
- Monitor VS and check for peripheral edema, especially in the morning.

CLIENT TEACHING

General

- Instruct the client not to take aspirin with other NSAIDs and, when taking an NSAID, not to take aspirin or acetaminophen.
- Instruct the client to avoid alcohol when taking NSAIDs. GI upset or gastric ulcer may result.
- Advise the client to inform the dentist or surgeon before a procedure when taking ibuprofen or other NSAIDs for a continuous period of time.
- Advise women not to take NSAIDs 1−2 d before menstruation to avoid heavy menstrual flow. If discomfort occurs, acetaminophen is usually prescribed.
- Advise women in the third trimester of pregnancy to avoid NSAIDs. If delivery occurs, excess bleeding might occur with NSAIDs.
- Inform the client that it may take several weeks to experience the desired drug effect of some NSAIDs.

Diet

- Instruct the client to take NSAIDs with meals or food to reduce GI upset.

Anti-inflammatory: Nonsteroidal Anti-inflammatory Drugs (NSAID)

Side Effects

• Advise the client of the common side effects of NSAIDs. Nausea, vomiting, peripheral edema, GI upset, purpura or petechiae, and/or dizziness might occur. Report occurrences of side effects.

EVALUATION

• Evaluate the effectiveness of the drug therapy, such as a decrease in pain and in swollen joints and an increase in mobility.

Anti-inflammatory: Nonsteroidal Anti-inflammatory Drugs

Generic (Brand)	Route and Dosage	Preg Cat	Interaction	t 1/2	PB	Onset	Peak	Duration
Salicylates								
Aspirin (ASA, Bayer, Ecotrin)	A: PO: 325–650 mg PRN See Prototype Drug— Aspirin—Analgesic	D: Near term	*Increase* risk of bleeding with anticoagulants; *increase* ulcerogenic effect with glucocorticoids *Lab: Increase* PT, bleeding time, uric acid	2–3 h (low dose)	90%	15–30 min	1–2 h	4–6 h
Diflunisal (Dolobid)	A: PO: Initially: 1 g (1,000 mg); maint: 500 mg q8–12h	C	*Increase* effects of acetaminophen, anticoagulants; may *increase* bleeding with warfarin *Decrease* diflunisal effects with antacids, steroids; may *decrease* effect of diuretics, anticoagulants	1 h	99%	1 h	2–3 h	8–12 h

continued

Generic (Brand)	Route and Dosage	Preg Cat	Interaction	t 1/2	PB	Onset	Peak	Duration
							Action	
Para-Chlorobenzoic Acid (Indoles)								
Indomethacin (Indocin)	A: PO: 25–50 mg b.i.d./ t.i.d. with food SR: 75 mg q.d./b.i.d.; max: 200 mg/d C: PO: 1–2 mg/kg/d in 2–4 divided doses; may increase to 4 mg/kg/d; max: 150–200 mg/d	B (D at near term)	May *increase* effect of digoxin, phenytoin, sulfonamides, warfarin, lithium; may *increase* bleeding time with aspirin, anticoagulants, alcohol May *decrease* effect of diuretics	3–120 h	90–99%	0.5–2 h	3 h	4–6 h
Sulindac (Clinoril)	A: PO: 150–200 mg b.i.d.	C	Same as indomethacin	7–18 h	93%	1–2 h	2 h or 4 h with food	10–12 h
Tolmetin (Tolectin)	A: PO: Initially: 400 mg t.i.d.; maint: 600–1800 mg/d in divided doses; max: 2 g/d C >2 y: PO: 20 mg/kg/d in divided doses; max: 30 mg/kg/d	B (D at near term)	Same as indomethacin *Lab:* Increase BUN, ALP, AST, hematocrit, bleeding time	1–1.5 h	99%	15–30 min	0.5–1 h	UK

	Dosage	Pregnancy Category	Drug-Lab-Food Interactions	$t\frac{1}{2}$	PB	Onset	Peak	Duration
Pyrazolone Phenylbutazone (Butazolidin)	A: PO: 100–400 mg/d in divided doses; max: 600 mg/d	C	May *increase* bleeding time with warfarin, aspirin, other NSAIDs, glucocorticoids; may *increase* lithium effect May *decrease* hypotensive effect of antihypertensives *Lab: Increase AST, ALT*	50–100 h	98%	UK	2 h	UK
Propionic Acid Fenoprofen calcium (Nalfon)	A: PO: 300–600 mg t.i.d./q.i.d.; max: 3.2 g/d	B (D at term)	Similar to ibuprofen	3 h	90%	30 min	1–2 h	4–6 h
Flurbiprofen sodium (Ansaid, Ocufen)	A: PO: 50–300 mg/d in 2–4 divided doses; max: 300 mg/d *Ophthalmic use:* 0.03% sol	C	*Increase* bleeding time with heparin, warfarin May *decrease* effects of aspirin, diuretics	5 h	UK	<2 h	1.5–2 h	6–8 h
Ibuprofen (Motrin, Advil, Nuprin, Medipren)	See Prototype Drug Chart							

continued

Generic (Brand)	Route and Dosage	Preg Cat	Interaction	t 1/2	PB	Onset	Peak	Duration
							Action	
Ketoprofen (Orudis)	*Inflammatory:* A: PO: 150–300 mg/d in 3–4 divided doses *Mild-moderate pain:* A: PO: 25–50 mg q6–8h PRN; max: 300 mg/d	B, D at near term	Similar to flurbiprofen	3–4 h	99%	1 h	1.5–2 h	4–6 h
Naproxen (Naprosyn)	A: PO: 250–500 mg b.i.d. C: PO: 5–10 mg/kg/d in 2 divided doses	B	Similar to ibuprofen	10–15 h	99%	1 h	2 h	7 h
Oxaprozin (Daypro)	A: PO: Initially: 1,200 mg/d; maint: 600 mg/d; max: 1800 mg/d in divided doses	C	*Increase* GI disturbance with aspirin, alcohol, steroids; *increase* effect of aspirin, warfarin *Decrease* antihypertensive effect with antihypertensive drugs	40 h	99%	UK	Up to 2–6 wk	UK
Anthranylic Acids (Fenamates) Meclofenamate (Meclomen)	A: PO: 200–400 mg in 3–4 divided doses	B, D at term	*Increase* bleeding time with anticoagulants; may *increase* effects of phenytoin, sulfonamides, sulfonylureas	3 h	99%	0.5–1 h	1–2 h	2–6 h

Drug	Dosage	Pregnancy category	Drug interactions	t½	Protein binding	Onset	Peak	Duration
Mefenamic acid (Ponstel)	A: PO: Initially: 500 mg; then 250 mg q6h PRN; max: 1 g/d	C	Same as meclofenamate	2–4 h	90%	1–2 h	2–4 h	6 h
Oxicams Piroxicam (Feldene)	A: PO: 10 mg b.i.d. or 20 mg q.d.	C	Similar to meclofenamate	30–86 h	99%	1 h	3–5 h	24–72 h
Phenylacetic Acid Diclofenac sodium (Voltaren)	A: PO: 25–50 t.i.d./q.i.d. or 75 mg b.i.d.	B	May *increase* digoxin levels; may *increase* bleeding time with warfarin; *increase* effects of phenytoin, sulfonamides, sulfonylurea *Decrease* antihypertensive effect with diuretics, beta blockers	2 h	90–99%	1 h	2–3 h	UK
Etodolac (Lodine)	A: PO: 200–400 mg q6–8h PRN; max: 1,200 mg/d	C	May *increase* serum levels with digoxin, lithium May *decrease* effects of diuretics, beta blockers (antihypertensive effect)	6–7 h	99%	0.5 h	1–2 h	4–12 h
Ketorolac (Toradol)	A: <50kg: IM: LD: 30 mg; maint: 15 mg q6h; A: >50kg: IM: LD: 30–60 mg; maint: 15–30 mg PRN	B	Similar to diclofenac	5–6 h	99%	15–45 min	1 h	6–8 h

KEY: For complete abbreviation key, see inside front cover.

139

Anti-inflammatory Agent: Gold

Auranofin

Auranofin
  (Ridaura)
Gold preparation
Pregnancy Category: C
Drug Forms:
Cap 3 mg

Dosage

A: PO: 6 mg/d in single or divided
  doses; may increase dose to
  9 mg/d

Contraindications

Severe renal or hepatic disease,
  colitis, systemic lupus
  erythematosus (SLE), pregnancy,
  blood dyscrasias
Caution: Diabetes mellitus, CHF

Drug-Lab-Food Interactions

With anticancer drugs, may cause
  bone marrow depression
Lab: Slightly *increase* liver enzyme
  tests

Pharmacokinetics

Absorption: PO: 25% absorbed
Distribution: PB: 60%
Metabolism: t 1/2: 26 d in blood;
  40–120 d in tissue
Excretion: >60% in urine (may appear
  for 15 mon); in feces

Pharmacodynamics

PO: Onset: UK
     Peak: 1–2 h
     Duration: Months

Therapeutic Effects/Uses: To alleviate inflammation and pain of rheumatoid arthritis.

Mode of Action: Inhibition of prostaglandin synthesis and decreased phagocytosis.

Side Effects

Anorexia, nausea, vomiting,
  diarrhea, stomatitis, abdominal
  cramps, pruritus, dizziness,
  headache, metallic taste, rash,
  dermatitis, photosensitivity

Adverse Reactions

Corneal gold deposits, urticaria,
  hematuria, proteinuria,
  bradycardia
Life-threatening: Nephrotoxicity,
  agranulocytosis,
  thrombocytopenia, interstitial
  pneumonitis

KEY: For complete abbreviation key, see inside front cover.

■ NURSING PROCESS: ANTI-INFLAMMATORY DRUGS: Gold

ASSESSMENT

• Obtain the client's health history. Usually, gold drugs such as auranofin are contraindicated if there is renal or hepatic dysfunction, marked hypertension, congestive heart failure, systemic lupus erythematosus (SLE), or uncontrolled diabetes mellitus.

• Check for proteinuria and hematuria before giving initial gold dose and during gold therapy.

• Observe the client for 30 min after gold injection for possible allergic reaction after the first and second injections. It takes approximately 10–15 min for a serious allergic reaction (anaphylaxis) to occur.

• Obtain baseline VS and hematology laboratory findings for future comparisons.

POTENTIAL NURSING DIAGNOSES

Impaired physical mobility
Pain
High risk for impaired skin integrity

PLANNING

• The client will be free of inflammation and pain while taking the gold treatment without adverse drug reaction.

NURSING INTERVENTIONS

• Monitor the client's VS. Report abnormal findings.

• Monitor laboratory tests, e.g., complete blood count (CBC). Report abnormal findings.

• Check periodically for signs of side effects and adverse reactions to gold therapy. Side effects may include anorexia, nausea, vomiting, diarrhea, gingivitis, stomatitis, rash, itching, and decreased urine output. Most gold drugs have a long half-life; thus, a cumulative effect can result. Auranofin causes less severe adverse reactions than other gold preparations.

CLIENT TEACHING

General

• Instruct the client to perform frequent dental hygiene, including brushing the teeth with a soft toothbrush and flossing to prevent or control gingivitis and stomatitis. Use of diluted hydrogen peroxide can be helpful with mild stomatitis.

• Instruct the client to adhere to scheduled laboratory blood tests and appointments with the health care provider so any adverse reactions can be monitored.

• Inform the client that the desired therapeutic effect may take as long as 3–4 mon to occur.

Diet

• Suggest high-fiber diet and/or antidiarrheal drugs to control diarrhea. If diarrhea is continuous or severe for a prolonged time, the gold drug is usually discontinued.

Anti-inflammatory Agent: Gold

Side Effects

- Explain to the client to report early symptoms of possible gold toxicity such as a metallic taste or pruritus. A rash may occur. These symptoms should be reported to the health care provider.
- Teach the client the side effects and to report them immediately. (See list of side effects and adverse reactions.)
- Instruct the client to avoid direct sunlight because the gold drug may cause photosensitivity. Use of sunblock is necessary.
- Instruct the client to report skin conditions such as dermatitis, bruising, and petechiae. Bleeding gums and blood in the stools should be reported to the health care provider.

EVALUATION

- Evaluate the effectiveness of the gold therapy by determining if the client has less pain and inflammation.
- Evaluate the client for present or repeated side effects. The gold therapy regimen may need to be changed or discontinued.

Generic (Brand)	Route and Dosage	Preg Cat	Interaction	t 1/2	PB	Action		
						Onset	Peak	Duration
Auranofin (Ridaura)	See Prototype Drug Chart							
Aurothioglucose (Solganal)	Increase dose weekly: A: IM: 10, 25, 50 mg (sol in oil)	C	*Increase* blood dyscrasias with immunosuppressants, cytotoxics, phenylbutazone, penicillamine	3–27 d	95%	2–3 h	4–6 h	6 mon
Gold sodium thiomalate (Myochrysine)	Increase dose weekly: A: IM: 10, 25, 50 mg (aqueous sol) until 1 g cumulative; maint: 25–50 mg q2–3wk	C	Same as aurothioglucose	3–27 d	95%	2–3 h	4–6 h	6 mon

KEY: For complete abbreviation key, see inside front cover.

Antigout

Allopurinol	Dosage
Allopurinol (Zyloprim) Uric acid biosynthesis inhibitor *Pregnancy Category:* C *Drug Forms:* Tab 100, 300 mg	A: PO: 200–300 mg/d (for mild gout) PO: 400–600 mg/d (for severe gout)

Contraindications	Drug-Lab-Food Interactions
Hypersensitivity, severe renal disease *Caution:* Hepatic disorder	*Increase* effect of warfarin, phenytoin, theophylline, anticancer drugs, ACE inhibitors; *increase* rash with ampicillin, amoxicillin; *increase* toxicity with thiazide diuretics *Decrease* allopurinal effect with antacids *Lab: Increase* AST, ALT, BUN

Pharmacokinetics	Pharmacodynamics
Absorption: PO: 80% absorbed *Distribution:* PB: UK *Metabolism:* t 1/2: Drug: 2–3 h Metabolite: 20–24 h *Excretion:* 10–20% in urine; 80–90% in feces	PO: Onset: 0.5–1 h Peak: 2–4 h Duration: 18–30 h

Therapeutic Effects/Uses: To treat gout and hyperuricemia; prevent urate calculi.

Mode of Action: Reduction of uric acid synthesis.

Side Effects	Adverse Reactions
Anorexia, nausea, vomiting, diarrhea, stomatitis, dizziness, headache, rash, pruritus, malaise, metallic taste	Cataracts, retinopathy *Life-threatening:* Bone marrow depression, aplastic anemia, thrombocytopenia, agranulocytosis, leukopenia

KEY: For complete abbreviation key, see inside front cover.

■ NURSING PROCESS: ANTIGOUT: Allopurinol (Zyloprim)

ASSESSMENT

- Obtain a medical history from the client of any gastric, renal, cardiac, or liver disorders. Antigout drugs are excreted via kidneys, so sufficient renal function is needed. Drug dosage and drug selection might need to be changed.
- Obtain a drug history. Report possible drug-drug interactions. (See drug-lab-food interaction list.)
- Assess the serum uric acid value to be used for future comparisons.
- Assess the urine output. Use the initial urine output for future comparisons.

Antigout

- Obtain laboratory tests (BUN, serum creatinine, ALP, AST, ALT, LDH) and compare with future laboratory test results.

POTENTIAL NURSING DIAGNOSES
Impaired tissue integrity
Pain

PLANNING
- Client's "gouty pain" is absent or controlled without side effects.

NURSING INTERVENTIONS
- Report GI symptoms, gastric pain, nausea, vomiting, or diarrhea when taking antigout drugs. Take these drugs with food to alleviate gastric distress.
- Monitor the client's urine output. Because the drugs and uric acid are excreted through the urine, kidney stones might occur, so both water intake and urine output should be increased.
- Monitor laboratory tests for renal and liver function, i.e., BUN, serum creatinine, ALP, AST, and ALT.

CLIENT TEACHING
General
- Encourage the client to keep medical appointments and to have regular scheduled laboratory tests for renal, liver, and blood cell (CBC) functions. Some antigout drugs may cause blood dyscrasias; blood tests should be monitored.
- Instruct the client to increase fluid intake; it will increase drug and uric acid excretion.

Diet
- Advise the client to avoid alcohol and caffeine because they can increase uric acid levels.
- Suggest to the client not to take large doses of vitamin C while taking allopurinol; kidney stones may occur.
- Instruct the client not to ingest foods that are high in purine content, such as organ meats, salmon and sardines, gravies, and legumes. Purine foods increase the uric acid levels.
- Instruct the client to report any gastric distress. Encourage the client to take antigout drugs with food or at mealtime.

Side Effects
- Instruct the client to report side effects of antigout drugs, such as anorexia, nausea, vomiting, diarrhea, stomatitis, dizziness, rash, pruritus, or metallic taste, to the health care provider.
- Advise the client to have yearly eye examination since visual changes can result from prolonged use of allopurinol.

EVALUATION
- Evaluate the client's response to the antigout drug. If pain persists, the drug regimen may need modification.
- Determine the presence of adverse reactions. Drug therapy for gout pain may need to be changed.

Generic (Brand)	Route and Dosage	Preg Cat	Interaction	t 1/2	PB	Action Onset	Action Peak	Action Duration
Anti-inflammatory Gout Drug Colchicine (Colsalide, Novocolchine)	A: PO: Initially: 0.5–1.2 mg; then 0.5–0.6 mg q1–2h for pain relief; max: 4 mg/d IV: Initially: 2 mg; then 0.5 mg q6h PRN; max: 4 mg/d	C	*Increase* effects of CNS depressants, adrenergics *Decrease* effect of vitamin B$_{12}$ *Lab: Increase AST, ALT*	20–30 min	10–30%	20 min	0.5–2 h	9 d
Uric Acid Biosynthesis Inhibitor Allopurinol (Zyloprim)	See Prototype Drug Chart							
Uricosurics Probenecid (Benemid)	A: PO: First week: 250 mg b.i.d.; maint: 500 mg b.i.d.; max: 2 g/d C <50 kg: PO: 25–40 mg/kg/d in 4 divided doses	B	*Increase* effect of anticoagulants; *increase* toxicity of NSAIDs *Decrease* probenecid effect with aspirin, alcohol, diuretics, diazoxides, nitrofurantoin; *decrease* effect of oral hypoglycemics	4–10 h	90%	30 min	2–4 h	8 h
Sulfinpyrazone (Anturane)	A: PO: First week: 100–200 mg b.i.d.; maint: 200–400 mg b.i.d.; max: 800 mg/d	C	Similar to probenecid	3 h	90%	30 min	2–4 h	4–6 h

KEY: For complete abbreviation key, see inside front cover.

ANTI-INFECTIVE AGENTS

Antibacterials:
Penicillins
Cephalosporins
Erythromycin
Tetracyclines
Aminoglycosides
Quinolones
Unclassified
Sulfonamides
Peptides

Antitubercular Agents

Antifungals

Antimalarials

Antivirals

Topical Anti-infectives:
Burns
Acne Vulgaris
Psoriasis

Antibacterials: Broad-Spectrum Penicillins

Amoxicillin trihydrate

Amoxicillin trihydrate
   (Amoxil)
Amoxicillin-clavulanate
   (Augmentin)
Broad-spectrum penicillin
Pregnancy Category: B
Drug Forms:
Cap 250, 500 mg
Tab (chewable) 125, 250 mg
Liq 62.5, 125, 250 mg/5 mL

Dosage

A: PO: 250–500 mg q8h
C: PO: 20–40 mg/kg/d in 3
   divided doses

Contraindications

Allergy to penicillin, severe renal
   disorder
Caution: Hypersensitivity to
   cephalosporins

Drug-Lab-Food Interactions

Increase effect with aspirin,
   probenecid
Decrease effect with tetracycline,
   erythromycin
Lab: Increase serum AST, ALT

Pharmacokinetics

Absorption: PO: >80% (intestine)
Distribution: PB: 20%
Metabolism: t 1/2: 1–1.5 h
Excretion: Amoxicillin: 70% in urine;
   clavulanate: 30–40% in urine

Pharmacodynamics

PO: Onset: 0.5 h
   Peak: 1–2 h
   Duration: 6–8 h

Therapeutic Effects/Uses: To treat respiratory tract infections, urinary tract infection, otitis media, and most gram-positive and gram-negative cocci and bacilli.

Mode of Action: Inhibition of the enzyme in cell wall synthesis. Bactericidal effect.

Side Effects

Nausea, vomiting, diarrhea, rash,
   stomatitis, edema

Adverse Reactions

Superinfections (vaginitis)
Life-threatening: Blood dyscrasias,
   bone marrow depression,
   hemolytic anemia, respiratory
   distress

KEY: For complete abbreviation key, see inside front cover.

■ NURSING PROCESS: ANTIBACTERIALS: Broad-Spectrum Penicillins

ASSESSMENT

• Assess for allergy to penicillin or cephalosporins. The client who is hypersensitive to amoxicillin should not take any type of penicillin products. Severe allergic reaction could occur. A small percentage of clients who are allergic to penicillin could also be allergic to a cephalosporin product.

• Check laboratory results, especially liver enzymes. Report elevated ALP, ALT, or AST.

• Assess urine output. If the amount is inadequate (<30 mL/h or <600 mL/d), drug and/or drug dosage may need to be changed.

POTENTIAL NURSING DIAGNOSES
High risk for infection
High risk for impaired tissue integrity
Noncompliance with drug regimen

PLANNING
• Client's infection will be controlled and later eliminated.

NURSING INTERVENTIONS
• Send a culture of the infectious area to the laboratory to determine antibiotic susceptibility (also known as C&S) before antibiotic therapy is started.
• Check for signs and symptoms of superinfection, especially for clients taking high doses of the antibiotic for a prolonged time. Signs and symptoms include stomatitis (mouth ulcers), genital discharge (vaginitis), and anal or genital itching.
• Check the client for allergic reaction to the penicillin product, especially after the first and second doses. This may be a mild reaction, such as a rash, or a severe reaction, such as respiratory distress or anaphylaxis.
• Have epinephrine available to counteract a severe allergic reaction.
• Check the client for bleeding if high doses of penicillin are being given; a decrease in platelet aggregation (clotting) may result.
• Monitor body temperature and infectious area.
• Dilute the antibiotic for IV use in an appropriate amount of solution as indicated in the drug circular.

CLIENT TEACHING
General
• Instruct the client to take all of the prescribed penicillin product such as amoxicillin until the bottle is empty. If only a portion of the penicillin is taken, drug resistance to that antibacterial agent may develop in the future.
• Advise the client who is allergic to penicillin to wear a medical alert (Medic-Alert) bracelet or necklace and carry a card that indicates the allergy. The client should notify the health care provider during history taking of his or her allergy to penicillin.
• Keep drugs out of reach of small children. Request child safety cap bottle.
• Inform the client to report any side effects or adverse reaction that may occur while taking the drug.
• Encourage the client to increase fluid intake; it will aid in decreasing the body temperature and in excreting the drug.
• Instruct the client or child's parent that chewable tablets must be chewed or crushed before swallowing.

Diet
• Advise the client to take medication with food to decrease gastric irritation.

EVALUATION
• Evaluate the effectiveness of the antibacterial agent by determining if the infection has ceased and no side effects, including superinfection, have occurred.

Generic (Brand)	Route and Dosage	Preg Cat	Interaction	t1/2	PB	Onset	Peak	Duration
							Action	
Basic Penicillins								
Penicillin G procaine (Crysticillin, Wycillin)	A: IM: 600,000–1.2 million U/d in 1–2 divided doses C: IM: 300,000–600,000 U/d in 1–2 divided doses NB: IM: 50,000 U/kg/d	B	Same as penicillin G sodium	0.5–1 h	65%	1–2 h	1–4 h	15–18 h
Penicillin G benzathine (Bicillin)	A: IM: 1.2 million U as a single dose C: IM: >27 kg: 900,000 U/dose IM: <27 kg: 50,000 U/kg/ dose or 300,000–600,000 U/dose	B	Same as penicillin G sodium	1 h	65%	Delayed	12–24 h	26 d
Penicillin G sodium/ potassium (Pentids, Pfizerpen)	A: PO: 200,000–500,000 U q6h IM: 500,000–5 million U/d in divided doses IV: 4–20 million U/d in divided doses, diluted in IV fluids C: PO: 25,000–90,000 U/d in divided doses IV: 50,000–100,000 U/kg/d in divided doses	B	*Increase* effect with aspirin, probenecid *Decrease* effect with tetracycline, erythromycin	0.5–1 h	65%	PO: 30 min IM: 15 min IV: Minutes	PO: 0.5–1 h IM: 15–30 min IV: 5–10 min	6 h

Drug	Route and Dosage	Pregnancy Category	Drug Interactions	t½	PB	Onset	Peak	Duration
Penicillin V potassium (V-Cillin K, Veetids, Betapen VK)	A: PO: 125–500 mg q6h C: PO: 15–50 mg/kg/d in 3–4 divided doses	B	Same as penicillin G *Decrease* effect with neomycin	30 min	80%	<30 min	0.5–1 h	6 h
Broad-Spectrum Penicillins								
Amoxicillin (Amoxil) Amoxicillin-clavulanate (Augmentin)	See Prototype Drug Chart See Prototype Drug Chart							
Ampicillin (Polycillin, Omnipen)	A: PO: 250–500 mg q6h IM/IV: 2–8 g/d in divided doses C: PO: 50–100 mg/kg/d in divided doses IM/IV: 50–200 mg/kg/d in divided doses	B	*Increase* ampicillin effect with aspirin, probenecid *Decrease* effect of oral contraceptives *Decrease* ampicillin effect with tetracycline, erythromycin	1–2 h	15–28%	Rapid	PO: 1–2 h IM: 1 h IV: 5 min	6–8 h
Ampicillin-sulbactam (Unasyn)	A: IV: 1.5–3.0 g q6h	B	Same as ampicillin	1–2 h	28–38%	Immediate	5 min	UK
Bacampicillin HCl (Spectrobid)	A: PO: 400–800 mg q12h C: PO: 25–50 mg/kg/d in divided doses	B	Similar to ampicillin	1 h	17–20%	UK	0.5–1 h	5–6 h
Cyclacillin (Cyclapen)	A: PO: 250–500 mg q6h C: PO: 50–100 mg/kg/d in divided doses	B	Similar to ampicillin	0.5–1 h	20%	UK	0.5–1 h	6–8 h

Continued

Antibacterials: Penicillins

Generic (Brand)	Route and Dosage	Preg Cat	Interaction	t 1/2	PB	Onset	Peak	Duration
Penicillinase-Resistant Penicillins								
Cloxacillin (Tegopen)	A: PO: 250–500 mg q6h C: PO: 50–100 mg/kg/d in 4 divided doses	B	Similar to ampicillin	0.5–1 h	90%	0.5 h	1–2 h	6 h
Dicloxacillin (Dynapen)	A: PO: 125–500 mg q6h C: PO: 12.5–25 mg/kg/d in 4 divided doses	B	Similar to ampicillin	0.5–1 h	95%	0.5 h	1–2 h	4–6 h
Methicillin (Staphcillin)	A: IM: 1 g q6h IV: 1–2 g q6h diluted in NSS C: IM/IV: 100–300 mg/kg/d in 4–6 divided doses	B	Similar to ampicillin	0.5–1 h	25–40%	IM: 20–30 min IV: Rapid	IM: 0.5–1 h IV: UK	IM: 4 h IV: 2 h
Nafcillin (Nafcin, Unipen)	A: PO: 250 mg–1 g q4–6h IM: 250–500 mg q6h IV: 500 mg–1 g q4–6h C: PO: 50–100 mg/kg/d in 4 divided doses IM: 25 mg/kg b.i.d. IV: 50–200 mg/kg/d in divided doses; max: 12 g/d	B	Similar to ampicillin	0.5–1.5 h	90%	PO: 1 h IM: <30 min	PO: 2 h IM: 0.5–1 h IV: Rapid	4–6 h

Generic (Trade)		Considerations	t½	Protein-Binding	Onset	Peak	Duration
Oxacillin (Prostaphlin, Bactocill)	A: PO: 250–1 g q4–6h; IM/IV: 500 mg–2 g q4h; max: IM/IV: 12 g; C: PO/IM/IV: 50–100 mg/kg/d in divided doses; max: IM/IV: 300 mg/kg/d	B	Similar to ampicillin	0.5–1 h	95%	PO/IM: 0.5 h IV: Rapid	PO/IM: 0.5–2 h IV: 15 min	PO/IM/IV: 4–6 h
Anti-*Pseudomonas* Penicillins								
Azlocillin (Azlin)	A: IV: 100–300 mg/kg/d or 3–4 g q4–6h; max: 24 g/d; C: IV: 75 mg/kg q4h; max: 24 g/d	B	Same as ampicillin *Increase* bleeding with anticoagulants	55–70 min	25–45%	UK	UK	UK
Carbenicillin disodium (Geocillin, Geopen)	A: PO: 1.5–3.0 g/d in divided doses IM: 1–2 g q6h or 200 mg/kg/d in 4 divided doses IV: 4–6 g q4–6h; C: PO: 30–50 mg/kg/d in divided doses; max: 2–3 g/d IM: 50–200 mg/kg/d in divided doses IV: 50–500 mg/kg/d in divided doses	B	Similar to ampicillin	1–1.5 h	50%	30 min	PO: 0.5–2 h IM: 45 min–1.5 h IV: 5–10 min	UK
Mezlocillin (Mezlin)	A: IM/IV: 3–4 g q6h or 100–300 mg/kg/d in 4 divided doses; max: 24 g/d C: IM/IV: 50 mg/kg q4h	B	Similar to ampicillin *Lab:* May *increase* BUN, AST, ALT, ALP, bilirubin	1 h	30–40%	Rapid	IV: 5–10 min	UK

Continued

Generic (Brand)	Route and Dosage	Preg Cat	Interaction	t 1/2	PB	Action			
						Onset	Peak	Duration	
Piperacillin (Pipracil)	A: IM/IV: 2–4 g q6h or 100–300 mg/kg/d in divided doses; max: 24 g/d C >12 y: IM/IV: 100–300 mg/kg/d in 4–6 divided doses	B	Similar to ampicillin	0.6–1.5 h	16–22%	Rapid	IM: 45 min–1 h IV: 5–10 min	UK	
Ticarcillin-clavulanate (Timentin)	A: IV: 3.1 g q6h C >12 y: IV: 200–300 mg/kg/d in 4–6 divided doses	B	Similar to ampicillin	1–1.5 h	45–65%	Rapid	IM: 1–2 h	UK	
Ticarcillin disodium (Ticar)	A: IM/IV: 1–2 g q6h C: IM/IV: 50–200 mg/kg/d in 4 divided doses Systemic infections: Dose is increased	C	Similar to ampicillin	1–1.5 h	45–65%	Rapid	IM: 1–2 h	May be present for 12 mo	

KEY: For complete abbreviation key, see inside front cover.

NOTES:

_____

_____

_____

_____

_____

_____

_____

_____

_____

_____

Antibacterials: Cephalosporins

Cefaclor

Cefaclor
  (Ceclor)
Second-generation cephalosporin
Pregnancy Category: B
Drug Forms:
Cap 250, 500 mg
Liq 125, 250, 325 mg/5 mL

Dosage

A: PO: 250–500 mg q8h; max: 4 g/d
C: PO: 20–40 mg/kg/d in 3 divided
  doses; max: 1 g/d

Contraindications

Hypersensitivity to cephalosporins
Caution: Hypersensitivity to
  penicillins; renal disease, lactation

Drug-Lab-Food Interactions

Increase effect with probenecid;
  increase toxicity of
  aminoglycosides, loop diuretics,
  colistin, vancomycin
Decrease effect with tetracyclines,
  erythromycin
Lab: May *increase* BUN, serum
  creatinine, AST, ALT, ALP, LDH,
  bilirubin

Pharmacokinetics

Absorption: PO: Well absorbed
Distribution: PB: 25%
Metabolism: t 1/2: 0.5–1 h
Excretion: 60–80% unchanged in
  urine

Pharmacodynamics

PO: Onset: Rapid
  Peak: 0.5–1 h
  Duration: UK

Therapeutic Effects/Uses: To treat respiratory, urinary, skin, and ear infections, or
cases resistant to ampicillin/amoxicillin.

Mode of Action: Inhibition of cell wall synthesis, causing cell death; bactericidal effect.

Side Effects

Anorexia, nausea, vomiting,
  diarrhea, weakness, headaches,
  vertigo, pruritus, maculopapular
  rash

Adverse Reactions

Superinfection (candidiasis),
  proteinuria, urticaria
Life-threatening: Renal failure

KEY: For complete abbreviation key, see inside front cover.

■ **NURSING PROCESS: Antibacterial: Cephalosporins**

ASSESSMENT

• Assess for allergy to cephalosporins. If allergic to one type or class of
cephalosporin, the client should not receive any other type of cephalosporin.
• Assess VS and urine output. Report abnormal findings, which may include
an elevated temperature or a decrease in urine output.

• Check laboratory results, especially those that indicate renal and liver function, such as BUN, serum creatinine, AST, ALT, ALP, and bilirubin. Report abnormal findings. Use these laboratory results for baseline values.

POTENTIAL DRUG DIAGNOSES
High risk for infection
Noncompliance with drug regimen

PLANNING
• Client's infection will be controlled and later eliminated.

NURSING INTERVENTIONS
• Culture the infectious area **before** cephalosporin therapy is started. The organism causing the infection can be determined by culture, and the antibiotics to which the organism is sensitive are determined by C&S. (Antibiotic therapy may be started before culture result is reported. The antibiotic may need to be changed after C&S test result.)
• Check for signs and symptoms of a superinfection, especially if the client is taking high doses of a cephalosporin product for a prolonged period of time. Superinfection is usually caused by the fungal organism *Candida* in the mouth (mouth ulcers) or in the genital area, such as the vagina (vaginitis).
• Refrigerate oral suspensions. For IV cephalosporins, dilute in an appropriate amount of IV fluids (50–100 mL) according to the drug circular.
• Administer IV cephalosporins over 30–45 min 2–4 times a day.
• Monitor VS, urine output, and laboratory results. Report abnormal findings.

CLIENT TEACHING
General
• Keep drugs out of reach of small children. Request child safety cap bottle.
• Instruct the client to report signs of superinfection, such as mouth ulcers or discharge from the anal or genital area.
• Advise the client to ingest buttermilk or yogurt to prevent superinfection of the intestinal flora with long-term use of a cephalosporin.
• Instruct the diabetic client not to use Clinitest tablets for urine glucose testing since false test results may occur. Tes-Tape or Clinistix may be used for urine testing, or Chemstrip bG may be used for blood glucose testing.
• Instruct the client to take the complete course of medication even when symptoms of infection have ended.

Diet
• Advise the client to take medication with food if gastric irritation occurs.

Side Effects
• Instruct the client to report any side effects from use of oral cephalosporin drug; they may include anorexia, nausea, vomiting, headache, dizziness, itching, and rash.

EVALUATION
• Evaluate the effectiveness of the cephalosporin by determining if the infection has ceased and no side effects, including superinfection, have occurred.

Generic (Brand)	Route and Dosage	Preg Cat	Interaction	t 1/2	PB	Action Onset	Action Peak	Action Duration
First Generation Cefadroxil (Duricef)	A: PO: 500 mg–2 g/d in 1–2 divided doses C: PO: 30 mg/kg/d in 2 divided doses	B	_Increase_ nephrotoxicity with aminoglycosides, loop diuretics, colistin _Decrease_ effect with tetracycline, erythromycin _Lab:_ May _increase_ BUN, AST, ALT, ALP	1–2 h	20%	Rapid	1 h	UK
Cefazolin sodium (Ancef, Kefzol)	A: IM/IV: 250 mg–2 g q6–8 h; max: 12 g/d C: IM/IV: 25–100 mg/kg/d in 3 divided doses; max: 6 g/d	B	Same as cefadroxil	1.5–2.5 h	75–85%	IM: Rapid IV: Immediate	IM: 0.5–2 h IV: 10–15 min	UK
Cephalexin (Keflex)	_Infection:_ A: PO: 250–500 mg q6h C: PO: 25–50 mg/kg/d in 3–4 divided doses _Otitis media:_ C: PO: 25–100 mg/kg/d in 4 divided doses; max: 3 g/d	B	Same as cefadroxil	0.5–1.2 h	10–15%	Rapid	1 h	UK
Cephalothin (Keflin)	A: IM/IV: 500 mg–1 g q4–6h C: IM/IV: 20–40 mg/kg q6h	B	Same as cefadroxil	30–50 min	65–80%	UK	IM: 30 min IV: 15 min	UK

Generic (Brand)	Route and Dosage	Pregnancy Category	Drug-Lab-Food Interactions	t½	PB	Onset	Peak	Duration
Cephapirin (Cefadyl)	A: IM/IV: 500 mg–1 g q4–6h C: IM/IV: 40–80 mg/kg/d in 4 divided doses	B	Same as cefadroxil	0.5–1 h	40–50%	Rapid	IM: 30 min IV: 5–10 min	UK
Cephradine (Velosef)	A: PO: 250–500 mg q6h or 500 mg–1 g q12h IM/IV: 500 mg–1 g q6–12 h C: PO: 25–50 mg/kg/d in 4 divided doses IM/IV: 50–100 mg/kg/d in 4 divided doses	B	Same as cefadroxil	1–2 h	20%	Rapid	PO: 1 h IM: 1–2 h IV: 5–10 min	UK
Second Generation								
Cefaclor (Ceclor)	See Prototype Drug Chart							
Cefamandole (Mandol)	A: IM/IV: 500 mg–1 g q4–8h	B	Similar to cefadroxil	45 min–1 h	60–75%	IM: Rapid IV: Rapid	IM: 0.5–2 h IV: 0.5 h	UK
Cefmetazole sodium (Zefazone)	A: IV: 2 g q6–12h	B	*Increase* effect with probenecid *Decrease* effect with erythromycin, tetracyclines *Lab:* May *increase* effect of ALP, AST, ALT, LDH, BUN, creatinine	1.5–3 h	68%	IV: Rapid	End of infusion	UK
Cefonicid sodium (Monocid)	A: IM/IV: 500 mg–2 g/d single dose or b.i.d.	B	Similar to cefadroxil	4.5 h	98%	Rapid	IM: 1 h IV: 5–10 min	UK
Ceforanide (Precef)	A: IM/IV: 500 mg–1 g q12h C: IM/IV: 20–40 mg/kg/d in 2 divided doses	B	Similar to cefadroxil	3 h	80%	Rapid	IM: 1 h IV: 30 min	UK

Continued

Antibacterials: Cephalosporins

Generic (Brand)	Route and Dosage	Preg Cat	Interaction	t 1/2	PB	Onset	Peak	Duration
							Action	
Cefoxitin sodium (Mefoxin)	A: IM/IV: 1–2 g q6–8h; max: 12 g/d C: IM/IV: 80–160 mg/kg/d in divided doses	B	Similar to cefadroxil	45 min–1 h	70%	Rapid	IIM: 20 min–1 h IV: 5–10 min	UK
Cefpodoxime (Proxetil, Vantin)	A: PO: 100–400 mg q12h × 1–2 wk C: 6 mo–12 y: PO: 10 mg/kg/d in 2 divided doses	B	*Decrease* effect with antacids	2–3 h	20–40%	1 h	UK	UK
Cefprozil monohydrate (Cefzil)	A: PO: 250–500 mg daily or q12h C: PO: 15 mg/kg q12h × 10 d	B	*Increase* effect with probenecid; *increase* toxicity with aminoglycosides, colistin *Decrease* effect of erythromycin, tetracyclines	1–2 h	99%	UK	1–2 h	UK
Cefuroxime (Ceftin, Zinacef)	A: PO: 250–500 mg q12h IM/IV: 750 mg – 1.5 g q8h C: PO: 125–250 mg q12h IM/IV: 50–100 mg/kg/d in divided doses	B	Similar to cefadroxil	1.5–2 h	50%	Rapid	PO: 2 h IM: 30 min	UK
Loracarbef (Lorabid)	A: PO: 200 mg qd × 7 d C: PO: 15 mg/kg q12h × 7 d	B	*Increase* effect with aminoglycosides, probenecid, furosemide, vancomycin	1 h	UK	30 min	45–60 min	UK

Third Generation

Drug		Dosage						
Cefixime (Suprax)	B	A: PO: 400 mg/d in 1–2 divided doses C: <12 y: PO: 8 mg/kg/d in 1–2 divided doses	Similar to cefadroxil	2.5–4 h	65%	Rapid	2–6 h	UK
Cefoperazone (Cefobid)	B	A: IM/IV: 2–4 g/d in 2 divided doses C: IV: 25–100 mg/kg q12h	Similar to cefadroxil	2.5 h	70–80%	IV: Rapid	IM: 1–2 h IV: 5–20 min	IM/IV: 6–8 h
Cefotaxime (Claforan)	B	A: IM/IV: 1–2 g q8–12h C: IM/IV: 50–200 mg/kg/d in 4–6 divided doses Life-threatening infection: 2 g q4h	Similar to cefadroxil	1–1.5 h	30–40%	UK	IM: 30 min IV: 5–10 min	UK
Cefotetan (Cefotan)	B	A: IM/IV: 500 mg–2 g q12h	Similar to cefadroxil	3–5 h	85%	Rapid	1.5–3 h	UK
Ceftazidime (Fortaz, Tazicef)	B	A: IM/IV: 500 mg–2 g q8–12h C: IV: 50 mg/kg q8h; max 6 g/d	Similar to cefadroxil	1–2 h	10–17%	Rapid	1 h	IV: End of infusion
Ceftriaxone (Rocephin)	B	A: IM/IV: 500 mg–2 g in single dose or q12h C: IM/IV: 50–75 mg/kg/d in 2 divided doses	Similar to cefadroxil	8 h	85–95%	Rapid	IM: 1–2 h IV: 10–15 min	UK
Ceftizoxime (Cefizox)	B	A: IM/IV: 500 mg–2 g q8–12h C: IV: 50 mg/kg q6–8h; max: 200 mg/kg/d	Similar to cefadroxil	2 h	30–60%	Rapid	IM: 1 h IV: 5–10 min	IV: End of infusion
Moxalactam disodium (Moxam)	C	A: IM/IV: 2–6 g/d in 2–3 divided doses C: IM/IV: 50 mg/kg q6–8h; max: 200 mg/kg/d	Similar to cefadroxil	2 h	25–50%	Rapid	IM: 0.5–2 h IV: 5–10 min	UK IV: End of infusion

KEY: For complete abbreviation key, see inside front cover.

Antibacterials: Erythromycin

Erythromycin

Erythromycin
  (E-Mycin, Erythrocin, Erythrocin
  Lactobionate [IV])
Macrolide antibiotic
Pregnancy Category: B
Drug Forms:
Various oral preparations (cap, tab,
  chewables, susp)
Inj 500 mg, 1 g

Dosage

A: PO: 250–500 mg q6h
  IV: 1–4 g/d in 4 divided doses

C: PO: 30–50 mg/kg/d in 4 divided
  doses
  IV: 20–50 mg/kg/d in 4–6 divided
  doses

Contraindications

Severe hepatic disease
Caution: Hepatic dysfunction,
  lactation

Drug-Lab-Food Interactions

Increase effect of digoxin,
  carbamazepine, theophylline,
  cyclosporine, warfarin, triazolam
Decrease effect of penicillins,
  clindamycin

Pharmacokinetics

Absorption: PO: Well absorbed
Distribution: PB: 65%
Metabolism: t 1/2: PO: 1–2 h
  IV: 3–5 h
Excretion: In bile, feces, and (small
  amount) urine

Pharmacodynamics

PO: Onset: 1 h
     Peak: 4 h
     Duration: 6 h
IV: Onset: UK
     Peak: UK
     Duration: UK

Therapeutic Effects/Uses: To treat gram-positive and some gram-negative organisms;
for clients who are allergic to penicillin.

Mode of Action: Inhibition of the steps of protein synthesis; bacteriostatic or bactericidal effect.

Side Effects

Anorexia, nausea, vomiting,
  diarrhea, tinnitus, abdominal
  cramps, pruritus, rash

Adverse Reactions

Superinfections, vaginitis, urticaria,
  stomatitis, hearing loss
Life-threatening: Hepatotoxicity,
  anaphylaxis

KEY: For complete abbreviation key, see inside front cover.

Antibacterials: Erythromycin

■ NURSING PROCESS: Antibacterials: Macrolides: Erythromycin

ASSESSMENT
- Assess VS and urine output. Report abnormal findings.
- Check laboratory tests for liver enzyme values to determine liver function. Liver enzyme tests should be periodically ordered for clients taking large doses of erythromycin for a continuous period of time.
- Obtain a history of drugs the client is currently taking. Erythromycin can increase the effects of digoxin, oral anticoagulants, theophylline, carbamazepine, and cyclosporine. Dosing for these drugs may need to be decreased.

POTENTIAL NURSING DIAGNOSES
High risk for infection
High risk for impaired tissue integrity

PLANNING
- Client's infection will be controlled and later eliminated.

NURSING INTERVENTIONS
- Obtain a culture from the infectious area and send to the laboratory for culture and (antibiotic) sensitivity (C&S) test *before* starting erythromycin therapy. Antibiotic can be initiated after culture has been obtained.
- Monitor VS, urine output, and laboratory results, especially liver enzymes: ALP, ALT, AST, and also bilirubin.
- Monitor the client for liver damage due to prolonged use and high dosage of macrolides, such as erythromycin. Signs of liver dysfunction include elevated liver enzyme levels and jaundice.
- Monitor bleeding times if the client is receiving an oral anticoagulant.
- Administer oral erythromycin 1 h before meals or 2 h after meals. Take with a full glass of water and not fruit juice. Take the drug with food if GI upset occurs. Chewable tablets should be chewed and not swallowed whole.
- For IV erythromycin, dilute in an appropriate amount of solution as indicated in the drug circular.

CLIENT TEACHING
General
- Instruct the client to take the full course of antibacterial agent as prescribed. Drug compliance is most important for all antibacterials (antibiotics).
Side Effects
- Instruct the client to report side effects, including adverse reactions. Encourage the client to report nausea, vomiting, diarrhea, abdominal cramps, and itching. Superinfection, a secondary infection due to drug therapy, such as stomatitis or vaginitis may occur.
- Instruct the client to report any symptoms of hearing impairment, such as tinnitus, vertigo, or roaring noises.

EVALUATION
- Evaluate the effectiveness of erythromycin by determining if the infection has been controlled or has ceased and no side effects, including superinfection, have occurred.

Antibacterials: Macrolides, Lincosamides, and Vancomycin

Generic (Brand)	Route and Dosage	Preg Cat	Interaction	t 1/2	PB	Action Onset	Action Peak	Action Duration
Macrolides								
Azithromycin (Zithromax)	A: PO: Initially: 500 mg × 1 dose; maint: 250 mg/d; max: 1.5 g	C	*Increase* effects of digoxin, theophylline, methylprednisolone *Decrease* absorption with antacids; *decrease* effect of clindamycin	11–55 h	50%	2 h	4–12 h	24 h
Clarithromycin (Biaxin)	A: PO: 250–500 mg q12h × 7–14 d	C	Same as azithromycin *Lab:* May *increase* BUN and serum ALP, ALT, AST, creatinine, LDH	3–6 h	65–75%	<2 h	2–4 h	12 h
Erythromycin base (E-Mycin, Ilotycin)	See Prototype Drug Chart							
Erythromycin estolate (Ilosone)								
Erythromycin ethylsuccinate (E.E.S., E-Mycin E, Pediamycin)								
Erythromycin lactobionate (Erythrocin Lactobionate IV)								
Erythromycin stearate (Erythrocin)								

Generic (Brand)	Route and Dosage	Pregnancy Category	Drug-Lab-Food Interactions	t½	PB	Onset	Peak	Duration
Lincosamides								
Clindamycin HCl (Cleocin)	A: PO: 150–450 mg q6–8h; max: 1,800 mg/d	B	*Decrease* effect with erythromycin, chloramphenicol *Lab:* May *increase* AST, ALT, ALP, CPK, bilirubin	2–3 h	94%	Rapid	PO: 1 h IM: 1.5 h IV: End of infusion	PO: 6 h
Clindamycin palmitate (Cleocin Pediatric)	C: PO: 25–40 mg/kg/d in 3–4 divided doses	B	Same as clindamycin HCl	2–3 h	94%	Rapid	PO: 1 h IM: 1.5 h IV: End of infusion	PO: 6 h
Clindamycin phosphate (Cleocin Phosphate)	A: IM/IV: 300–900 mg q6–8h; max: 2,700 mg/d C: IM/IV: 20–30 mg/kg/d in 3–4 divided doses	B	Same as clindamycin HCl	2–3 h	94%	Rapid	IM: 1–3 h	IM: 8–12 h
Lincomycin (Lincorex)	A: PO: 500 mg q6–8h; max: 8 g/d IM: 600 mg daily–q12h IV: 600 mg–1 g q8–12h; dilute in 100 mL of IV fluids C: PO: 30–60 mg/kg/d in 3–4 divided doses IV: 10–20 mg/kg/d in 2–3 divided doses, dilute in IV fluids	B	Similar to clindamycin HCl	4–6 h	70–75%	UK	PO: 2–4 h IM: 30 min IV: 15 min	PO: 6–8 h IM: 8–12 h IV: 10–14 h
Vancomycin								
Vancomycin HCl (Vancocin)	A: IV: 500 mg q6h or 1 g q12h C: IV: 40 mg/kg/d in 4 divided doses; dilute in IV fluids; run for 1–1.5 h	C	*Increase* nephrotoxicity effect with aminoglycosides, amphotericin B, colistin	5–11 h	10%	Rapid	30–45 min after infusion	12 h

KEY: For complete abbreviation key, see inside front cover.

Antibacterials: Tetracyclines

Tetracycline

Tetracycline
(Achromycin, Tetracyn, Panmycin,
Sumycin)
Pregnancy Category: D (includes child
<8 y)
Drug Forms:
Tab 250, 500 mg
Cap 100, 250, 500 mg
Susp 125 mg/5 mL

Dosage

Systemic infection:
A: PO: 250–500 mg q6–12h
IM: 250 mg/d; 300 mg/d in 2–3
divided doses
C: >8 y: PO: 25–50 mg/kg/d in 4
divided doses
IM: 15–25 mg/kg/d in 2–3
divided doses; max: 250 mg/dose

Contraindications

Hypersensitivity, pregnancy, severe
hepatic or renal disease
Caution: History of allergies, renal
and hepatic dysfunction,
myasthenia gravis

Drug-Lab-Food Interactions

May *increase* or *decrease* effects of
anticoagulants
Decrease tetracycline absorption with
antacids, iron, and zinc; *decrease*
effects of oral contraceptives
Food: Dairy products (milk, cheese)
decrease effect
Lab: *Decrease* serum potassium level

Pharmacokinetics

Absorption: PO: 75–80% absorbed
Distribution: PB: 20–60 h
Metabolism: t 1/2: 6–12 h
Excretion: Unchanged in the urine

Pharmacodynamics

PO: Onset: 1–2 h
Peak: 2–4 h
Duration: 6 h
IV: Onset: Rapid
Peak: 0.5–1 h
Duration: UK

Therapeutic Effects/Uses: To treat uncommon gram-positive and gram-negative organisms, skin infections or disorders, chlamydia, gonorrhea, syphilis, rickettsial infection.

Mode of Action: Inhibition of the steps of protein synthesis. Bacteriostatic or bactericidal effect.

Side Effects

Nausea, vomiting, diarrhea, rash,
flatulence, abdominal discomfort,
headache, photosensitivity,
pruritus, epigastric distress,
heartburn

Adverse Reactions

Superinfection (candidiasis)
Life-threatening: Blood dyscrasias,
hepatotoxicity, nephrotoxicity,
exfoliative dermatitis, intracranial
hypertension

KEY: For complete abbreviation key, see inside front cover.

■ **NURSING PROCESS: Antibacterials: Tetracyclines**

ASSESSMENT

● Assess VS and urine output. Report abnormal findings.
● Check laboratory results, especially those that indicate renal and liver function, such as BUN, serum creatinine, AST, ALT, APT, and bilirubin.

Antibacterials: Tetracyclines

- Obtain a history of dietary intake and drugs the client is currently taking. Dairy products and antacids will decrease drug absorption.

POTENTIAL NURSING DIAGNOSES

High risk for infection
Noncompliance with drug regimen
High risk for impaired skin integrity

PLANNING

- Client's infection will be controlled and later eliminated.

NURSING INTERVENTIONS

- Obtain a culture from the infectious area and send to the laboratory for C&S test. Antibiotic therapy can be started after the culture has been taken.
- Administer tetracycline 1 h before meals or 2 h after meals for absorption.
- Monitor laboratory values for liver and kidney functions; these include liver enzymes, BUN, and serum creatinine.
- Monitor VS and urine output.

CLIENT TEACHING

General

- Instruct the client to store tetracycline out of the light and extreme heat. Tetracycline decomposes in light and heat, causing the drug to become toxic.
- Advise the client to check the expiration date on the bottle of tetracycline; out-of-date tetracycline can be toxic.
- Advise a woman contemplating pregnancy who has an infection to inform her health care provider and to avoid taking tetracycline because of possible teratogenic effect.
- Inform parents that children less than 8 years old should not take tetracycline because it can cause discoloration of permanent teeth.
- Instruct the client to take the complete course of tetracycline as prescribed.

Diet

- Instruct the client to avoid milk products, iron, and antacids. Tetracycline should be taken 1 h before meals or 2 h after meals with a full glass of water. If GI upset occurs, drug can be taken with food except milk products.

Side Effects

- Instruct the client to use sunblock/protective clothing during sun exposure. Photosensitivity is associated with tetracycline.
- Instruct the client to report signs of a superinfection (mouth ulcers, anal or genital discharge).
- Advise client to use additional contraceptive techniques and not to rely on oral contraceptives when taking drug because effectiveness may decrease.
- Advise the client to use effective oral hygiene several times a day to prevent or alleviate mouth ulcers (stomatitis).

EVALUATION

- Evaluate the effectiveness of tetracycline by determining if the infection has been controlled or has ceased and no side effects have occurred.

Antibacterials: Tetracyclines

Generic (Brand)	Route and Dosage	Preg Cat	Interaction	t 1/2	PB	Action Onset	Action Peak	Action Duration
Demeclocycline HCl (Declomycin)	A: PO: 150 mg q6h or 300 mg q12h C: >8 y: PO: 6–12 mg/kg/d in 2–4 divided doses	D	May *increase* risk of digoxin toxicity *Decrease* effect with antacids, iron, calcium, magnesium, sodium bicarbonate, cimetidine *Food: Decrease* effect with dairy products	10–17 h	35–90%	1.5–3 h	3–6 h	>24 h
Doxycycline hyclate (Vibramycin)	A: PO: 100 mg q12–24 h IV: 100–200 mg/d C: >8 y: PO/IV: 2–4 mg/kg/d in 1–2 divided doses	D	Same as demeclocycline *Increase* effect of anticoagulants *Decrease* effects of penicillins, oral contraceptives	15–24 h	25–92%	1 h	1.5–4 h	UK
Minocycline HCl (Minocin)	A: PO/IV: 100 mg q12h or 50 mg q6h C: >8 y: PO/IV: 4 mg/kg/d in 2 divided doses	D	Same as doxycycline	11–20 h	55–88%	1 h	2–3 h	UK

Drug	Dosage			6–10 h	20–40%	1–2 h	2–4 h	PO: 6 h
Oxytetracycline HCl (Terramycin)	A: PO: 250–500 mg q6–12h IM: 200–300 mg/d in 2–3 divided doses IV: 250–500 mg in 2 divided doses C: >8 y: PO: 25–50 mg/kg/d in 4 divided doses IM: 15–25 mg/kg/d in 2–3 divided doses; max: 250 mg/dose IV: 10–20 mg/kg/d in 2 divided doses	D	Same as demeclocycline					
Tetracycline (Achromycin, Tetracyn, Sumycin, Panmycin)	See Prototype Drug Chart							

KEY: For complete abbreviation key, see inside front cover.

169

Antibacterials: Aminoglycosides

Gentamicin Sulfate

Gentamicin sulfate
(Garamycin)
Aminoglycoside
Pregnancy Category: C
Drug Forms:
Inj 10, 40 mg/mL
Intrathecal 2 mg/mL
Available for topical and ophthalmic
use

Dosage

A: IM: 3 mg/kg/d in 3–4 divided
doses
IV: 3–5 mg/kg/d in 3–4 divided
doses
C: IM/IV: 2–2.5 mg/kg q8–12h
TDM: 5–10 μg/mL; peak: 10–12
μg/mL; trough: 0.5–2 μg/mL

Contraindications

Hypersensitivity, severe renal
disease, pregnancy and breast
feeding
Caution: Renal disease,
neuromuscular disorders
(myasthenia gravis, parkinsonism),
heart failure, elderly, neonates

Drug-Lab-Food Interactions

Increase risk of ototoxicity with loop
diuretics, methoxyflurane; *increase*
risk of nephrotoxicity with
amphotericin B, polymyxin,
cisplatin, furosemide, vancomycin
Lab: *Increase* AST, ALT, LDH,
bilirubin, BUN, serum creatinine
Decrease serum potassium and
magnesium

Pharmacokinetics

Absorption: IM: Well absorbed
Distribution: PB: UK
Metabolism: t 1/2: 2 h
Excretion: Unchanged in urine

Pharmacodynamics

IM/IV: Onset: Rapid
Peak: 1–2 h
Duration: 6–8 h

Therapeutic Effects/Uses: To treat serious infections caused by gram-negative organisms, such as *Pseudomonas aeruginosa*, *Proteus*; to treat pelvic inflammatory disease (PID); and to treat methicillin-resistant *Staphylococcus aureus* infections.

Mode of Action: Inhibition of bacterial protein synthesis. Bactericidal effect.

Side Effects

Anorexia, nausea, vomiting, rash,
numbness, tremors, tinnitus,
pruritus, muscle cramps or
weakness, photosensitivity

Adverse Reactions

Oliguria, deafness, urticaria,
palpitation, visual disturbances,
superinfection
Life-threatening: Thrombocytopenia,
ototoxicity, nephrotoxicity,
neuromuscular blockade,
agranulocytosis, liver damage

KEY: For complete abbreviation key, see inside front cover.

■ NURSING PROCESS: Antibacterials: Aminoglycosides

ASSESSMENT

• Assess VS and urine output. Compare these results with future VS and urine output. An adverse reaction to most aminoglycosides is nephrotoxicity.

• Assess laboratory results to determine renal and liver functions, including BUN, serum creatinine, ALP, ALT, AST, and bilirubin. Serum electrolytes should also be checked. Aminoglycosides may decrease the serum potassium and magnesium levels.

• Obtain a medical history related to renal or hearing disorders. Large doses of aminoglycosides could cause nephrototoxicity or ototoxicity.

POTENTIAL NURSING DIAGNOSES
High risk for infection
High risk for impaired tissue integrity
High risk for altered tissue perfusion: renal

PLANNING
• Client's infection will be controlled and later eliminated.

NURSING INTERVENTIONS
• Send a culture of the infectious area to the laboratory to determine organism and antibiotic sensitivity, (C&S) before aminoglycoside is started.
• Monitor intake and output. Urine output should be at least 600 mL/d. Immediately report if urine output is decreased. Urinalysis may be ordered daily. Check results for proteinuria, casts, blood cells, or appearance.
• Check for hearing loss. Aminoglycosides can cause ototoxicity.
• Check laboratory results and compare with baseline values. Report abnormal results.
• Monitor VS. Note if body temperature has decreased.
• For IV use, dilute the aminoglycoside in 50–200 mL of NSS or D_5W solution and administer in 30–60 min.
• Check that the TDM has been ordered for peak and trough drug levels. The TDM for gentamicin is 5–10 μg/mL. Blood should be drawn 45–60 min after drug has been administered for peak levels and minutes before the next drug dosing for trough levels. Drug peak values should be 10–12 μg/mL, and trough values should be 0.5–2 μg/mL.
• Monitor for signs and symptoms of superinfection, such as stomatitis (mouth ulcers), genital discharge (vaginitis), and anal or genital itching.

CLIENT TEACHING
General
• Unless fluids are restricted, encourage the client to increase fluid intake.
• Instruct the client never to take leftover antibiotics.

Side Effects
• Instruct the client to report side effects resulting from the aminoglycosides, including nausea, vomiting, tremors, tinnitus, pruritus, and muscle cramps.
• Instruct the client to use sunblock lotion and protective clothing during sun exposure. Photosensitivity can be caused by aminoglycosides.

EVALUATION
• Evaluate the effectiveness of the aminoglycoside by determining if the infection has ceased and no side effects have occurred.

Antibacterials: Aminoglycosides

Generic (Brand)	Route and Dosage	Preg Cat	Interaction	t 1/2	PB	Onset	Peak	Duration
							Action	
Amikacin SO$_4$ (Amikin)	A&C: IM/IV: 15 mg/kg/d in 2–3 divided doses; max: 1.5 g/d NB: IV: 7.5 mg/kg q12h TDM: Peak: 15–30 mg/mL; trough: 5–10 mg/mL	C	May *increase* nephrotoxicity with cephalosporins, amphotericin B, furosemide, cyclosporine *Lab:* May *increase* BUN, AST, ALT, bilirubin May *decrease* electrolyte concentrations	2–3 h	4–11%	Rapid	1–2 h	UK
Gentamicin SO$_4$ (Garamycin)	See Prototype Drug Chart							
Kanamycin SO$_4$ (Kantrex)	A: PO: 1 g q6h *Hepatic coma:* 8–12 g/d in divided doses IM/IV: 15 mg/kg/d in 2 divided doses C: IV: Same as adult	D	Similar to amikacin	2–3 h	10%	Rapid	1–2 h	UK
Neomycin SO$_4$ (Mycifradin)	A: PO: GI surgery: 1 g qh for 4 doses; then 1 g q4h for 24 h or other regimens	C	May *decrease* effects of penicillin V, digoxin	2–3 h	10%	PO: UK IM: Rapid	1–2 h 1–4 h	PO: UK IM: 6–8 h

Drug	Dosage	Pregnancy Category	Drug-Lab Interactions	t½	PB	Onset	Peak	Duration
	Hepatic coma: 4–12 g/d in divided doses IM: 15 mg/kg/d in 4 divided doses; max: 1 g/d C: PO: 10 mg/kg in q4–6 h for 3 d							
Netilmicin (Netromycin)	A: IM/IV: 3–6 mg/kg/d in 3 divided doses C: IM/IV: 5–8 mg/kg/d in 3 divided doses TDM: Peak: 0.5–10 µg/mL; trough: <4 µg/mL	D	Similar to amikacin	2–3 h	10%	Rapid	0.5–1 h	UK
Paromomycin (Humatin)	*Intestinal amebiasis:* A&C: PO: 25–35 mg/kg/d in 3 divided doses for 5–10 d	C	*Increase* effect of oral anticoagulants *Decrease* effect of methotrexate, digoxin *Lab:* Decrease cholesterol with prolonged use	Not absorbed into systemic circulation	UK	UK	UK	UK
Streptomycin SO₄	*Tuberculosis:* A: IM: 1 g daily for 2–3 mo; then 1 g 3 × wk *Endocarditis:* A: IM: 1 g q12h for 1 wk; dose may be decreased	C	May *increase* anticoagulant effect with warfarin	2–3 h	30%	Rapid	1–2 h	UK
Tobramycin SO₄ (Nebcin)	A: IM/IV: 3–5 mg/kg/d in 3 divided doses C: IM/IV: 6–7.5 mg/kg/d in 3–4 divided doses TDM: Peak: 10–12 µg/mL; trough: 0.5–2 µg/mL	D	Similar to amikacin	2–3 h	10%	Rapid	1–1.5 h	8 h

KEY: For complete abbreviation key, see inside front cover.

Antibacterials: Quinolones

Ciprofloxacin

Ciprofloxacin
  (Cipro)
Quinolone, Fluoroquinoline
Pregnancy Category: C (X at term),
  breast feeding
Drug Forms:
Tab 250, 500, 750 mg
Inj 200-, 400-mg vials

Dosage

A: PO: 250–500 mg q12h
Severe infections:
A: PO: 500–750 mg q12h
  IV: 200 mg q12h
Mild to moderate infections:
A: IV: 400 mg q12h

Contraindications

Severe renal disease, hypersensitivity
  to other quinolones, pregnancy
  and breast feeding
Caution: Seizure disorders, renal
  disorders, children <14 y, elderly,
  clients receiving theophylline

Drug-Lab-Food Interactions

Increase effect with probenecid;
  increase effect of theophylline,
  caffeine
Decrease drug absorption with
  antacids, iron
Lab: Increase AST, ALT

Pharmacokinetics

Absorption: PO: 70% absorbed
Distribution: PB: 20%
Metabolism: t 1/2: 3–4 h
Excretion: 50% unchanged in urine

Pharmacodynamics

PO: Onset: 0.5–1 h
     Peak: 1–2 h
     Duration: UK

Therapeutic Effects/Uses: To treat lower respiratory, renal, bone, and joint infections.

Mode of Action: Interference with the enzyme DNA gyrase, which is needed for bacterial DNA synthesis. Bactericidal effect.

Side Effects

Nausea, vomiting, diarrhea,
  abdominal cramps, flatulence,
  headache, dizziness, fatigue,
  restlessness, insomnia, rash,
  flushing, tinnitus, photosensitivity

Adverse Reactions

Urticaria, oral candidiasis,
  crystalluria, hematuria, seizures

KEY: For complete abbreviation key, see inside front cover.

■ NURSING PROCESS: Antibacterials: Quinolones

ASSESSMENT

• Assess VS and intake and urine output. Compare these results with future VS and urine output. Fluid intake should be at least 2,000 mL/d.

• Assess laboratory results to determine renal function: BUN and serum creatinine.

- Obtain a drug and diet history. Antacids and iron preparations decrease absorption of quinolones such as ciprofloxacin (Cipro). Ciprofloxacin can increase the effects of theophylline and caffeine.

POTENTIAL NURSING DIAGNOSES
High risk for infection
High risk for impaired tissue integrity
Noncompliance with drug regimen

PLANNING
- Client's infection will be controlled and later eliminated.

NURSING INTERVENTIONS
- Culture the infectious site and send specimen to the laboratory for C&S.
- Monitor intake and output. Urine output should be at least 750 mL/d. Client should be well hydrated, and fluid intake should be >2,000 mL/d to prevent crystalluria. Urine pH should be <6.7.
- Monitor VS. Report abnormal findings.
- Check laboratory results, especially BUN and serum creatinine. Elevated values may indicate renal dysfunction.
- Administer ciprofloxacin 1 h before or 2 h after meals or 2 h before or after antacids and iron products for absorption. Take with a full glass of water. If GI distress occurs, drug may be taken with food.
- For IV ciprofloxacin, dilute the antibiotic in an appropriate amount of solution as indicated in the drug circular. Infuse over 60 min.
- Check for signs and symptoms of superinfection such as stomatitis (mouth ulcers), furry **black** tongue, anal or genital discharge, and itching.
- Monitor serum theophylline levels. Ciprofloxacin can increase theophylline levels. Check for symptoms of CNS stimulation: nervousness, insomnia, anxiety, and tachycardia.

CLIENT TEACHING
General
- Instruct the client to drink at least 6–8 glassfuls (8 oz) of fluid daily.
- Instruct the client to avoid caffeinated products.

Side Effects
- Advise the client to avoid operating hazardous machinery or operating a motor vehicle while taking the drug or until drug stability has occurred due to possible drug-related dizziness.
- Advise the client that photosensitivity is a side effect of most quinolones. The client should use sunglasses, sunblock, and protective clothing when in the sun.
- Instruct the client to report side effects, such as dizziness, nausea, vomiting, diarrhea, flatulence, abdominal cramps, tinnitus, and rash. Older adults are more likely to develop side effects.

EVALUATION
- Evaluate the effectiveness of the quinolone by determining if the infection has ceased and the body temperature has returned within normal range.

Generic (Brand)	Route and Dosage	Preg Cat	Interaction	t 1/2	PB	Onset	Peak	Duration
							Action	
						Onset	Peak	Duration
Quinolones								
Cinoxacin (Cinobac)	A: PO: 1 g/d in 2–4 divided doses for 1–2 wk C >12 y: Same as adult	B	*Increase* effect with probenecid	1.5 h	60–80%	1–1.5 h	2–3 h	6–12 h
Ciprofloxacin HCl (Cipro)	See Prototype Drug Chart							
Enoxacin (Penetrex)	A: PO: 200–400 mg b.i.d. 7–14 d	C	*Increase* effects of probenecid; *increase* toxicity with theophylline *Decrease* enoxacin effect with antacids	3–6 h	40%	1 h	1–3 h	UK
Lomefloxacin HCl (Maxaquin)	A: PO: 200–400 mg/d ×7–14 d	C	*Increase* effects of warfarin; *increase* effect with cimetidine, probenecid *Decrease* effect with antacids, sucralfate, nitrofurantoin	6–8 h	UK	1 h	1–2 h	UK
Nalidixic acid (NegGram)	A: PO: 1 g q.i.d. for 1–2 wk; 1 g b.i.d. for long-term use C: PO: 55 mg/kg/d in 4 divided doses for 1–2 wk; 33 mg/kg/d for long-term use	B	*Increase* effects of anticoagulants	2–6 h	95%	<1 h	1–2 h	UK

Drug	Route and Dosage	Pregnancy Category	Drug Interactions	$t_{1/2}$	Protein Binding	Onset	Peak	Duration
Norfloxacin (Noroxin)	A: PO: 400 mg b.i.d., a.c. or p.c. for 1–3 wk	C	*Decrease* absorption with iron, antacids *Lab:* May *increase* AST, ALT, ALP	3–4 h	10–15%	45 min–1 h	1–2 h	UK
Ofloxacin (Floxin)	A: PO: 200–400 mg q12h × 10 d	C	Similar to lomefloxacin	5–8 h	20%	1 h	1–2 h	UK
Unclassified Aztreonam (Azactam)	*Urinary tract infections:* A: IM/IV: 0.5–1.0 g q8–12h *Severe infections:* A: IM/IV: 1.0–2.0 g q6–8h; max: 8 g/d	B	*Decrease* effects of cefoxitin, imipenem	1.7–2.1 h	56%	IM/IV: Rapid	IM: 1 h IV: Rapid	IM/IV: 8 h
Chloramphenicol (Chloromycetin)	A&C: PO/IV: 50 mg/kg/d in 4 divided doses (q6h) NB: 25 mg/kg/d in 4 divided doses (q6h)	C	*Increase* effects of barbiturates, oral hypoglycemics, oral anticoagulants, Cytoxan, phenytoin *Decrease* effects of penicillins, iron, folic acid	1.5–4 h	50–60% Neonate: 30%	PO: 1 h IV: Rapid	PO: 1–3 h IV: 1 h	PO: 8 h
Imipenem-cilastatin (Primaxin)	A: IM: 500–750 mg q12h IV: 250 mg–1 g q6–8h C: IV: 15–25 mg/kg q6h	C	*Decrease* effect with cephalosporins, penicillins **Not** to be mixed with other antibacterials	1 h	20%	Immediate	0.5–1 h	UK
Spectinomycin HCl (Trobicin)	A: IM: 2–4 g as single dose	B	None noted	1–3 h	10%	1 h	1–2 h	8–12 h

KEY: For complete abbreviation key, see inside front cover.

Antibacterials: Sulfonamides (Trimethoprim-Sulfamethoxazole)

Co-Trimoxazole

Co-trimoxazole
(Bactrim, Septra)
Sulfonamide: trimethoprim-
sulfamethoxazole

Pregnancy Category: C

Drug Forms:
Tab 80 mg (T)/400 mg (S)
Susp 40 mg (T)/200 mg (S)/5 mL
Inj 16 mg (T)/80 mg (S)/mL

Dosage

A: PO: 160/800 mg q12h (160 mg
[T]/800 mg [S])
C: PO: 8/40 mg q12h (8 mg [T]/40
mg [S])

Contraindications

Severe renal or hepatic disease,
hypersensitivity to sulfonamides

Drug-Lab-Food Interactions

Increase anticoagulant effect with
warfarin

Lab: *Increase* BUN, serum creatinine

Pharmacokinetics

Absorption: PO: Well absorbed
Distribution: PB: 50–65%; crosses
placenta
Metabolism: t 1/2: 8–12 h
Excretion: In urine as metabolites

Pharmacodynamics

PO: Onset: 0.5–1 h
     Peak: 2–4 h
     Duration: UK
IV: Onset: Immediate
     Peak: 0.5–1 h
     Duration: UK

Therapeutic Effects/Uses: To treat urinary tract infection, otitis media, bronchitis,
pneumonia, *Pneumocystis carinii*, rheumatic fever, burns.

Mode of Action: Inhibition of protein synthesis of nucleic acids. Bactericidal effect.

Side Effects

Anorexia, nausea, vomiting,
diarrhea, rash, stomatitis, fatigue,
depression, headache, vertigo,
photosensitivity

Adverse Reactions

Life-threatening: Leukopenia,
thrombocytopenia, increased bone
marrow depression, hemolytic
anemia, aplastic anemia,
agranulocytosis, Stevens-Johnson
syndrome, renal failure

KEY: T: trimethoprim, S: sulfamethoxazole; for complete abbreviation key, see inside
front cover.

■ NURSING PROCESS: Antibacterials: Sulfonamides

ASSESSMENT

• Assess the client's renal function by checking urinary output (>600 mL/d), BUN (normal, 8–25 mg/dL), and serum creatinine (normal, 0.5–1.5 mg/dL).
• Obtain a medical history from the client. Sulfonamides such as co-trimoxazole (trimethoprim-sulfamethoxazole [Bactrim, Septra]) are contraindicated for clients with severe renal or liver disease.
• Assess if the client is hypersensitive to sulfonamides. An allergic reaction can include rash, skin eruptions, and itching. A severe hypersensitivity reaction includes erythema multiforme (erythematous macular, papular, or vesicular eruption; if severe, can cover the entire body) or exfoliative dermatitis (desquamation, scaling, and itching of skin).
• Obtain a history of drugs the client is currently taking. Oral antidiabetic drugs (sulfonylureas) with sulfonamides increase the hypoglycemic effect; the use of warfarin with sulfonamides increases the anticoagulant effect.
• Assess baseline laboratory results, especially CBC. Blood dyscrasias may occur due to high doses of sulfonamides over a continuous period of time, causing life-threatening conditions.

POTENTIAL NURSING DIAGNOSES

High risk for infection
High risk for impaired tissue integrity
Altered patterns of urinary elimination

PLANNING

• Client's infection will be controlled and later alleviated.

NURSING INTERVENTIONS

• Administer sulfonamides with a full glass of water. Extra fluid intake can prevent crystalluria and kidney stone formation.
• Monitor the client's intake and output. Urine output should be at least 1,200 mL/d to decrease the risk of crystalluria. The sulfonamides sulfadiazine and sulfamethoxazole are more likely to cause crystalluria than are sulfisoxazole (Gantrisin) and combination drugs. Fluid intake should be at least 2,000 mL/d.
• Monitor VS. Note if the temperature has decreased.
• Observe the client for hematologic reaction that may lead to life-threatening anemias. Early signs are sore throat, purpura, and decreasing white blood cell and platelet counts. Check the client's CBC and compare with baseline findings.
• Check for signs and symptoms of superinfection (secondary infection caused by a different organism than the primary infection). Symptoms include stomatitis (mouth ulcers), furry **black** tongue, anal or genital discharge, and itching.

CLIENT TEACHING

General

• Instruct the client to drink several quarts of fluid daily while taking sulfonamides to avoid the complication of crystalluria.
• Advise a pregnant woman to avoid sulfonamides during the last 3 mo of pregnancy.

Antibacterials: Sulfonamides (Trimethoprim-Sulfamethoxazole)

- Instruct the client not to take antacids with sulfonamides because antacids decrease the absorption rate.
- Advise the client who has an allergy to one sulfonamide that all sulfonamide preparations should be avoided, with the health care provider's approval, due to the possibility of cross-sensitivity. Observe the client for rash or any skin eruptions.

Skill

- Instruct the client to take the sulfonamide 1 h before or 2 h after meals with a full glass of water.

Side Effects

- Instruct the client to report bruising or bleeding that could be caused from drug-induced blood disorder. Advise the client to have blood cell count monitored.
- Advise the client to avoid direct sunlight and to use sunblock and protective clothing to decrease the risk of photosensitive reactions.

EVALUATION

- Evaluate the effectiveness of the sulfonamide by determining if the infection has been alleviated and the blood cell count is within normal range.

Generic (Brand)	Route and Dosage	Preg Cat	Interaction	t 1/2	PB	Action Onset	Action Peak	Action Duration
Short Acting								
Sulfadiazine (Microsulfon)	A: PO: LD: 2–4 g; then 2–4 g/d in 4 divided doses C: PO: LD: 75 mg or 2 g/m²; then 150 mg/kg/d in 4–6 divided doses	C	*Increase* hypoglycemic effect with oral antidiabetics; *increase* anticoagulant effect with warfarin *Decrease* effect of oral contraceptives	8–12 h	20–30%	0.5–1 h	3–6 h	Short acting
Sulfamethizole (Sulfasol, Thiosulfil Forte)	A: PO: 0.5–1 g in 3–4 divided doses C: PO: 30–45 mg/kg/d in 4 divided doses	C	Same as sulfadiazine	1.5 h	90%	Rapid	2 h	Short acting
Sulfisoxazole (Gantrisin)	A: PO: LD: 2–4 g; then 4–8 g/d in 4–6 divided doses C: PO: LD: 75 mg/kg or 2 g/m²; then 150 mg/kg/d in 4–6 divided doses	C	Same as sulfadiazine	4.5–7.5 h	85–95%	Rapid	2–4 h	Short acting

continued

Antibacterials: Sulfonamides—Continued

Generic (Brand)	Route and Dosage	Preg Cat	Interaction	t 1/2	PB	Onset	Peak	Duration
							Action	
						Onset	Peak	Duration
Intermediate Acting Sulfamethoxazole (Gantanol)	A: PO: LD: 2 g; then 2–3 g/d in 2–3 divided doses for 7–10 d C: PO: LD: 50–60 mg; then 25–30 mg/kg q12h; max: 75 mg/d	C	Same as sulfadiazine	7–12 h	60–70%	1 h	3–4 h	UK
Sulfasalazine (Azaline, Azulfidine, Salazoprin)	A: PO: Initially: 1 g q6–8h; maint: 2 g q6h C >2 y: PO: Initially: 40–60 mg/kg/d in 4–6 divided doses; maint: 20–30 mg/kg/d in 4 divided doses; max: 2 g/d	B (D, near term)	*Increase* effects of oral anticoagulants, folic acid; *increase* hypoglycemic effect with oral antidiabetics	5.5 h	99%	1 h	1.5–6 h	UK
Trimethoprim-sulfamethoxazole (Bactrim, Septra)	See Prototype Drug Chart							

KEY: For complete abbreviation key, see inside front cover.

Generic (Brand)	Route and Dosage	Preg Cat	Interaction	t 1/2	PB	Action			
						Onset	Peak	Duration	
Bacitracin (Bactrin USP)	A: PO: 20,000–25,000 U q6h A: IM: 40,000–100,000 U/d in 4 divided doses Infant: IM: 900 U/kg/d in 2–3 divided doses	C	Similar to polymyxin B	UK	<20%	IM: Rapid	1–2 h	6–12 h	
Colistin (PO) (ColyMycin S, Polymyxin E)	A&C: PO: 5–15 mg/kg/d in 3 divided doses	C	Similar to polymyxin B Lab: May increase BUN, creatinine	2–3 h	UK	IM: UK IV: Rapid	IM: 1–2 h IV: End of infusion	IM: 8–12 h IV: UK	
Colistimethate sodium (IM/IV) (Coly-Mycin M)	IM/IV: 2.5–5 mg/kg/d in divided doses		Same as colistin						
Polymyxin B SO₄ (Aerosporin)	A: IM: 25,000 U/kg/d in divided doses IV: 15,000–25,000 U/kg/d in 2 divided doses (q12h) C >2 y: Same as adult	B	May cause nephrotoxicity with aminoglycosides, amphotericin B	4.5–6 h	UK	IM: Rapid IV: Rapid	IM: 2 h IV: End of infusion	UK	

KEY: For complete abbreviation key, see inside front cover.

Antitubercular Drugs

Isoniazid

Isoniazid
  (INH, Nydrazid)
Antituberculars
Pregnancy Category: C
Drug Forms:
Tab 50, 100, 300 mg
Liq 50 mg/5 mL
Inj 100 mg/mL

Dosage

A: PO/IM: 5–10 mg/kg/d in a single
  dose; max: 300 mg/d
Prophylaxis: 300 mg/d
C: PO/IM: 10–20 mg/kd/d in a
  single dose; max: 500 mg/d
Prophylaxis: 10 mg/kg/d in a single
  dose

Contraindications

Severe renal or hepatic disease,
  alcoholism, diabetic retinopathy

Drug-Lab-Food Interactions

Increase effect with alcohol, rifampin,
  cycloserine

Pharmacokinetics

Absorption: PO: Well absorbed
Distribution: PB: 10%
Metabolism: t 1/2: 1–4 h
Excretion: 50% unchanged in urine

Pharmacodynamics

PO: Onset: 0.5 h
    Peak: 1–2 h
    Duration: PO: 6–8 h
         IM: 6 h

Therapeutic Effects/Uses: To treat tuberculosis; prophylactic measure against tuberculosis.
Mode of Action: Inhibition of bacterial cell wall synthesis.

Side Effects

Drowsiness, tremors, rash, blurred
  vision, photosensitivity

Adverse Reactions

Psychotic behavior, peripheral
  neuropathy, vitamin B_6 deficiency
Life-threatening: Blood dyscrasias,
  thrombocytopenia, seizures

KEY: For complete abbreviation key, see inside front cover.

Antitubercular Drugs

■ **NURSING PROCESS: Antitubercular Drugs**

ASSESSMENT
- Obtain a history from the client of any past instances of tuberculosis, last purified protein derivative (PPD) tuberculin test and reaction, last chest x-ray and result, and allergy to any of the antitubercular drugs if taken previously.
- Obtain a medical history from the client. Most antitubercular drugs are contraindicated if the client has a severe hepatic disease.
- Check laboratory tests for liver enzyme values, bilirubin, BUN, and serum creatinine. These baseline values can be compared with future laboratory test results.
- Assess the client for signs and symptoms of peripheral neuropathy, such as numbness or tingling of the extremities.
- Check the client for hearing changes if the antitubercular drug regimen includes streptomycin. Ototoxicity is an adverse reaction to streptomycin.

POTENTIAL NURSING DIAGNOSES
High risk for infection
High risk for impaired tissue integrity

PLANNING
- Client's sputum test for acid-fast bacilli will be negative in 2–3 mo after the prescribed antitubercular therapy.

NURSING INTERVENTIONS
- Administer the commonly ordered antitubercular drug isoniazid (INH) 1 h before or 2 h after meals. Food decreases absorption rate.
- Administer pyridoxine (vitamin B_6) as prescribed with isoniazid to prevent peripheral neuropathy.
- Monitor serum liver enzyme levels, especially if the client is taking isoniazid and/or rifampin. Elevated levels may indicate liver toxicity.
- Collect sputum specimens for acid-fast bacilli early in morning. Usually three consecutive morning sputum specimens are sent to the laboratory, and the routine is repeated several weeks later.
- Have eye examinations performed on clients taking isoniazid and ethambutol. Visual disturbances may result in clients taking these antitubercular drugs.
- Emphasize the importance of complying with drug regimen.

CLIENT TEACHING
General
- Instruct the client to take the antitubercular drug such as isoniazid 1 h before meals or 2 h after meals for better absorption.
- Instruct the client to take the antitubercular drugs as prescribed. Ineffective treatment of tuberculosis might occur if the drugs are taken intermittently or discontinued when symptoms are decreased or when the client is feeling better. Compliance with the drug regimen is a must.
- Instruct the client not to take antacids while taking antitubercular drug(s) because they decrease the drug absorption. The client should also avoid alcohol because it may increase the risk of hepatotoxicity.
- Advise the client to keep medical appointments and to participate in spu-

tum testing. Sputum testing is important to determine the effectiveness of the drug regimen.

• Advise the woman contemplating pregnancy to first check with her health care provider about taking the antitubercular drugs ethambutol and rifampin.

Side Effects

• Instruct the client to report any numbness, tingling, or burning of the hands and feet. Peripheral neuritis is a common side effect of isoniazid. Vitamin B_6 prevents peripheral neuropathy. Neuritis may not occur if the client eats a balanced diet daily.

• Advise the client to avoid direct sunlight to decrease the risk of photosensitivity. Client should use sunblock while in the sun.

• Inform the client taking rifampin that urine, feces, saliva, sputum, sweat, and tears may be a harmless red-orange color. Soft contact lenses may be permanently stained.

• Advise the client receiving ethambutol to take daily single doses to avoid visual problems. Divided doses of ethambutol may cause visual disturbances.

EVALUATION

• Evaluate the effectiveness of the antitubercular drug(s). Sputum specimen for acid-fast bacilli should be negative after taking antitubular drugs for several weeks to months.

Generic (Brand)	Route and Dosage	Preg Cat	Interaction	t 1/2	PB	Onset	Peak	Duration
							Action	
Aminosalicylate sodium P.A.S. sodium	A: PO: 14–16 g/d in 2–3 divided doses C: PO: 275–420 mg/kg/d in 3–4 divided doses; take with food	C	*Decrease* effect of digoxin, vitamin B_{12}	1 h	Normal renal function: 15%	UK	1–2 h	UK
Ethambutol HCl (Myambutol)	A: PO: 15 mg/kg as a single dose *Retreatment* A: PO: 25 mg/kg as a single dose for 2 mo; then decrease to 15 mg/kg/d C >12 y: Same as adult	C	*Increase* nephrotoxicity with aminoglycosides, cisplatin	3–4 h Renal dysfunction: 8 h	10–20%	Rapid	2–4 h	UK
Isoniazid (INH, Nydrazid)	See Prototype Drug Chart							
Rifabutin (Mycobutin)	A: PO: 300 mg/d in 1 or 2 divided doses	B	Similar to rifampin	16–69 h	85%	UK	2–4 h	UK
Rifampin (Rifadin, Rimactane)	A: PO: 600 mg/d as a single dose C: PO: 10–20 mg/kg/d as a single dose; max: 600 mg/d	C	*Decrease* effect with barbiturates, corticosteroids, oral hypoglycemics, digoxin, oral contraceptives	3 h	85–90%	1–2 h	2–4 h	>24 h
Streptomycin SO_4	A: IM: 1 g daily or 7–15 mg/kg/d for 2–3 mo, then 2–3 × wk C: IM: 20–40 mg/kg/d in divided doses	C	May *increase* anticoagulant effect with warfarin	2–3 h	30%	Rapid	1–2 h	UK

KEY: For complete abbreviation key, see inside front cover.

187

Antifungals

Nystatin	Dosage

Nystatin
  (Mycostatin)
Antifungal
Pregnancy Category: C
Drug Forms:
Tab 500,000 U
Susp 100,000 U
Vaginal tab 100,000 U
	A: Topical use as directed
	Intestinal infections:
	A: PO: 500,000–1,000,000 U t.i.d. or
	  q8h
	Oral candidiasis:
	A: PO: 400,000–600,000 U q6–8h
	Neonate (<7 d): PO: 100,000 U q.i.d.
	C: PO: 250,000–500,000 U q.i.d.

Contraindications	Drug-Lab-Food Interactions
Hypersensitivity Vag: Pregnancy	None significant known

Pharmacokinetics	Pharmacodynamics

Absorption: PO: Poorly absorbed
Distribution: PB: UK
Metabolism: t 1/2: UK
Excretion: In feces unchanged
	PO: Onset: Rapid
	    Peak: UK
	    Duration: 6–12 h
	Vaginally: Onset: 24–72 h
	    Peak: UK
	    Duration: UK

Therapeutic Effects/Uses: To treat *Candida* infections.
Mode of Action: Increase permeability of the fungal cell membrane.

Side Effects	Adverse Reactions

PO: Anorexia, nausea, vomiting,
  diarrhea (large doses), stomach
  cramps, rash
Vag: Rash, burning sensation
	None known

KEY: For complete abbreviation key, see inside front cover.

■ NURSING PROCESS: Antifungals

ASSESSMENT

• Obtain a medical history from the client of any serious renal or hepatic disorder. Antifungal agents such as amphotericin B, fluconazole (Diflucan), flucytosine (Ancobon), and ketoconazole (Nizoral) are contraindicated if the client has a serious renal or liver disease.

• Check laboratory tests for liver enzyme values (ALP, ALT, AST, GGT), BUN, bilirubin, and serum creatinine. Elevated levels can indicate liver or renal dysfunction. These test results may be used for future comparisons.

• Obtain baseline VS for future comparison.

POTENTIAL NURSING DIAGNOSES
High risk for infection
High risk for impaired tissue integrity

PLANNING
• Client's fungal infection will be resolved.

NURSING INTERVENTIONS
• Obtain a culture to determine the fungus, e.g., *Candida*.
• Monitor the client's urinary output; many of the antifungal drugs may cause nephrotoxicity.
• Monitor the laboratory results and compare with baseline findings, i.e., BUN, serum creatinine, ALP, ALT, AST, bilirubin, and electrolytes. Certain antifungals could cause hepatotoxicity as well as nephrotoxicity when taking high doses over a prolonged period of time.
• Monitor VS. Compare with baseline findings.
• Observe for side effects and adverse reactions to antifungal drugs (antimycotics), such as nausea, vomiting, headache, phlebitis, and signs and symptoms of electrolyte imbalance (hypokalemia with amphotericin B).

CLIENT TEACHING
General
• Instruct the client to take the drug as prescribed. Compliance is of utmost importance since discontinuing the drug too soon may result in a relapse.
• Advise the client to obtain laboratory testing as indicated. Serum liver enzymes, BUN, creatinine, and electrolytes should be monitored.
• Advise the client taking ketoconazole not to consume alcohol.

Skill
• Instruct the client on the administration of nystatin (Mycostatin) suspension. Place the nystatin dose, usually 1–2 teaspoons, in the mouth. Swish the solution in the mouth and swallow (swish and swallow), or after swishing, have the client expectorate the solution (check with health care provider).

Side Effects
• Advise the client to avoid operating hazardous equipment or a motor vehicle when taking amphotericin B, ketoconazole, or flucytosine because these drugs may cause visual changes, sleepiness, dizziness, or lethargy.
• Instruct the client to report side effects, such as nausea, vomiting, diarrhea, dermatitis, rash, dizziness, tinnitus, edema, and flatulence. These symptoms may occur when taking certain antifungal drugs.

EVALUATION
• Evaluate the effectiveness of the antifungal (antimycotic) drug by noting the absence of the fungal infection, e.g., decreased itching, redness, and rawness.

Antifungals

Generic (Brand)	Route and Dosage	Preg Cat	Interaction	t 1/2	PB	Onset	Peak	Duration
Polyenes Amphotericin B (Fungizone)	*Test dose:* A: IV: 0.25–1.0 mg in 20 mL of D₅W infused over 20–30 min A: IV: 0.25–1.0 mg/kg/d in D₅W or 1.5 mg/kg q.o.d.; max: 1.5 mg/kg/d C: IV: Same as adult, except dilution and infuse time differ	B	May *increase* effect of digoxin, skeletal muscle relaxants; may *increase* risk of nephrotoxicity with aminoglycosides; *increase* hypokalemia with corticosteroids	Initially: 24 h Final: 15 d	90%	Rapid	1–2 h after infusion	20 h
Nystatin (Mycostatin)	See Prototype Drug Chart							
Imidazoles Fluconazole (Diflucan)	A: PO/IV: 50–400 mg/d; maint: 100–200 mg/d C: PO/IV: 3–6 mg/kg/d	C	Same as miconazole May *increase* effect of phenytoin	20–40 h	12%	PO: UK IV: Rapid	PO: 1–2 h IV: End of infusion	UK
Itraconazole (Sporanox)	A: PO: Loading dose: 200 mg q8h × 3d; maint: 200 mg/d; max: 400 mg/d in 2 divided doses	C	May *increase* effect of phenytoin *Decrease* effect of rifampin; may *decrease* effect of warfarin	21–42 h	99%	UK	1.5–5 h Steady state: 12 h	UK

Drug	Dose	Preg. Cat.	Drug Interactions	$t_{1/2}$	Protein Binding	Onset	Peak	Duration
Ketoconazole (Nizoral)	A: PO: 200–400 mg/d as a single dose C: PO: 3.3–6.6 mg/kg/d as single dose C <20 kg: PO: 50 mg daily	C	*Increase* effect with cyclosporine *Decrease* absorption with antacids, anticholinergics, H_2 blockers	Initially: 2 h Final: 8 h	95%	1 h	1–2 h	UK
Miconazole nitrate (Monistat, Micatin)	A: IV: 200–3,600 mg/d in D_5W in 3 divided doses; infuse IV over 30–60 min C: IV: 20–40 mg/kg/d in divided doses; max: 15 mg/kg/inf A: Supp: 100 mg vag h.s. for 7 d Available: Vaginal cream 2%; lotion	B	*Increase* effect of anticoagulants; may *increase* hypoglycemic reaction with oral hypoglycemics	Triphasic: 40 min, 2 h, 24 h	92%	Rapid	End of infusion	UK
Antimetabolites Terbinafine HCl (Lamisil)	A&C: Topical: Cream 1%, apply 1–2× per day	B	None significant known	NA	NA	UK	UK	UK
Flucytosine (Ancobon)	A: PO: 50–150 mg/kg/d in 4 divided doses C <50 kg: PO: 1.5–4.5 g/m²/d in 4 divided doses	C	Synergistic effect with amphotericin B	3–8 h	5%	Rapid	2–6 h	UK
Antiprotozoal Atovaquone (Mepron)	A: PO: 750 mg t.i.d. with food × 21 d	C	*Increase* effect with other highly protein-bound drugs	2–3 d	99%	UK	2 peaks First: 1–8 h Second: 2–3 d	6–20 wk

KEY: For complete abbreviation key, see inside front cover.

Antimalarials

Generic (Brand)	Route and Dosage	Preg Cat	Interaction	t 1/2	PB	Action			
						Onset	Peak	Duration	
Chloroquine HCl (Aralen HCl)	*Acute malaria:* A: PO: 600 mg base/dose; then 6 h later: 300 mg/dose; then at 24 and 48 h: 300 mg/dose IM: 200 mg/base q6h PRN C: PO: 10 mg base/kg/dose, then 6 h later: 5 mg base/kg/dose; 24–48 h later: 5 mg base/kg/dose. IM: 5 mg base/kg q12h *Prophylaxis:* 2 wk before and 6–8 wk after exposure A&C: PO: 5 mg/kg/wk; max: 300 mg base/wk	C	*Increase* effects of digoxin, anticoagulants, neuromuscular blocker *Decrease* absorption with antacids	2.5–5 d Terminal: 1–2 mo	50–65%	PO, IM: Rapid	3.5 h IV/IM: 0.5 h	Days to weeks	
Hydroxychloroquine SO$_4$ (Plaquenil SO$_4$)	*Acute malaria:* A: PO: 800 mg/dose; 6 h: 400 mg (2 tab); 24 h: 400 mg (2 tab); 48 h: 400 mg (2 tab) C: PO: 10 mg base/kg/dose, 6 h: 5 mg base/kg; 24 h: 5 mg base/kg; 48 h: 5 mg base/kg/dose	C	Similar to chloroquine HCl	2.5–5 d	55%	<1 h	1–2 h	UK	

Drug	Dosage		Drug Interactions	t½	PB	Onset	Peak	Duration
Mefloquine HCl (Lariam)	*Prophylaxis:* 1 wk before and 6–8 wk after exposure A&C: PO: 5 mg base/kg/wk; max: 300 mg base/wk	C	*Increase* ECG abnormalities with antidysrhythmics, beta blockers May *decrease* effect of valproic acid	21 d	98%	UK	7–24 h	UK
Primaquine phosphate	*Malaria prophylaxis:* A: PO: 15 mg/d for 14 d (single doses) C: PO: 0.3 mg/kg/d for 14 d (single doses)	C	*Increase* toxicity of quinacrine	3.7–9.6 h	UK	UK	1–6 h	UK
Pyrimethamine (Daraprim)	*Malaria prophylaxis:* A&C >10 y: PO: 25 mg/wk C <4 y: PO: 6.25 mg/wk C 4–10 y: PO: 12.5 mg/wk	C	*Decrease* effect of folic acid	1.5–2 d	80%	UK	>2 h	2 wk
Quinacrine HCl (Atabrine HCl)	*Malaria suppression:* A: PO: 100 mg/d C: PO: 50 mg/d	C	*Increase* toxicity with primaquine	UK	UK	UK	8 h	4 wk
Quinine SO_4 (Quin-260, Quiphile)	*Acute malaria:* A: PO: 650 mg q8h for 3–7 d C: PO: 25 mg/kg/d in 3 divided doses (q8h) for 3–7 d	X	*Similar* to chloroquine HCl	6–14 h	70–95%	<1 h	1–3 h	6–8 h

KEY: For complete abbreviation key, see inside front cover.

Antivirals

Acyclovir sodium

Acyclovir sodium
   (Zovirax)
Antiviral
Pregnancy Category: C
Drug Forms:
Cap 200 mg
Inj 500 mg/vial

Dosage

A: PO: 200 mg q4h 3–5×/d
   IV: 5 mg/kg q8h × 5d (diluted in
   D_5W)
C <12 y: IV: 250 mg/m^2 q8h × 5d;
   infuse over 1 h

Contraindications

Hypersensitivity, severe renal or
   hepatic disease
Caution: Electrolyte imbalance,
   lactation

Drug-Lab-Food Interactions

Increase nephroneurotoxicity with
   aminoglycosides, probenecid,
   interferon
Lab: May *increase* AST, ALT, BUN

Pharmacokinetics

Absorption: PO: Slowly absorbed
Distribution: PB: 10–30%
Metabolism: t 1/2: 2–3 h
Excretion: 95% unchanged in urine

Pharmacodynamics

PO: Onset: UK
       Peak: 1.5–2 h
       Duration: 4–8 h
IV: Onset: Rapid
     Peak: 1–2 h
     Duration: 4–8 h

Therapeutic Effects/Uses: To treat herpes simplex I, genital herpes II.
Mode of Action: Interference with synthesis by the virus of DNA.

Side Effects

Nausea, vomiting, diarrhea,
   headache, tremors, lethargy, rash,
   pruritus, increased bleeding time,
   phlebitis at IV site

Adverse Reactions

Urticaria, anemia, gingival
   hyperplasia
Life-threatening: Nephrotoxicity (large
   doses), neuropathy, bone marrow
   depression, granulocytopenia,
   thrombocytopenia, leukopenia,
   seizure, acute renal failure

KEY: For complete abbreviation key, see inside front cover.

■ NURSING PROCESS: Antivirals

ASSESSMENT

- Obtain a medical history of any serious renal or hepatic disease.
- Obtain baseline VS and a complete blood count. Use these findings for comparison with future results.
- Assess baseline laboratory results, particularly BUN, serum creatinine, liver enzymes, bilirubin, and electrolytes. Use these results for future comparisons.
- Assess baseline VS and urine output. Report abnormal findings.

POTENTIAL NURSING DIAGNOSES
High risk of infection
High risk for impaired tissue integrity

PLANNING
- Symptoms of viral infections will be eliminated or diminished.

NURSING INTERVENTIONS
- Monitor the client's complete blood count (CBC). Report abnormal results, such as leukopenia, thrombocytopenia, and low hemoglobin and hematocrit.
- Monitor other laboratory tests, such as BUN, serum creatinine, and liver enzymes, and compare with baseline values.
- Monitor the client's urinary output. An antiviral drug such as acyclovir can affect renal function.
- Monitor VS, especially blood pressure. Acyclovir and amantadine may cause orthostatic hypotension.
- Observe for signs and symptoms of side effects. Most antiviral drugs have many side effects; see Prototype Drug Chart.
- Check for superimposed infection (superinfection) due to high dose and prolonged use of an antiviral drug such as acyclovir.
- Administer oral acyclovir as prescribed. Oral dose can be taken at mealtime.
- For IV use, dilute the antiviral drug in an appropriate amount of solution as indicated in the drug circular. Administer the IV drug over 60 min. **Never** give acyclovir as a bolus (IV push).

CLIENT TEACHING
General
- Advise the client to maintain an adequate fluid intake to ensure adequate hydration for drug therapy and to increase urine output.
- Instruct the client with genital herpes to avoid spreading the infection by sexual abstinence or the use of a condom. Advise these women to have a Pap test done every 6 mo or as indicated by the health care provider. Cervical cancer is more prevalent in women with genital herpes simplex.
- Instruct clients taking zidovudine to have blood cell count monitored.

Side Effects
- Instruct the client to perform oral hygiene several times a day. Gingival hyperplasia (red, swollen gums) can occur with prolonged use of antiviral drugs.
- Instruct the client to report adverse reactions, including decrease in urine output and CNS changes such as dizziness, anxiety, or confusion.
- Advise the client with dizziness due to orthostatic hypotension to arise slowly from a sitting to a standing position.
- Instruct the client to report any side effects associated with the antiviral drug, such as nausea, vomiting, diarrhea, increased bleeding time, rash, urticaria, or menstrual abnormalities.

EVALUATION
- Evaluate the effectiveness of the antiviral drug in eliminating the virus or in decreasing symptoms.
- Determine if side effects are absent.

Generic (Brand)	Route and Dosage	Preg Cat	Interaction	t 1/2	PB	Action			
						Onset	Peak	Duration	
General									
Amantadine HCl (Symmetrel)	*Influenza A:* A: PO: 200 mg/d in 1–2 divided doses C 1–8 y: PO: 4.4–8.8 mg/kg/d in 2–3 divided doses C 9–12 y: PO: 100–200 mg/d in 1–2 divided doses	C	May *increase* anticholinergic effect; *increase* CNS action with CNS stimulants	24 h	UK	10–15 min	1–4 h	UK	
Rimantadine HCl (Flumadine)	A: PO: 200 mg/d in 1 or 2 divided doses C: PO: 5–7 mg/kg/d	C	Similar to amantadine HCl	33 h	40%	UK	3–6 h	UK	
Antimetabolites									
Acyclovir (Zovirax)	See Prototype Drug Chart								
Didanosine (Videx)	*HIV infections:* A >75 kg: PO: 300 mg q12h 50–75 kg: 200 mg q12h 35–50 kg: 125 mg q12h C: PO: tab: 1.1–1.4 m²: 100 mg b.i.d. Pedi Powder: 0.8–1 m²: 75 mg q12h 0.5–0.7 m²: 50 mg q12h <0.4 m²: 25 mg q12h	B	Avoid taking with tetracyclines, ciprofloxacin	1.5 h	UK	UK	0.6–1 h	UK	

			Increase effect of digoxin	UK	UK	UK	UK	UK
Famciclovir (Famvir)	*Herpes zoster:* A: PO: 500 mg q8h × 7 d			2.5–6 h	1–2%	3–8 d	12–14 d	>14 d
Ganciclovir sodium (Cytovene)	A&C: IV: Initially: 5 mg/kg q12h × 14–21 d; maint: 5 mg/kg/d × 7 d or 6 mg/kg/d × 5 d	C	May *increase* toxicity with cytotoxic drugs May *increase* seizures with imipenem-cilastatin *Lab:* May *increase* BUN, creatinine; may *decrease* blood glucose					
Ribavirin (Virazole)	A&C: By aerosol inhalation administration	X	May antagonize effect of zidovudine	24 h	NA	UK	1–1.5 h	UK
Vidarabine monohydrate (Vira-A)	A: IV: 10–15 mg/kg/d infused over 12–24 h	C	*Increase* CNS side effects with allopurinol	1.5–3 h	20–30%	Rapid	End of infusion	UK
Zalcitabine (Hivid)	*HIV infections:* A: PO: 0.75 mg q8h given with zidovudine 200 mg q8h	C	May cause peripheral neuropathy with aminoglycosides, amphotericin, cisplatin, INH, nitrofurantoin, phenytoin, vincristine, disulfiram	1.2–2 h	<4%	UK	1–2 h	UK
Zidovudine (Retrovir)	A: PO: 100–200 mg q4h IV: 1–2 mg/kg q4h; max: 1,200 mg/d C: PO: 90–180 mg/m² q6h; max: 200 mg q6h	C	May *increase* toxicity with aspirin, acetaminophen, H$_2$ blockers, lorazepam	1 h	25–38%	Rapid	0.5–1.5 h	UK

KEY: For complete abbreviation key, see inside front cover.

Topical Anti-infectives: Burns

Mafenide acetate	Dosage
Mafenide acetate (Sulfamylon) Anti-infective, sulfonamide derivative *Pregnancy Category:* C *Drug Form:* Cream 85 mg/g as acetate	A&C: Topical: Apply ¹⁄₁₆-inch layer evenly to affected area daily/b.i.d; reapply as necessary

Contraindications	Drug-Lab-Food Interactions
Hypersensitivity, inhalation injury	None known

Pharmacokinetics	Pharmacodynamics
Absorption: Some absorbed *Distribution:* PB: UK *Metabolism:* t 1/2: UK *Excretion:* In urine	Onset: On contact Peak: 2–4 h Duration: As long as applied

Therapeutic Effects/Uses: To treat second- and third-degree burns; to prevent organism invasion of burned tissue areas; to treat burn infections.

Mode of Action: Inhibits bacterial cell wall synthesis.

Side Effects	Adverse Reactions
Rash, burning sensation, urticaria, pruritus, swelling	Metabolic acidosis, respiratory alkalosis, blistering, superinfection *Life-threatening:* Bone marrow suppression, fatal hemolytic anemia

KEY: For complete abbreviation key, see inside front cover.

■ NURSING PROCESS: Topical Anti-infectives: Burns

ASSESSMENT

- Assess burned tissue for infection. Culture an oozing wound.
- Check client's VS. Report abnormal findings such as an elevated temperature.

POTENTIAL NURSING DIAGNOSES

High risk for infection related to loss of skin integrity
Pain related to thermal injury

PLANNING

- Aseptic technique will be enforced when caring for burned tissue, and tissue will be free from infection.

NURSING INTERVENTIONS

- Administer prescribed analgesia before application, if needed.
- Cleanse burned tissue sites using aseptic technique.
- Apply topical antibacterial drug and dressing with sterile technique.
- Monitor client's fluid balance and renal function.
- Monitor client for side effects of and adverse reactions to topical drug.
- Monitor client's VS and be alert for signs of infection. Use with caution in client with acute renal failure.
- Closely monitor client's acid-base balance, especially in the presence of pulmonary or renal dysfunction.
- Store drug in dry place at room temperature.

CLIENT TEACHING

General

- Instruct client and family about changes in respiratory status.

Skill

- Explain to client and family the care given to the burned tissue areas, using aseptic technique.
- Instruct client and family to apply topical agent and dressings to the burned areas.

EVALUATION

- Evaluate effectiveness of treatment interventions to burned tissue areas by determining if healing is proceeding and sites are free from infection.

Generic (Brand)	Route and Dosage	Preg Cat	Interaction	t 1/2	PB	Onset	Peak	Duration
							Action	
						Onset	Peak	Duration
Burns								
Nitrofurazone (Furacin)	0.2% cream, ointment, sol *Adjunctive therapy:* Apply directly or to dressing daily for 2°–3° burns; q4–5d for 2° burns with scant exudate	C	None significant reported	NA	NA	UK	UK	UK
Mafenide acetate (Sulfamylon)	See Prototype Drug Chart							
Silver nitrate	0.5 sol; 10%, 25% sticks; apply only to affected area 2–3×/wk for 2–3 wk	C	Do not use with alkalis, phosphates, thimerosal, benzalkonium chloride, halogenated acids	NA	NA	UK	UK	UK
Silver sulfadiazine (Silvadene, SSD)	1% cream, apply daily–b.i.d. in 1/16-inch layer	C	May inactivate topical proteolytic enzymes concurrently applied	NA	NA	On contact	UK	As long as applied
Acne Vulgaris: Keratolytics								
Benzoyl peroxide (Bezac, Persa-Gel, Desquam)	2.5–10% daily–q.i.d. (cream, gel, or lotion)	C	*Increase* skin irritation with tretinoin	NA	NA	UK	UK	UK
Salicylic acid (Sebulex, Freezone)	*Antiacne/antiseborrheic:* 2–10% cream, gel shampoo Use as directed	C	Avoid use by aspirin-sensitive clients	NA	NA	UK	UK	UK
Resorcinol and sulfur	2% resorcinol + 5% sulfur 2% resorcin + 8% sulfur Use as directed	C	Avoid use with other acne preparations	NA	NA	UK	UK	UK

Drug	Dosage	Preg Category	Drug Interactions					
Acne Vulgaris: **Antibiotics** Tetracycline, erythromycin, clindamycin (Cleocin), and meclocycline (Meclan)	As directed	B, C	None significant known	NA	NA	UK	UK	UK
Tretinoin (Retin-A)	Cream: 0.05–0.1% Gel: 0.025–0.1% Liquid: 0.05% daily h.s.	B	*Increase* irritation with salicylic acid, resorcinol, benzoyl peroxide	NA	NA	UK	UK	UK
Psoriasis Methoxsalen (8-MOP [hard gelatin], Oxsoralen-Ultra [soft gelatin] Do *not* interchange hard and soft capsules	A&C >12 y: PO: 10–20 mg 2 h before exposure to therapeutic ultraviolet rays Topical application before exposure to ultraviolet rays	C	*Increase* effects with phenothiazines, tetracyclines, thiazides, sulfonamides	2 h	80–90%	≥10 wk	UK	8 h Sensitive to sun
Etretinate (Tegison)	A: PO: 0.5–0.75 mg/kg/d in divided doses; max: 1.5 mg/kg/d	X	*Increase* absorption with milk, high-fat foods; alcohol increases triglycerides	4–8 d	99%	Weeks	Weeks– months	Years

KEY: For complete abbreviation key, see inside front cover.

URINARY AGENTS

Urinary Anti-infectives

Urinary Analgesic

Urinary Stimulant

Urinary Antispasmodics

Urinary Anti-infectives

Nitrofurantoin

Nitrofurantoin
   (Furadantin, Furalan, Furan,
   Macrodantin)
Antibacterial
Pregnancy Category: B
Drug Forms:
Cap 25, 50, 100 mg
Tab 50, 100 mg
Susp 25 mg/5 mL

Dosage

Initial/Recurrent UTI:
A: PO: 50–100 mg q.i.d. with meals
   and h.s.; take with food
C: PO: >1 mo: 5–7 mg/kg in 4
   divided doses
Long-term Prophylaxis:
A: PO: 50–100 mg q.i.d.
C: PO: 1–2 mg/kg in 1–2 divided
   doses

Contraindications

Hypersensitivity, moderate to severe
   renal impairment, oliguria, anuria,
   Cl_{cr} <40 mL/min, infants <1 mo,
   term pregnancy, lactation with
   infant suspected of having G-6-PD
   deficiency
Caution: Vitamin B deficiency,
   electrolyte imbalance, diabetes
   mellitus

Drug-Lab-Food Interactions

Decrease effect with probenecid;
   decrease absorption with antacids

Pharmacokinetics

Absorption: Well absorbed from GI
   tract; enhanced with food
Distribution: PB: 40%; Crosses
   placenta and enters breast milk
Metabolism: t 1/2: 20–60 min
Excretion: In urine; small amounts in
   bile

Pharmacodynamics

PO: Onset: UK
     Peak: 30 min
     Duration: UK

Therapeutic Effects/Uses: To treat acute and chronic UTIs.
Mode of Action: Inhibits bacterial enzymes and metabolism.

Side Effects

Anorexia, nausea, vomiting,
   rust/brown discoloration of urine,
   diarrhea, rash, pruritus, dizziness,
   headache, drowsiness

Adverse Reactions

Superinfection, peripheral
   neuropathy, hemolytic anemia,
   agranulocytosis
Life-threatening: Anaphylaxis,
   hepatotoxicity, Stevens-Johnson
   syndrome

KEY: For complete abbreviation key, see inside front cover.

■ NURSING PROCESS: Nitrofurantoin

ASSESSMENT

• Obtain a history from the client of clinical problems with urinary tract infection (UTI) or other urinary tract disorders.

Urinary Anti-infectives

- Assess the client for signs and symptoms of UTI, such as pain or burning sensation on urination and frequency and urgency of urination.
- Assess CBC on clients with long-term therapy; monitor regularly.
- Assess renal and hepatic function.
- Assess urine pH; 5.5 is desired; however, alkalinization of the urine is *not* recommended.

POTENTIAL NURSING DIAGNOSES
Altered comfort; pain
High risk for infection

PLANNING
- Client will be free of signs and symptoms of UTI within 10 d.

NURSING INTERVENTIONS
- Monitor the client's output. Careful attention to output is required when administering urinary anti-infectives to clients with anuria and oliguria. Report promptly any decrease in urine output.
- Before the start of drug therapy, obtain a urine culture to determine the organism causing the UTI.
- Observe the client for side effects of and adverse reactions to urinary anti-infectives drugs. Peripheral neuropathy (tingling, numbness of extremities) may result from renal insufficiency (inability to excrete drug) or long-term use of nitrofurantoin. Peripheral neuropathy may be irreversible.
- Dilute IV nitrofurantoin in 500 mL of IV solution before administering; constitute in sterile water without preservative.

CLIENT TEACHING
General
- Advise the client not to crush tablets or open capsules.
- Advise the client to rinse mouth thoroughly after taking oral nitrofurantoin. This drug can stain the teeth.
- Avoid antacids because they interfere with drug absorption.
- Instruct client to shake suspension well before taking and protect it from freezing.
- Advise client not to drive a motor vehicle or operate dangerous machinery; drug may cause drowsiness.
- Advise the diabetic client not to use Clinitest to test for glucose because a false-positive may result.

Diet
- Instruct the client to increase fluids and take the drug with food; this minimizes GI upset.

Side Effects
- Advise the client that urine may turn a harmless brown.
- Advise the client to report any signs of secondary fungal or bacterial infection (superinfection), such as stomatitis or anogenital discharge or itching.

EVALUATION
- Evaluate the effectiveness of the urinary anti-infectives in alleviating the UTI. Client is free of side effects and adverse reactions to drug.

Generic (Brand)	Route and Dosage	Preg Cat	Interaction	t 1/2	PB	Action			
						Onset	Peak	Duration	
Methenamine mandelate (Mandelamine)	A: PO: 1 g q.i.d. p.c. C 6–12 y: PO: 0.5 g q.i.d. p.c. C <6 y: PO: 50 mg/kg in 4 divided doses p.c.	C	May precipitate sulfonamides; may *decrease* effectiveness with urinary alkalinizers	3–6 h	UK	UK	2 h	UK
Trimethoprim (Proloprim, Trimpex)	A: PO: 100 mg q12h or 200 mg q24h; if Cl$_{cr}$ is 15–30 mL/min: 50 mg q12h; if Cl$_{cr}$ <15 mL/min: do not use	C	*Increase* risk of bone marrow depression with antineoplastics/radiation; *increase* elimination with rifampin *Lab: Increase* BUN, AST, ALT	8–11 h	44%	Rapid	1–4 h	UK
Quinolones								
Cinoxacin (Cinobac)	A: PO: 1 g/d in 2–4 doses for 1–2 wk; *Renal dysfunction:* Initially: 500 mg; if Cl$_{cr}$ is >80 mL/min: 500 mg b.i.d.; 80–50 mL/min: 250 mg t.i.d.; 50–20 mL/min: 250 mg b.i.d.; <20 mL/min: 250 mg q.d. Not recommended for infants or prepubertal children	C, although *not* recommended during pregnancy	*Decrease* effect with probenecid *Lab: Increase* AST, ALT, BUN, alkaline phosphatase, creatinine	1.5 h Impaired renal function: ≥10 h	60–80%	UK	2–4 h	6–8 h

Drug	Dosage	Pregnancy category	Drug interactions	t½	Protein binding	Onset	Peak	Duration
Ciprofloxacin (Cipro)	A: PO: mild to moderate: 250 mg q12h; severe/complicated: 250–500 mg q12h *Renal dysfunction:* If Cl$_{cr}$ >50 mL/min (PO), >30 mL/min (IV): Usual dose 30–50 mL/min: 250–500 mg q12h 5–29 mL/min: 250–500 mg q18h (PO); 200–400 mg q18–24h (IV) *Hemo or peritoneal dialysis:* 250–500 mg q24h after dialysis	C	*Increase* levels of drug with probenecid, theophylline *Decrease* absorption with antacids *Lab: Increase* AST, ALT, BUN	4–6 h	20–40%	PO: Rapid IV: Rapid	1–2 h End of infusion	6–8 h UK
Methenamine hippurate (Hiprex, Urex)	A: PO: 1 g b.i.d. C 6–12 y: 0.5–1 g b.i.d.	C	*Decrease* effect with urinary alkalinizers May precipitate sulfonamides	3–6 h	UK	UK	2 h	UK
Nalidixic acid (NegGram)	A: PO: 1 g q.i.d. for 1–2 wk; 1 g b.i.d. for long-term use C: PO: 55 mg/kg/d in 4 divided doses for 1–2 wk; 33 mg/kg/d for long-term use C <3 mo: *Do not use*	B	*Increase* effects of oral contraceptives *Decrease* effects of antacids	1–2 h Elderly: 12 h	93%	1–2 h	1–2 h	UK

continued

Urinary Anti-infectives continued

Generic (Brand)	Route and Dosage	Preg Cat	Interaction	t 1/2	PB	Onset	Peak	Duration
							Action	
Norfloxacin (Noroxin)	A: PO: 400 mg b.i.d. for 1–2 wk on empty stomach *Uncomplicated cystitis due to E. coli, K. pneumoniae, P. mirabilis:* 400 mg b.i.d. ×3d *Uncomplicated due to any other organism:* 400 mg b.i.d. ×7–10d *Complicated:* 400 mg b.i.d. ×10–21d *Renal impairment (Cl$_{cr}$ <30 mL/min):* 400 mg q.d.	C	*Increase* toxicity with theophylline *Decrease* absorption with sucralfate iron, antacids; *decrease* effects with nitrofurantoin *Lab: Increase* AST, ALT, BUN, alkaline phosphatase	3–4 h	10–15%	UK	1–3 h	UK
Other								
Aztreonam (Azactam)	A: IM/IV: 500 mg–1 g q8–12h	B	*Increase* effects with furosemide, probenecid, cefoxitin, imipenem	1.5–2 h	56–60%	IM: Rapid IV: Rapid	1 h End of infusion	UK UK
Co-trimoxazole or sulfamethoxazole-trimethoprim (Bactrim, Septra)	See Anti-infectives: Sulfonamides							

Drug	Uses and Dosage	Pregnancy Category	Drug Interactions					
Enoxacin (Penetrex)	*Uncomplicated UTI:* A: PO: 200 mg q12h for 7 d *Complicated or severe UTI:* A: PO: 400 mg q12h for 14 d If Cl_cr <30 mL/min, reduce dose by 50%	C Pregnant, X	*Increase* effects of oral anticoagulants, probenecid, theophylline *Decrease* absorption with antacids, oral iron, sucralfate	3–6 h	UK	UK	1–2 h	UK
Imipenem/cilastatin sodium (Primaxin)	A: IV: 250 mg–1 g q6–8h; max: 4 g/d or 50 mg/kg/d, whichever is the lesser amount C: Safety and efficacy not established Dosing adjustment with renal impairment	C	*Increase* risk of seizures with ganciclovir *Decrease* effects with cephalosporins, penicillins, aztreonam	1 h	I: 20% C: 40%	UK	I: 2 h C: 1 h	UK UK
Methylene blue (Urolene Blue)	*Cystitis, urethritis:* A: PO: 60–125 mg b.i.d./t.i.d. p.c. with glass of water	C	None significant	UK	UK	UK	UK	UK
Nitrofurantoin (Furadantin; Furalan, Macrodantin)	See Prototype Drug Chart							
Polymyxin B SO₄ (Aerosporin)	A&C: IV: 15,000–25,000 U/kg/d in divided doses q12h	B	*Increase* nephrotoxicity with vancomycin, aminoglycosides, amphotericin B; *increase* effects of neuromuscular blockers	4–6 h	UK	Rapid	2 h	UK

KEY: For complete abbreviation key, see inside front cover.

Urinary Analgesic

Phenazopyridine

Phenazopyridine
  (Pyridium, Urodine)
Antipruritic, local anesthetic
Pregnancy Category: B
Drug Forms:
Tab 100, 200 mg

Dosage

A: PO: 100–200 mg t.i.d. p.c.
C: PO: 12 mg/kg in 3 divided doses

Contraindications

Severe liver or renal disease,
  pregnancy or breast feeding

Drug-Lab-Food Interactions

May interfere with urinalysis color
  reactions, urinary glucose, ketones,
  proteins, steroids

Pharmacokinetics

Absorption: PO: Well absorbed
Distribution: PB: UK
Metabolism: t 1/2: UK
Excretion: In urine

Pharmacodynamics

PO: Onset: UK
     Peak: 5–6 h
     Duration: 6–8 h

Therapeutic Effects/Uses: For relief of UTI from infection, trauma, and surgery (use with urinary antiseptic).

Mode of Action: Produces analgesia/local anesthesia on urinary tract mucosa. Exact mechanism of action unknown.

Side Effects

Anorexia, nausea, vomiting,
  diarrhea, heartburn, red-orange
  discoloration of urine, rash,
  pruritus, headache, vertigo

Adverse Reactions

Life-threatening: Agranulocytosis,
  hepatotoxicity, nephrotoxicity,
  thrombocytopenia, leukopenia,
  hemolytic anemia

KEY: For complete abbreviation key, see inside front cover.

■ NURSING PROCESS: Urinary Analgesic: Phenazopyridine (Pyridium)

ASSESSMENT

- Obtain a history from the client of clinical problems with the urinary tract.
- Obtain a drug history; report probable drug-drug interactions.
- Assess the client for signs and symptoms of UTI such as pain or burning sensation on urination and frequency and urgency of urination.
- Assess hepatic function studies, especially serum liver enzymes, with long-term therapy.

POTENTIAL NURSING DIAGNOSES

Altered patterns of urinary elimination
Pain due to renal problem

PLANNING

- The client will be free of urinary tract pain within 3 d.

NURSING INTERVENTIONS

- Administer drug with food or milk to decrease gastric distress. Chewable tablets should be chewed.
- Observe client for side effects of and adverse reaction to urinary analgesic.

CLIENT TEACHING

General

- Instruct client to take medication exactly as ordered; not to exceed recommended dosage. Advise to take with food or milk.

Side Effects

- Advise the client that urine will be harmless reddish orange but does permanently stain clothing and contact lens.
- Instruct client to report signs of hepatotoxicity, including yellowing of skin or sclera, clay-colored stools, abdominal pain, diarrhea, dark urine, or fever.

EVALUATION

- Evaluate the effectiveness of the drug in alleviating the urinary tract pain. Client is free of side effects and adverse reactions to drug.

Urinary Analgesic, Stimulant, and Antispasmodics

Generic (Brand)	Route and Dosage	Preg Cat	Interaction	t 1/2	PB	Action		
						Onset	Peak	Duration
Urinary Analgesic Phenazopyridine HCl (Pyridium, Urodine)	See Prototype Drug Chart							
Urinary Stimulant Bethanechol Cl (Urecholine, Duvoid, Urabeth)	A: PO: 10–50 mg b.i.d./t.i.d./q.i.d. 1 h a.c. or 2 h p.c. SC: 2.5–10 mg t.i.d./q.i.d. PRN C: PO: 0.6 mg/kg/d in 3–4 divided doses	C	*Increased* effect with cholinergics *Decrease* action with procainamide, quinidine Hypotension with ganglionic blockers	UK	UK	PO: 30–90 min SC: 5–15 min	1 h 15–30 min	6 h 2 h

Urinary
Antispasmodics

Drug	Route and Dosage						
Dimethyl sulfoxide (DMSO, Rimso-50)	*Bladder instillation:* 50 mL of 50% sol retained for 15 min; repeat q2wk until relief	C	None significant	UK	UK	UK	4–8 h	UK
Flavoxate HCl (Urispas)	A: PO: 100–200 mg t.i.d. or q.i.d.	B	None significant	UK	UK	1 h	UK	UK
Oxybutynin Cl (Ditropan)	A: PO: 5 mg b.i.d. or t.i.d. C >5 y: PO: 5 mg b.i.d. C 1–5 y: PO: 0.2 mg/kg b.i.d./q.i.d.	B	None significant	1–3 h	UK	PO: 30–60 min	3–6 h	7–10 h
Propantheline bromide (Pro-Banthine)	A: PO: 15 mg t.i.d. 30 min a.c and 30 mg h.s.; max: 120 mg/d Elderly: 7.5 mg t.i.d./q.i.d. C: PO: 10 mg/m² q.i.d.	C	*Increase* chance of extrapyramidal reactions *Decrease* absorption of ketoconazole	1.5 h	UK	30–45 min	2–6 h	6 h

KEY: For complete abbreviation key, see inside front cover.

ANTINEOPLASTIC AGENTS

Alkylating Drugs

Antimetabolites

Miscellaneous Anticancer Drugs

Biologic Response Modifiers:
    Epoetin Alfa
    Granulocyte Colony–Stimulating Factor
    Granulocyte Macrophage Colony–Stimulating Factor
    Interferons

Antineoplastic: Alkylating Drug

Cyclophosphamide

Cyclophosphamide
  (Cytoxan)
Alkylating drug
Pregnancy Category: D
Drug Forms:
Inj IV (powder) 100, 200, 500 mg;
  1, 2 g
Tab 25, 50 mg

Dosage

A: PO: Initially: 1–5 mg/kg over
  2–5 d; maint: 1–5 mg/kg/d
  IV: Initially: 45–50 mg/kg in
  divided doses over 2–5 d
C: PO/IV: Initially: 2–8 mg/kg in
  divided doses for 6 d; maint:
  10–15 mg/kg every 7–10 d
If bone marrow depression occurs,
  dosage adjustment is necessary

Contraindications

Hypersensitivity, severe bone
  marrow depression
Caution: Pregnancy, liver or kidney
  disease

Drug-Lab-Food Interactions

Thiazides, anticoagulants, digoxin,
  phenobarbital, rifampin
Lab: Uric acid, Pap test, purified
  protein derivative (PPD), mumps,
  candida

Pharmacokinetics

Absorption: PO: Well absorbed
Distribution: PB: 50%
Metabolism: t 1/2: 3–12 h
Excretion: 25–40% in urine
  unchanged; 5–20% in feces

Pharmacodynamics

Effects on blood count:
PO/IV: Onset: 7 d
  Peak: 10–14 d
  Duration: 21 d

Therapeutic Effects/Uses: To treat breast, lung, ovarian cancers; Hodgkin's disease; leukemias; and lymphomas; an immunosuppressant agent.

Mode of Action: Inhibition of protein synthesis through interference with DNA replication by alkylation of DNA.

Side Effects

Nausea, vomiting, diarrhea, weight
  loss, hematuria, alopecia,
  impotence, sterility, ovarian
  fibrosis, headache, dizziness,
  dermatitis

Adverse Reactions

Hemorrhagic cystitis, secondary
  neoplasm
Life-threatening: Leukopenia,
  thrombocytopenia, cardiotoxicity
  (very high doses), hepatotoxicity
  (long term)

KEY: For complete abbreviation key, see inside front cover.

■ NURSING PROCESS: Cyclophosphamide

ASSESSMENT

• Assess CBC, differential, and platelet count weekly. Withhold drug if platelets < 75,000 cells/mm^3 or WBC < 4,000 cells/mm^3; notify health care provider.
• Assess results of pulmonary function tests, chest x-rays, and renal and liver function studies during therapy.
• Assess temperature; fever may be early sign of infection.

POTENTIAL NURSING DIAGNOSES
High risk for infection
Body image disturbance

PLANNING
- Client will experience improved blood count status indicative of improvement/remission of the specific cancer growth.

NURSING INTERVENTIONS
- Hydrate client with IV and/or oral fluids before chemotherapy starts.
- Administer antacid before oral drug.
- Administer antiemetic 30–60 min before giving drug.
- Monitor IV site frequently for irritation and phlebitis.
- Increase fluids to 2–3 L/d to reduce risk of hemorrhagic cystitis, urate deposition, or calculus formation.
- Store drug in airtight container at room temperature.

CLIENT TEACHING
General
- Advise women who are contemplating pregnancy while taking antineoplastics to first seek medical advice. There may be teratogenic effects to the fetus. Pregnancy should be avoided for 3–4 mo after completing antineoplastic therapy in most situations. Some sources recommend that both men and women avoid conception for 2 y after completing treatment.
- Remind client to consult health care provider before administration of any vaccination.

Diet
- Advise client to follow diet low in purines (organ meats, beans, and peas) to alkalize urine.
- Advise client to avoid citric acid.

Side Effects
- Instruct client about good oral hygiene with soft toothbrush for stomatitis; do not use toothbrush when platelet count is <50,000 cells/mm^3.
- Emphasize with client protective isolation precautions. Advise the client not to visit anyone with any type of respiratory infection. A decreased WBC puts the client at high risk for acquiring an infection.
- Instruct client to report promptly signs of infection (fever, sore throat), bleeding (bleeding gums, petechiae, bruises, hematuria, blood in the stool), and anemia (increased fatigue, dyspnea, orthostatic hypotension).
- Remind client that she may experience amenorrhea, menstrual irregularities, or sterility and that he may experience impotence.
- Advise client of possible hair loss; recommend consideration of wig or hairpiece.

EVALUATION
- Client will be free of cancer as indicated by improved blood counts and free of side effects of drug.

Generic (Brand)	Route and Dosage*	Preg Cat	Interaction	t1/2	PB	Onset	Peak	Duration
							Action	
Nitrogen Mustards								
Chlorambucil (Leukeran)	A: PO: 0.1–0.2 mg/kg/d	D	*Increase* toxicity with other antineoplastics and radiation	1.5 h	99%	WBC: 7–14 d	7–14 d	12–28 d
Cyclophosphamide (Cytoxan)	See Prototype Drug Chart							
Estramustine phosphate sodium (Emcyt)	*Palliation prostate cancer:* A: PO: 10–16 mg/kg/d in 3–4 divided doses for 28–90 d; determine if response occurred	C	*Increase* toxicity with hepatotoxic agents, smoking, virus vaccines *Decrease* absorption with calcium-rich foods and supplements, milk	20 h	UK	Effect tumor spread 30–90 d	2–3 h	Hemotologic effects: 6 wk
Ifosfamide (Ifex)	A: IV: 1–2 g/m²/d for 5 d q21–28 d C: IV: 1,800 mg/m²/d for 3–5 d q21–28 d	D	*Increase* toxicity with antineoplastics, radiation, live virus vaccines, phenobarbital, phenytoin, chloral hydrate	High dose: 12–15 h Low dose: 4–8 h	UK	UK	UK	UK
Mechlorethamine HCl (Mustargen)	A: IV: 0.4 mg/kg/dose or 6–10 mg/m² as single dose or in divided doses	D	Similar to chlorambucil	<1 min	UK	24 h	7–12 d	10–21 d
Melphalan (Alkeran)	A: PO: 6 mg/d	D	Similar to chlorambucil	1.5 h	≤30%	4–5 d	2–3 wk	5–6 wk
Uracil mustard	*Palliation chronic lymphocytic leukemia, non-Hodgkin's lymphoma:* A: PO: 0.15 mg/kg/wk for 4 wk C: PO: 0.30 mg/kg/wk for 4 wk	X	*Increase* toxicity with antineoplastics, radiation, virus vaccines; dosage adjustment of antigout agents *Lab: Increase* blood uric acid	UK	UK	UK	UK	2 h

Nitrosoureas							
Carmustine (BiCNU)	A: IV: 75–100 mg/m²/d for 2 d or 200 mg/m² q6 wk as single dose or divided into 2 doses on successive days; next course is dependent on blood count	D	*Increase* bone marrow toxicity with cimetidine; hepatic dysfunction with etoposide	15–30 min	UK	Platelets: 3–5 d	3–5 wk	6 wk
Lomustine (CeeNu)	A: PO: 130 mg/m²/d as single dose	D	Similar to ifosfamide	1–2 d	50%	UK	4–6 wk	1–2 wk
Streptozocin (Zanosar)	A: IV: 500 mg/m²/d for 5 d or 1 g/m²/wk	C	*Increase* toxicity with antineoplastics and radiation	35–45 min	UK	Tumor response: 15 d	35 d	UK
Alkyl Sulfonates							
Busulfan (Myleran)	A: PO: 4–8 mg/d; max: 12 mg/d C: PO: 0.06–0.12 mg/kg/d	D	Similar to streptozocin	UK	UK	10–14 d	3 wk	<1 mo
Alkylating-like							
Altretamine (Hexalen)	A: PO: 4–12 mg/kg/d in 3–4 divided doses for 28–90 d	D	*Increase* toxicity with MAOIs; may cause severe orthostatic hypotension *Decrease* effect with phenobarbital	13 h	6%	Effect on blood counts: UK	3–4 wk	6 wk
Carboplatin (Paraplatin)	A: IV: 360 mg/m² q4 wk	D	*Increase* bone marrow depression with nephrotoxic agents	2–6 h	0%	UK	21 d	28 d
Cisplatin (Platinol)	A: IV: 20 mg/m²/d for 5 d; then 50–70 mg/m² q3 wk or 100 mg/m² q4 wk	D	Similar to streptozocin *Increase* toxicity with aminoglycosides, loop diuretics, phenytoin	alpha: 30–60 min beta: 60–72 h	>90%	Effect on blood count: UK	18–21 d	35–40 d

continued

Generic (Brand)	Route and Dosage*	Preg Cat	Interaction	t1/2	PB	Onset	Peak	Duration
							Action	
Dacarbazine (DTIC)	*Hodgkin's disease:* A: IV: 150 mg/m² daily for 5 d; repeat course q28d or 375 mg/m² on day 1 of combination therapy: repeat course q15d *Metastatic malignant melanoma:* A: IV: 2–4.5 mg/kg daily for 10 d; repeat q28d	C	*Increase* toxicity with antineoplastics, radiation, virus vaccines, phenobarbital, phenytoin	5 h	5–10%	WBC: 18–24 d Platelets: UK	21–25 d 14–16 d	3–5 d 3–5 d
Pipobroman (Vercyte)	*Chronic myelocytic leukemia:* A: PO: Initially: 1.5–2.5 mg/kg/d for 30 d; maint: 10–175 mg/d	D	Similar to cyclophosphamide	UK	UK	UK	UK	UK
Procarbazine HCl (Matulane)	A: PO: Initially: 2–4 mg/kg/d in divided doses for 7 d; then increase to 4–6 mg/kg/d until desired leukocyte/platelet counts	D	*Increase* CNS depression with phenothiazines, narcotics, barbiturates; *increase* toxicity with tyramine-rich foods	10 min	UK	14 d	2–8 wk	4–6 wk
Triethylenethio-phosphoramide (thiotepa)	A: IV: 0.2 mg/kg/d for 4–5 d; then 0.3–0.4 mg/kg at 2- to 4- wk intervals	D	Similar to carboplatin; *increase* toxicity with antineoplastics or radiation, neuromuscular blocking agents (e.g., succinylcholine)	1.5–2 h	UK	10 d	14 d	20 d

KEY: For complete abbreviation key, see inside front cover.
*Refer to individual protocol.

NOTES:

_____

_____

_____

_____

_____

_____

_____

_____

_____

_____

Antineoplastic: Antimetabolite

Fluorouracil

Fluorouracil
  (Adrucil, 5-FU)
Pregnancy Category: D
Antimetabolite
Drug Forms:
Inj IV 50 mg/mL
Sol/cream 2%, 5%

Dosage

A: IV: 12 mg/kg/d ×4d; max:
  800 mg/d; repeat with 6 mg/kg on
  day 6, 8, 10, and 12
Maint: 10–15 mg/kg/wk as single
  dose; max: 1 g/wk
Topical: 1–2% sol/cream b.i.d. to
  head/neck lesions; 5% to other
  body areas
Refer to specific protocol.

Contraindications

Hypersensitivity, pregnancy, severe
  infection, myelosuppression,
  marginal nutritional status

Drug-Lab-Food Interactions

Bone marrow depressants, live virus
  vaccines, cimetidine, calcium
Lab: Liver function studies, albumin,
  AST, ALT

Pharmacokinetics

Absorption: Topical: 5–10%
Distribution: PB: UK
Metabolism: t 1/2: 10–20 min
Excretion: In urine and expired
  carbon dioxide

Pharmacodynamics

Effects on blood count:
IV: Onset: 1–9 d
  Peak: 9–21 d
  Duration: 30 d
Topical: Onset: 2–3 d
       Peak: 2–6 wk
       Duration: 4–8 wk

Therapeutic Effects/Uses: To treat cancer of breast, cervix, colon, liver, ovary, pancreas, stomach, and rectum. In combination with levamisole after surgical resection in clients with Duke's Stage C colon cancer.

Mode of Action: Prevention of thymidine production, thereby inhibiting DNA and RNA synthesis. Not phase specific.

Side Effects

Nausea, vomiting, diarrhea,
  stomatitis, alopecia, rash

Adverse Reactions

Anemia
Life-threatening: Thrombocytopenia,
  myelosuppression, hemorrhage,
  renal failure

KEY: For complete abbreviation key, see inside front cover.

■ NURSING PROCESS: Fluorouracil

ASSESSMENT

- Assess the client's VS and use for future comparison.
- Assess CBC and platelet count weekly. Notify health care provider and withhold drug if WBC is <3,500/mm^3 or platelet count is <100,000 cells/mm^3.
- Assess renal function studies before and during drug therapy.
- Assess temperature every 4–6 h; fever may be early sign of infection.

POTENTIAL NURSING DIAGNOSES
High risk for infection
Altered nutrition; less than body requirements
Body image disturbance

PLANNING
- Client will have blood tests with values in the desired range.
- Client will be free of adverse reactions to drug therapy.
- Client's neoplasm will decrease in size.

NURSING INTERVENTIONS
- Handle drug with care during preparation; avoid direct skin contact with anticancer drugs. (Follow protocols.) Solution is colorless to light yellow.
- Administer IV dose over 1–2 min. Apply firm prolonged pressure to injection site if thrombocytopenia is present.
- Monitor IV site frequently. Extravasation produces severe pain. If this occurs, apply ice pack and notify health care provider.
- Administer antiemetic 30–60 min before drug to prevent vomiting.
- Offer the client food and fluids that may decrease nausea, such as cola, crackers, or ginger ale.
- Administer antibiotics prophylactically for infection, analgesics for pain, and antispasmodics for diarrhea, as ordered.
- Maintain strict medical asepsis.
- Encourage fluid intake of 2–3 L/d, unless contraindicated, to prevent dehydration.
- Support good oral hygiene; brush teeth with soft toothbrush and use waxed dental floss.
- Monitor fluid intake and output and nutritional intake. GI effects are common on the fourth day of treatment.

CLIENT TEACHING
General
- Emphasize protective precautions, as necessary.
- Teach the client to examine mouth daily and report stomatitis (ulceration in mouth). Good oral hygiene several times a day is essential. If stomatitis occurs, rinse mouth with baking soda or saline. Do not use a toothbrush when the platelet count is <50,000/mm^3.
- Advise women who are contemplating pregnancy while taking antineoplastics to first seek medical advice. Teratogenic effects to the fetus can occur from antineoplastics. Pregnancy should be avoided for 3–4 mo after completing antineoplastic therapy in most situations. Some sources recommend that both men and women avoid conception for 2 y after completion of treatment.
- Advise the client not to visit anyone with any type of respiratory infection. A decreased WBC count puts the client at high risk for acquiring an infection.

Side Effects
- Advise the client to promptly report signs of bleeding, anemia, and infection to the health care provider.

EVALUATION
- The client's tumor size will be decreased.
- Evaluate the client's blood tests results.
- Evaluate for side effects or adverse reactions to drug therapy.

Antineoplastics: Antimetabolites

Generic (Brand)	Route and Dosage*	Preg Cat	Interaction	t1/2	PB	Onset	Peak	Duration
							Action	
Folic Acid Antagonist								
Methotrexate (Mexate)	A: PO/IM: 3.3 mg/m²/d for 4–6 wk	D	*Increase* toxicity of drug with NSAIDs, 5-FU, sulfonamides, live virus vaccines	8–16 h	50%	5–7 d	7–14 d	21 d
Pyrimidine Analogs								
Cytarabine HCl (Cytosar-U, ara-C)	A: IV: 100–200 mg/m²/d or 3 mg/kg/d as continuous 12- or 24-h infusion	D	*Decrease* absorption of po digoxin	1–3 h	15%	24 h	7–10 d	12 d
Floxuridine (FUDR)	A: Intra-arterial: 0.1–0.6 mg/kg/d for 14 d IV: 0.5–1 mg/kg/d for 7–15 d	D	*Increase* bone marrow depression with radiation or antineoplastics	20 h	UK	1–10 d	10–21 d	30 d
5-Fluorouracil (Adrucil, 5-FU)	See Prototype Drug Chart							
Purine Analogs								
Cladribine (Leustatin)	*Hairy cell leukemia:* A: IV: 0.09 mg/kg/d for 7 d	D	*Increase* bone marrow depression with radiation or other antineoplastics	5.5 h	20%	UK	UK	UK

Drug							
Fludarabine (Fludara)	D	*Increase* toxicity with myelosuppressive agents *Lab: Increase* uric acid	9 h	UK	Blood counts: UK	14–16 d	UK
A: IV: 25 mg/m² over 30 min daily for 5 consecutive d; repeat course q28d C: IV: 10 mg/m² bolus over 15 min; then 30 mg/m²/d over 5 d							
6-Mercaptopurine (Purinethol) A&C: PO: 1.5–2.5 mg/kg/d; max: 5 mg/kg	D	Allopurinol *increases* bone marrow depression	A: 45 min C: 20 min	19%	5–10 d	14 d	21 d
Thioguanine A&C: PO: 2–3 mg/kg/d	D	Similar to 5-fluorouracil hepatotoxicity with busulfan	2–11 h	UK	Effect on blood count 7–10 d	14 d	21 d
Ribonucleotide Reductase Inhibitor Hydroxyurea (Hydrea) *Palliation:* A: PO: 20–30 mg/kg/d or 80 mg/kg q3d C: No dosage regimens established	D	*Increase* toxicity with cytotoxic agents, radiation; *increase* neurotoxicity with fluorouracil *Lab: Increase* uric acid, BUN, creatinine	3–4 h	UK	Blood counts: 7 d	10 d	21 d

KEY: For complete abbreviation key, see inside front cover.
*Refer to specific protocol.

Generic (Brand)	Route and Dosage*	Preg Cat	Interaction	t 1/2	PB	Action Onset	Action Peak	Action Duration
Antimicrotubule Paclitaxel (Taxol)	*Ovarian cancer:* A: IV: 135 mg/m² for 24 h q3wk; shortened infusions approved for refractory breast cancer	D	*Decrease* metabolism of drug with ketoconazole	5–17 h	80–90%	UK	11 d	3 wk
Enzyme Inhibitor Pentostatin (Nipent)	*Hairy cell leukemia:* A: IV: 4 mg/m² every other wk	D	*Increase* toxicity with fludarabine	6 h	UK	5 mo	UK	>8 mo
Podophyllotoxin Derivative Etoposide (VePesid, VP-16)	A: IV: 50–100 mg/m²/d on days 1–5	D	*Increase* bone marrow depression with radiation or other antineoplastics, sodium salicylate, tolbutamide	4–11 h	97%	7 d	14 d	20 d
Antitumor Antibiotics Bleomycin SO₄ (Blenoxane)	A: IM/IV: 10–20 U/m²/wk or 0.25–0.5 U/kg/wk Reduce dose with renal impairment	D	*Increase* toxicity with other antineoplastics *Decrease* effects of digoxin, phenytoin	2 h	1%	7 d	14 d	21 d

Dactinomycin (Actinomycin D, Cosmegen)	A: IV: 500 µg/m²/d for 5 d; max: 15 mg/kg/d; may repeat q3–6 wk	C	*Increase* effects of radiation therapy; may interfere with antibacterial drug levels; not compatible with heparin	36 h	80–90%	7 d	14 d	21 d
Daunorubicin HCl (Cerubidine)	*Leukemias:* A: IV: 30–60 mg/m²/d for 2–3 d; repeat dose in 3–4 wk. Reduce dose with hepatic/renal impairment	D	Severe local tissue necrosis with extravasation	19 h	80%	7–10 d	14 d	21 d
Doxorubicin (Adriamycin)	*Solid tumors:* A: IV: 30–75 mg/m²; repeat q21d. Reduce dose with hepatic impairment	D	*Increase* effects of barbiturates, digoxin, radiation	3–22 h	80–90%	7–10 d	14 d	21 d
Idarubicin (Idamycin)	*Solid tumor:* A: IV: 12–15 mg/m²/d for 3 d *Leukemia:* A: IV: 10–12 mg/m²/d for 3–4 d; repeat q3 wk. Reduce dose with hepatic/renal impairment	D	Similar to daunorubicin	22 h	97%	UK	UK	UK
Mitomycin (Mutamycin)	A: IV: 10–20 mg/m² q6–8wk. Reduce dose with renal impairment	D	*Increase* toxicity with vinca alkaloids; cardiotoxicity with doxorubicin	17 min	UK	4 wk	8 wk	10 wk

continued

Antineoplastic: Miscellaneous

Generic (Brand)	Route and Dosage*	Preg Cat	Interaction	t1/2	PB	Onset	Peak	Duration
							Action	
Plicamycin (Mithracin, mithramycin)	*Testicular tumor:* A: IV: 25–30 µg/kg/d for 8–10 d *Hypercalcemia:* A: IV: 15–25 µg/kg/d for 3–4 d Reduce dose with renal impairment	X	*Increase* toxicity with aspirin, glucogen, calcium products, etidronate	2–8 h	0%	Calcium decrease 24 h	48–72 h	5–15 d
Vinca Alkaloids Teniposide (Vumon, VM 26)	*Leukemia:* A: IV over ≥30–60 min: 165 mg/m² and cytarabine 300 mg/m² 2×wk for 8–9 doses	D	Increase toxicity with tolbutamide, sodium salicylate, sulfamethizole	10–38 h	>99%	UK	16–18 d	15 d
Vinblastine SO₄ (Velban)	A&C: IV: 0.1–0.5 mg/kg/wk or 3.7 mg/m²/wk or q2 wk	D	*Increase* toxicity with mitomycin-C *Decrease* effect of phenytoin	1–25 h	75%	5 d	10 d	14 d
Vincristine SO₄ (Oncovin)	A: IV: 0.4–1.4 mg/m²/wk; max: 2 mg/dose C: IV: 1–2 mg/m²/wk; max: 2 mg/dose	D	*Increase* toxicity with digoxin, L-asparaginase *Decrease* effect of phenytoin	19–155 h	75%	7 d	14 d	21 d

Androgens

Drug		Uses and Dosage	Drug Interactions	t½	PB	Onset	Peak	Duration
Testolactone (Teslac) CSS III	C	*Palliation breast carcinoma:* A: PO (females): 250 mg q.i.d.	*Increase* effects of oral anticoagulants *Lab: Increase* calcium, creatinine	UK	UK	Clinical effects: 6–12 wk	UK	UK
Trimetrexate glucuronate (Neutrexin)	D	A: IV: Inf: 8–12 mg/m² daily for 5 d Leucovorin must be given concurrent with Rx daily for 72 h p Rx Administer drugs through separate lines	Alter P-450 enzyme system with erythromycin, rifampin, ketoconazole	13.6 h	86–94%	UK	UK	UK
Other Aldesleukin (Interleukin-2, Proleukin)	C	*Metastatic renal cell carcinoma:* A: IV: 0.037 mg/kg/d q8h (15 min IV); treatment: two 5-d cycles with 9-d rest between; max: 28 doses per course	*Increase* toxicity with analgesics, antiemetics, sedatives, narcotics, tranquilizers; nephrotoxic, hepatotoxic, and myelotoxic agents; *increase* hypotension with beta blockers	20–120 mo	UK	UK	UK	UK
Aminoglutethimide (Cytadren)	D	A: PO: 250 mg q6h; increased q2 wk to 2 g/d in 2–3 divided doses to decrease nausea and vomiting	*Decrease* effect of digitoxin, warfarin, dexamethasone, theophylline *Lab: Decrease* thyroxine	7–15 h	20–25%	*Adrenal* suppression: 3–5 d	UK	36–72 h; 1 yr after long term

KEY: For complete abbreviation key, see inside front cover.
*Refer to specific protocol.

229

Antineoplastic: Miscellaneous

Generic (Brand)	Route and Dosage*	Preg Cat	Interaction	t 1/2	PB	Action Onset	Action Peak	Action Duration
Other								
Asparaginase (Elspar)	Start with intradermal skin test A: IV/IM: 6,000 U/m² q.o.d. for 3–4 wk or 1,000–20,000 U/m² for 10–20 d	C	*Increase* toxicity with vincristine, prednisone *Decrease* effect of methotrexate	8–30 h	30%	Immediate	IM: 14–24 h IV: UK	24–36 d
Flutamide (Eulexin)	A: PO: 250 mg q8h *Note:* Give simultaneously with LHRH analog therapy, e.g., leuprolide acetate, 7.5 mg IM/mo	D	None known	5–6 h Elderly: 10 h	94–96%	UK	UK	UK
Goserelin acetate (Zoladex)	*Palliation prostate cancer:* A: SC: 3.6 mg into upper abdomen q28d	X	None known *Lab: Decrease* after initial increase in follicle-stimulating hormone, testosterone, luteinizing hormone	4–6 h	UK	UK	12–15 d	29 d
Mitotane (Lysodren)	*Palliation adrenal cortical carcinoma:* A: PO: 1–6 g/d in divided doses; increasing to 8–10 g/d in 3–4 divided doses; max: 18 g/d	C	*Increase* toxicity with CNS depressants *Decrease* effect of phenytoin, warfarin, barbiturates	20–160 d	UK	*Decrease* adrenocortical function 2–3 d	TR: 6 wk	UK

Megestrol acetate	*Breast cancer:* A: PO: 40 mg q.i.d. *Endometrial cancer:* A: PO: 40–320 mg/d in divided doses; max: 800 mg/d	X	*Decrease* effects with bromocriptine *Lab:* Altered liver function and thyroid tests	15–20 h	UK	response 6–8 wk	1–3 h	3–12 mo
Mitoxantrone (Novantrone)	*Solid tumor:* A: IV: 12 mg/m^2/d × 3; dilute with 50 mL NSS or D$_5$W over 15–30 min	D	Similar to daunorubicin	6 d	78%	7–10 d	14 d	21 d
Polyestradiol PO$_4$ (Estradurin)	*Palliation prostate cancer:* A: IM: 40 mg q2–4 wk; max: 80 mg	X	Unknown	UK	UK	UK	UK	UK
Progesterone (Gesterol 50, Progestaject, Progestasert)	*Endometrial and breast carcinoma:* A: IM: 5–10 mg/d for 6–8 d	X	*Lab:* Altered thyroid, liver function, coagulation tests	5 min	UK	UK	UK	24 h
Tamoxifen citrate (Nolvadex)	*Palliation/adjunctive treatment of breast carcinoma:* A: PO: 10–20 mg b.i.d	D	*Increase* toxicity of warfarin, cyclosporine, allopurinol *Lab: Increase* T$_4$	7 d	UK	Tumor response: 4–10 wk	3–6 mo	UK

KEY: For complete abbreviation key, see inside front cover.
Refer to specific protocol.

Biologic Response Modifiers

Epoetin Alfa (Erythropoietin [EPO])

Epoetin Alfa (Erythropoietin [EPO])
(Epogen, Procrit)
Pregnancy Category: C
Drug Forms:
Inj 2,000, 4,000 U/mL

Dosage

A: 50–100 U/kg 3 × wk
  IV: Dialysis clients
IV/SC: Nondialysis, CRF clients
IV/SC: 100 U/kg 3 × wk for 8 wk in
  AZT-treated HIV-infected clients
Initial dose to those with EPO levels
  <500 mU/mL and receiving
  <4,200 mg of AZT/wk. Clients
  with EPO level >500 mU/mL are
  unlikely to respond to EPO
  therapy.

Contraindications

Uncontrolled hypertension,
  hypersensitivity to mammalian
  cell–derived products or human
  albumin
Caution: Pregnancy, lactation,
  porphyria; safety in children not
  known

Drug-Lab-Food Interactions

Drug: None known
Lab: Increase hematocrit, decreased
  plasma volume

Pharmacokinetics

Absorption: UK
Distribution: PB: UK
Metabolism: t 1/2: 4–13 h in clients
  with CRF; 20% less in those with
  normal renal function
Excretion: In urine

Pharmacodynamics

IV: Onset: 1 wk to 10 d
  Peak: 2–4 wk
  Duration: UK
SC: Onset: 1 wk to 10 d
  Peak: 5–24 h
  Duration: UK

Therapeutic Effects/Uses: To treat anemia secondary to CRF or AZT (zidovudine) treatment of HIV infections. Use in clients with anemia secondary to cancer or its treatment is under investigation.

Mode of Action: Increased production of RBCs, triggered by hypoxia or anemia.

Side Effects

Sense of well-being, hypertension,
  arthralgias, nausea, edema, fatigue,
  injection site reaction, rash,
  diarrhea, shortness of breath

Adverse Reactions

Seizures, hyperkalemia
Life-threatening: Cerebral vascular
  accident, MI

KEY: For complete abbreviation key, see inside front cover.

■ NURSING PROCESS: Biologic Response Modifiers

ASSESSMENT

- Obtain baseline information about the client's physical status, including height, weight, VS, laboratory values (CBC, uric acid, electrolytes, BUN, creatinine, and liver function tests), cardiopulmonary assessment, intake and output, skin assessment, daily activities status (ability to perform activities of daily living, sleep-rest cycle), nutritional status, presence or absence of underlying symptoms of disease, and the use of current or past medication and treatment.
- Assess CBC and platelet count (with **filgrastim** and **sargramostim**) before therapy and biweekly throughout therapy to avoid leukocytosis. Assess renal and hepatic function tests in clients with dysfunction (liver enzymes, BUN, serum creatinine). With **erythropoietin**, assess blood pressure before start and especially early in therapy. Most clients will need supplemental iron. Desired levels are >100 ng/mL for serum ferritin and >20% for serum iron transferrin saturation.
- Obtain baseline data regarding the client's psychosocial status, including educational level, ability and desire to learn, support systems, past coping strategies, presence or absence of emotional difficulties, and self-care abilities.
- Assess the client for signs and symptoms of biologic response modifiers (BRM), such as fatigue, chills, diarrhea, and weakness. With **filgrastim**, be alert to changes in clients with preexisting cardiac conditions.
- Assess the client's and family's ability to administer subcutaneous BRM.
- Determine the client's and family's understanding of BRM and related side effects.

POTENTIAL NURSING DIAGNOSES

Altered nutrition; less than body requirements
High risk for infection
High risk for fluid volume deficit
Altered oral mucous membrane
Fatigue
Body image disturbance
Anxiety
Fear
High risk for caregiver role strain

PLANNING

- Client and family will verbalize an understanding of the importance of reporting BRM-related side effects.
- Client and family will demonstrate correct and safe BRM administration.
- Client and family will identify strategies to deal with BRM-related side effects.
- Client will remain free of infection (**filgrastim** and **sargramostim**).

NURSING INTERVENTIONS

- Monitor the client's temperature at the onset of chills.
- Administer prescribed meperidine 25–50 mg IV to decrease rigors.
- Premedicate the client with acetaminophen to reduce chills and fever and with diphenhydramine to reduce nausea.
- Cover the client with blankets to promote warmth during chills.

(text continues on page 235)   **233**

Granulocyte Colony–Stimulating Factor

Filgrastim

Filgrastim
  (Neupogen)
Granulocyte colony–stimulating
  factor (G-CSF)
Pregnancy Category: C
Drug Forms:
Vial 300 µg/mL; 480 µg/1.6 mL

Dosage

A: IV inf/SC: 5 µg/kg/d
C: 5–10 µg/kg/d
Refer to specific protocols.

Contraindications

Hypersensitivity to *E. coli*–derived
  proteins; 24 h before or after
  cytotoxic chemotherapy
Caution: Pregnancy, lactation; safety
  in children not known

Drug-Lab-Food Interactions

Drug: None known
Lab: Increase lactic acid, LDH, alkaline
  phosphatase; transient *increase* in
  neutrophils

Pharmacokinetics

Absorption: SC: Well absorbed
Distribution: PB: UK
Metabolism: t 1/2: 2–3.5 h
Excretion: Probably in urine

Pharmacodynamics

IV/SC: Onset: 24 h
        Peak: 3–5 d
        Duration: 4–7 d

Therapeutic Effects/Uses: To decrease incidence of infection in clients receiving myelosuppressive chemotherapeutic agents; adjunct to chemotherapy for both solid tumor and hematologic malignancies.

Mode of Action: Increases production of neutrophils and enhances their phagocytosis.

Side Effects

Nausea, vomiting, skeletal pain,
  alopecia, diarrhea, fever, skin rash,
  anorexia, headache, cough, chest
  pain, sore throat, constipation

Adverse Reactions

Neutropenia, dyspnea,
  splenomegaly, psoriasis, hematuria
Life-threatening: Thrombocytopenia,
  myocardial infarction, adult
  respiratory distress syndrome in
  clients with sepsis

KEY: For complete abbreviation key, see inside front cover.
See page 233 for Nursing Process.

- Encourage the client to rest when tired and to notify health care provider if profound fatigue or anorexia occurs.
- Encourage the client to drink at least 2 L of fluid a day to promote excretion of cellular breakdown products.
- Administer antiemetic as necessary. Premedicate the client with antiemetic and administer antiemetic around the clock for 24 h after BRM administration to further delay nausea or vomiting.
- Consult the dietitian, social worker, and physical or occupational therapist as necessary.
- Provide the client and family the opportunity to discuss the effect of BRM therapy on the quality of life.
- Refer the client and family to a financial counselor if reimbursement of BRM therapy is problematic.
- Administer BRM at bedtime to decrease the consequences of fatigue.
- Continue with the same brand of BRM, and notify the health care provider if you are considering changing the brand.
- Remember, with **sargramostim**, use only one dose per vial; be alert for expiration date. Avoid shaking vial. Reconstituted solutions are clear; use within 6 h and discard unused portion. Recall that albumin may be added, depending on drug concentration, to prevent adsorption of drug to components of the drug delivery system.
- Remember, with **filgrastim**, drug vials are for one-time use; any vial left at room temperature for more than 6 h should be discarded. Drug vials are preservative free. Store in refrigerator at 2–8°C. Avoid shaking vials.

CLIENT AND FAMILY TEACHING

General

- Explain to the client and family the rationale for BRM therapy.
- Explain the frequency and rationale for studies and procedures during BRM therapy.
- Inform the client and family that most BRM side effects disappear within 72–96 h after discontinuation of therapy.
- Instruct clients of childbearing age to use contraceptives during BRM therapy and for 2 y after completion of therapy.
- Provide the client with information regarding the effect on sexuality of BRM-related fatigue.

Side Effects

- Advise the client to report episodes of difficulty in concentration, confusion, or somnolence.
- Report weight loss.
- Report dyspnea, palpitations, and signs of infection or bleeding.

Skill

- Demonstrate correct drug administration techniques.
- Provide the client and family with written or video instructions regarding BRM self-administration.

EVALUATION

- Evaluate the client's and family's education strategies by asking them to discuss the potential effect of BRM therapy on the quality of life.
- Evaluate the client's and family's BRM self-administration technique.

(text continues on page 237)

Granulocyte Macrophage Colony–Stimulating Factor

Sargramostim

Sargramostim
(Leukine, Prokine)
Granulocyte macrophage
colony–stimulating factor
(GM-CSF)

Pregnancy Category: C

Drug Forms:
Powder in vial 250 μg (Leukine only)
and 500 μg of sargramostim

Dosage

A: IV: 250 μg/m²/d as a 2-h inf for 21
d after autologous BMT; a
maximum tolerated dose has not
been determined
Some protocols use SC
administration.

Contraindications

Within 24 h of chemotherapy
administration or within 12 h after
last dose of radiation therapy,
excessive leukemia myeloid blast
cells in bone marrow,
hypersensitivity to GM-CSF, yeast-
derived products

Caution: Pregnancy, lactation,
congestive heart failure; safety in
children not established; not FDA
approved for children

Drug-Lab-Food Interactions

Lithium and steroids may *increase*
effect
Lab: Increase in WBC and platelet
counts

Pharmacokinetics

Absorption: IV: Essentially complete
Distribution: PB: UK
Metabolism: t 1/2: 2 h
Excretion: Probably in urine

Pharmacodynamics

IV: Onset: 7–14 d
   Peak: UK
   Duration: Baseline WBC by 1 wk
   after administration

Therapeutic Effects/Uses: To accelerate growth and development of bone marrow
and circulating blood cell activity in autologous BMT.

Mode of Action: Increased production and functional activity of eosinophils,
macrophages, monocytes, and neutrophils.

Side Effects

Generally well tolerated; diarrhea,
fatigue, chills, weakness, local
irritation at injection site,
peripheral edema, rash

Adverse Reactions

Pleural/pericardial effusion, rigors,
GI hemorrhage, dyspnea

KEY: For complete abbreviation key, see inside front cover.
See pages 233, 235, 237 for Nursing Process.

- Evaluate periodically the client's and family's management of BRM-related side effects.
- There will be a decreased incidence of infection in clients after autologous bone marrow transplant.

Biologic Response Modifiers: Interferons

Generic (Brand)	Route and Dosage	Preg Cat	Interaction	t1/2	PB	Onset	Peak	Duration
							Action	
Interferon alfa-2a (Roferon-A)	*Hairy cell leukemia, condylomata acuminata:* A: SC/IM: 3 million IU daily for 16–24 wk	C	*Increase* toxicity with vinblastine; *increase* effects of theophylline, cimetidine	IM/IV: 2–3 h SC: 3 h	UK	Myelosuppression: 7–10 d	6–8 h Nadir: 14 d	Recovery: 21 d
Interferon alfa-2b (Intron-A)	A: SC: 2 million IU/m² 3 × wk *Kaposi sarcoma:* A: IM/SC/IV: Initially: 36 million IU daily for 10–12 wk; maint: 36 million IU 3 × wk	C	*Increase* toxicity effect with vinblastine, cimetidine	IM/IV: 2 h SC: 3 h	UK	7–10 d	14 d	21 d
Interferon gamma-1b (Actimmune)	*Body surface area >0.5 m²:* A: SC: 50 µg/m² 3 × wk *Body surface area <0.5 m²:* A&C <1 y: SC: 1.5 µg/kg 3 × wk	C	*Increase* bone marrow depression with other antineoplastics or radiation therapy	SC: 6 h IM: 3 h IV: 0.5 h	UK	UK	SC: 7 h IM: 4 h IV: UK	UK
Interferon alfa-N3 (Alferon N)	*Condylomata acuminata:* A: Inject into wart: 250,000 U (0.05 mL) twice weekly; max: 8 wk Do *not* repeat for >3 mo after end of therapy	C	Similar to interferon alfa-2a	UK	UK	7–10 d	14 d	21 d
Interferon beta-1b (Betaseron)	*Reduce number of clinical exacerbations of multiple sclerosis:* A >18 y: SC: 8 million U q.o.d. C: Not recommended	C	Not fully evaluated; none significant known	0.5–4 h	UK	UK	1–8 h	UK

KEY: For complete abbreviation key, see inside front cover.

NOTES:

RESPIRATORY AGENTS

Antihistamines

Antitussives and Expectorants

Decongestants

Bronchodilators:
Adrenergic
Methylxanthine

Antihistamine

Diphenhydramine HCl

Diphenhydramine HCl
 (Benadryl)
Antihistamine
Pregnancy Category: B
Drug Forms:
Cap 25, 50 mg
Tab 50 mg
Elix, syrup 12.5 mg/5 mL
Inj 10, 50 mg/mL
Topical 1–2% cream, lotion

Dosage

A: PO: 25–50 mg q6–8h
A: IM/IV: 10–50 mg as single dose;
 max: 400 mg/d
C: PO/IM/IV 5 mg/kg/d in 4
 divided doses; max: 300 mg/d

Contraindications

Acute asthmatic attack, severe liver
 disease, lower respiratory disease,
 neonate
Caution: Narrow-angle glaucoma,
 benign prostatic hypertrophy,
 pregnancy, newborn or premature
 infant, breast feeding; sinus
 infection

Drug-Lab-Food Interactions

Increase CNS depression with alcohol,
 narcotics, hypnotics, barbiturates;
 avoid use of MAOIs
Decrease effects of oral anticoagulants

Pharmacokinetics

Absorption: PO: Well absorbed
Distribution: PB: 82%
Metabolism: t 1/2: 2–7 h
Excretion: In urine as metabolites

Pharmacodynamics

PO: Onset: 15–45 min
 Peak: 1–4 h
 Duration: 4–8 h
IM: Onset: 15–30 min
 Peak: 1–4 h
 Duration: 4–7 h
IV: Onset: Immediate
 Peak: 0.5–1 h
 Duration: 4–7 h

Therapeutic Effects/Uses: To treat allergic rhinitis, itching; to prevent motion sickness; sleep aid

Mode of Action: Blocks histamine, thereby decreasing allergic response. Effects respiratory system, blood vessels, and GI system.

Side Effects

Drowsiness, dizziness, fatigue,
 nausea, vomiting, urinary
 retention, constipation, blurred
 vision, dry mouth and throat,
 reduced secretions, hypotension,
 epigastric distress, vision and
 hearing disturbances; excitation in
 children

Adverse Reactions

Life threatening: Agranulocytosis,
 hemolytic anemia,
 thrombocytopenia

KEY: For complete abbreviation key, see inside front cover.

■ NURSING PROCESS: Diphenhydramine

ASSESSMENT
- Obtain baseline VS.
- Obtain drug history; report if drug-drug interaction is probable.
- Assess for signs and symptoms of urinary dysfunction, including retention, dysuria, and frequency.
- Assess CBC during drug therapy.
- Assess cardiac and respiratory status.
- If allergic reaction, obtain history of environmental exposures, drugs, recent foods, and stress.

POTENTIAL NURSING DIAGNOSES
Fluid volume deficit, potential
Sleep pattern disturbance

PLANNING
- Client will have improvement of histamine-associated (allergy) effects.
- Client will have improved sleep, if used as a sleep aid.

NURSING INTERVENTIONS
- Give with food to decrease gastric distress.
- Administer IM in large muscle. Avoid SC injection.

CLIENT TEACHING
General
- Instruct client to avoid driving a motor vehicle and other dangerous activities if drowsiness occurs or until stabilized on drug.
- Avoid alcohol and other CNS depressants.
- Instruct client to take drug as prescribed. Notify health care provider if confusion or hypotension occurs.
- For prophylaxis of motion sickness, take drug 30 min before offending event and then before meals and h.s. during the event.

EVALUATION
- Evaluate effectiveness of drug in relieving allergic symptoms or as a sleep aid.

Antihistamines for Treatment of Allergic Rhinitis

Generic (Brand)	Route and Dosage	Preg Cat	Interaction	t 1/2	PB	Action: Onset	Action: Peak	Action: Duration
Antihistamines Chlorpheniramine maleate (Chlor-Trimeton, Kloromin, Phenetron, Telechlor, Teldrin)	A: PO: 2–4 mg q4–6h; max: 24 mg/24 h SR: 8–12 mg q8–12 h C: 6–12 y: PO: 2 mg q4–6h	C	*Increase* effect of drug with MAOIs; *increase* CNS depression *Decrease* effects of oral anticoagulants, heparin	20–24 h	72%	20–60 min	6 h	8–12 h
Diphenhydramine (Benadryl)	See Prototype Drug Chart							
Phenothiazines (Antihistamine Action) Promethazine HCl (Phenergan, Prometh, Prorex, V-Gan)	A: PO/IM: 12.5–25 mg q4–6h PRN a.c. & h.s. C: PO/IM: 0.5 mg/kg q4–6h Tab & suppository not recommended <2 y	C	Similar to chlorpheniramine	UK	UK	PO: 20 min IM: 3–5 min	UK	4–6 h
Trimeprazine tartrate (Temaril)	*Non-SR:* A: PO: 2.5 mg q.i.d. C 3–12 y: PO: 2.5 mg t.i.d. C 0.5–3 y: 1.25 mg t.i.d. *SR:* A: PO: 5 mg q12h C >6 y: PO: 5 mg/d	C	Similar to chlorpheniramine	5 h	UK	15–60 min	4 h	UK
Piperazine Derivative Hydroxyzine (Atarax, Vistaril)	A: PO: 25–100 mg t.i.d./q.i.d. C >6 y: 50–100 mg/d in divided doses *For pruritus:* C: <6 y: PO: 50 mg/d in divided doses	C	*Increase* CNS depression with alcohol, analgesics, barbiturates, narcotics *Decrease* effects of epinephrine	3 h	UK	15–30 min	<2 h	4–6 h

	Dosage	Pregnancy Category	Drug Interactions	Half-Life	Protein Binding	Onset	Peak	Duration
Butyrophenone Derivative								
Terfenadine (Seldane)	A: PO: 60 mg b.i.d. C >6 y: PO: 30 mg b.i.d. C 3–6 y: PO: 15 mg b.i.d.	C	Cardiotoxic effects with erythromycin, ketoconazole; *Increase* effects with pseudoephedrine	20 h	97%	60–90 min	3–4 h	>12 h
Ethanolamine Derivative								
Carbinoxamine and pseudoephedrine (Carbiset, Carbodec, Rondec, Filmtab)	A: PO: 5 mL q.i.d. or 1 tab q.i.d. C <18 mo: PO: 0.25–1 mL q.i.d. C 1.5–6 y: PO: 2.5 mL t.i.d./q.i.d. C >6 y: PO: 5 mL b.i.d./q.i.d.	C	*Increase* toxicity of tricyclic antidepressants, barbiturates; *increase* toxicity with MAOIs	10–20 h	UK	15–60 min	UK	UK
Clemastine fumarate (Tavist)	A: PO: 1.5–2.5 mg b.i.d./t.i.d.; max: 8 mg/d C <12 y: PO: 0.4–1 mg b.i.d.	C	*Increase* toxicity with tricyclic antidepressants, CNS depressants, MAOIs, phenothiazines	UK	UK	15–60 min	5–7 h	12 h
Ethylenediamine Derivative								
Tripelennamine HCl	A: PO: 25–50 mg q4–6h or SR: 100 mg q8–12h; max: 600 mg/d C: PO: 5 mg/kg/d in 4–6 divided doses; max: 300 mg/d Note: 5 mL of tripelennamine citrate elix = 25 mg HCl	B	*Increase* CNS depression with alcohol, CNS depressants; *increase* anticholinergic effects with MAOIs	UK	UK	15–30 min	2–3 h	4–6 h SR: 8 h

continued

Antihistamines for Treatment of Allergic Rhinitis *Continued*

Generic (Brand)	Route and Dosage	Preg Cat	Interaction	t 1/2	PB	Onset	Peak	Duration
							Action	
						Onset	Peak	Duration
Piperidine Derivatives								
Azatadine maleate (Optimine)	A: PO: 1–2 mg b.i.d.	B	*Increase* effect/toxicity with CNS depressants, alcohol, tricyclic antidepressants, procarbazine	9–12 h	UK	Rapid	4 h	12 h
Cyproheptadine HCl	A: PO: 4–20 mg/d divided q8h; max: 0.5 mg/kg/d C >6 y: PO: 4 mg q8–12h; max: 16 mg/d	B	*Increase* toxicity with MAOIs	UK	UK	15–60 min	UK	8 h
Propylamine Derivatives								
Brompheniramine maleate (Bromphen, Dimetane, Histaject, Nasahist B, Oraminic II)	A: PO: 4 mg q4–6h or SR: 8 mg q8–12h; max: 12 mg/d IM/IV/SC: 10 mg q6–12h; max: 40 mg/d C 6–12 y: PO: 2–4 mg q6–8h; max: 12–16 mg/d	C	*Increase* toxicity with MAOIs, tricyclic antidepressants, CNS depressants	25–36 h	UK	15–60 min	3–9 h	4–25 h
Dexchlorpheniramine maleate (Dexchlor, Poladex, Polaramine, Polargen)	A: PO: 2 mg q4–6h or SR: 4–6 mg q8–10h or h.s. C >6 y: PO: 1 mg q4–6h or SR: 4 mg h.s.	B	*Increase* toxicity with MAOIs, tricyclic antidepressants, CNS depressants, phenothiazines, guanabenz	UK	UK	15–60 min	3 h	3–6 h
Triprolidine and pseudoephedrine	A: PO: 2–5 mg q4–6h; max: 10 mg/d C >6 y: PO: 1.25 mg q6–8h	B	*Increase* effect with MAOIs	3 h	UK	15–60 min	2–3 h	4–8 h

Drug	Dosage		Drug interactions					
Triprolidine HCl (Actidil, Myidyl)	A: PO: 2.5 mg b.i.d./t.i.d.; max: 10 mg/d C 6–12 y: PO: 1.25 mg b.i.d./t.i.d.; max: 5 mg/d C 2–5 y: PO: 0.6 mg t.i.d./q.i.d.; max: 2.5 mg/d C 4 mo–2 y: PO: 0.3 mg t.i.d./q.i.d.; max: 1.25 mg/d	C	*Increase* effects with alcohol, CNS depressants, MAOIs	3 h	UK	Rapid	3–5 h	8 h
Other								
Cromolyn sodium (Intal)	*Prophylaxis bronchial asthma:* A&C >5 y: Inhal: 2 metered sprays or PO: 20 mg ≤1 h before exercise *Allergic rhinitis:* A&C >5 y: 1 spray per nostril t.i.d./q.i.d.; max: 6 per day	B	None significant reported *Not* used for acute asthma attacks	90 min	UK	PO: UK Inhal: <1 wk Spray: <1 wk	2–3 wk 2–4 wk 2–4 wk	UK UK UK
Miscellaneous								
Astemizole (Hismanal)	A: PO: 30 mg on day 1; 20 mg on day 2, 10 mg on day 3; take on empty stomach C 6–12 y: PO: 5 mg/d C <6 y: PO: 0.2 mg/kg/d	C	*Increase* toxicity with CNS depressants; cardiotoxicity with triazole antifungals, macrolide antibiotics	2.5 d	96%	2–3 d	9–12 d	Weeks after discontinuing drug
Cetirizine	A: 5–10 mg/d	C	Caution with erythromycin, ketoconazole	8 h	93%	15–60 min	1 h	UK
Loratadine (Claritin)	A: PO 10 mg daily	B	None significant reported	8–11 h	UK	30 min	4–6 h	>24 h
Methdilazine HCl (Tacaryl)	A: PO: 8 mg b.i.d./q.i.d. C >3 y: PO: 4 mg b.i.d./q.i.d.	C	*Increase* toxicity with CNS depressants	UK	UK	15–60 min	UK	6–12 h

KEY: For complete abbreviation key, see inside front cover.

Antitussive

Dextromethorphan hydrobromide

Dextromethorphan hydrobromide
 (Robitussin DM, Romilar, Sucrets
 Cough Control, PediCare 1,
 Benylin DM, and others)
OTC preparation
Antitussive
Pregnancy Category: C
Drug Forms:
Lozenge 5 mg
Sol 5, 7.5, 10, 15 mg/mL

Dosage

A: PO: 10–30 mg q4–8h; max:
 120 mg/24 h
C 6–12 y: PO: 5–10 mg q4–6h; max:
 60 mg/d
C 2–5 y: PO: 2.5–7.5 mg q4–8h; max:
 30 mg/d
Sustained Action Liquid (Delsym):
A: 60 mg q12h
C 6–12 y: 30 mg q12h
C 2–5 y: 15 mg q12h

Contraindications

Chronic obstructive pulmonary
 disease, chronic productive cough,
 hypersensitivity, clients taking
 MAOIs

Drug-Lab-Food Interactions

Increase effect/toxicity with MAOIs,
 narcotics, sedative-hypnotics,
 barbiturates, antidepressants,
 alcohol

Pharmacokinetics

Absorption: PO: Rapidly absorbed
Distribution: PB: UK
Metabolism: t 1/2: UK
Excretion: In urine, UK

Pharmacodynamics

PO: Onset: 15–30 min
 Peak: UK
 Duration: 3–6 h

Therapeutic Effects/Uses: To provide temporary suppression of a nonproductive cough; to reduce viscosity of tenacious secretions.
Mode of Action: Inhibition of the cough center in the medulla.

Side Effects

Nausea, dizziness, drowsiness,
 sedation

Adverse Reactions

Hallucinations at high doses
Life threatening: None known

KEY: For complete abbreviation key, see inside front cover.

■ **NURSING PROCESS: Dextromethorphan Hydrobromide**

ASSESSMENT
- Obtain baseline VS. Report and document abnormal findings.

POTENTIAL NURSING DIAGNOSES
Fatigue
Sleep deprivation due to chronic coughing
High risk for infection

PLANNING
- Client will be free of nonproductive cough. A secondary bacterial infection does not occur.

NURSING INTERVENTIONS
- Monitor VS.
- Observe color of secretions.

CLIENT TEACHING
General
- Instruct the client to maintain adequate fluid intake.
- Advise the client not to drive a motor vehicle or operate dangerous machinery.
- Instruct the client to avoid environmental pollutants, smoking, and dust.
- Instruct the client to get adequate rest.
- Instruct the client not to take a cold remedy near or at bedtime. Insomnia may occur if it contains a decongestant.
- Instruct the client/parents to have child perform three effective coughs before bedtime to promote uninterrupted sleep.
- Instruct the client/parents to keep the drug stored out of reach of small children; request child safety caps.
- Advise the client to contact the health care provider if cough persists for >1 wk or is combined with chest pain, fever, or headache.

Skill
- Instruct the client to cough effectively, to take deep breaths before coughing and be in the upright position.

EVALUATION
- Evaluate the effectiveness of the drug therapy. Determine that the client is free of a nonproductive cough, has adequate fluid intake and rest, and is afebrile.

Generic (Brand)	Route and Dosage	Preg Cat	t1/2	PB	Onset	Peak	Duration
						Action	
					Onset	Peak	Duration
Narcotic Antitussives							
Codeine CSS II	A: PO: 10–20 mg q4–6h; max: 120 mg/d C 6–12 y: 5–10 mg q4–6h; max: 60 mg/d C 2–6 y: 2.5–5 mg q4–6h; max: 30 mg/d	C	2–4 h	7%	15–30 min	1–2 h	4–6 h
Guaifenesin and codeine (Cheracol, Medi-Tuss A-C, Robitussin A-C) CSS V	*Temporary relief of cough due to minor irritation:* A: PO: 5–10 mL q6–8h	C	UK	UK	15–30 min	UK	UK
Hydrocodone (Hycodan) CSS III	A: PO: 5–10 mg q6–8h C: PO: 0.6 mg/kg/d in 3–4 divided doses, not to exceed 10 mg/single dose	C	3–4 h	UK	30–60 min	UK	3–6 h
Nonnarcotic Antitussives							
Benzonatate (Tessalon)	*Relief of nonproductive cough:* A: PO: 100 mg t.i.d. or q4h; max: 600 mg/d	C	UK	UK	15–30 min	UK	3–8 h

Interaction column:
- Codeine: *Increase* CNS depression with alcohol, narcotics, barbiturates, antipsychotics, muscle relaxants
- Guaifenesin and codeine: *Increase* sedation with CNS depressants
- Hydrocodone: *Increase* CNS depression with alcohol barbiturates, antipsychotics, general anesthesia, tricyclic antidepressants
- Benzonatate: *Increase* sedation with CNS depressants

Drug	Route and Dosage	Pregnancy Category	Drug Interactions					
Dextromethorphan hydrobromide (Benylin, Romilar, Sucrets cough control, and others)	See Prototype Drug Chart							
Diphenhydramine (Benadryl)	See Prototype Drug Chart							
Promethazine with dextromethorphan	A: PO: 5 mL q4–6h; max: 30 mL/d C 6–12 y: PO: 2.5–5 mL q4–6h; max: 20 mL/d	C	*Increase* sedation with CNS depressants	UK	UK	15–30 min	UK	6–12 h
Expectorants								
Guaifenesin (Robitussin)	A: PO: 100–400 mg q4h; max: 2.4 g/d C 6–12 y: PO: 100–200 mg q4h; max: 1.2 g/d C 2–5 y: PO: 50–100 mg q4h; max: 600 mg/d	C	None significant	UK	UK	30 min	UK	4–6 h
Iodinated glycerol (Iophen, Organidin)	A: PO: 60 mg q.i.d.; sol: 20 gtt q.i.d.; elix: 5 mL q.i.d. C: PO: Up to half adult dose according to weight	X	*Increase* toxicity with MAOIs, lithium, CNS depressants	UK	UK	UK	UK	UK
Potassium iodide (SSKI)	A: PO: 300–650 mg t.i.d/q.i.d. C: PO: 60–250 mg q6–8h	D	*Increase* toxicity with lithium	UK	UK	UK	UK	UK
Antitussive/ Expectorant								
Guaifenesin and dextromethorphan (Robitussin-DM)	A: PO: 10 mL q6–8h	C	*Increase* toxicity with MAOIs	UK	UK	15–30 min	UK	4–6 h

KEY: For complete abbreviation key, see inside front cover.

Systemic and Nasal Decongestants (Sympathomimetic Amines)

Generic (Brand)	Route and Dosage	Preg Cat	Interaction	t 1/2	PB	Onset	Peak	Duration
							Action	
Ephedrine SO$_4$ (Ectasule, Vicks Vatronol)	A: PO: 25–50 mg t.i.d./q.i.d. PRN SC/IM/IV: 25–50 mg; may repeat q10min; max: 150 mg/24 h	C	May cause hypertensive crises with MAOIs *Increase* adverse reactions to theophylline	3–6 h	UK	PO: 15–60 min IM: 30–60 min	UK	3–5 h 12 h
Naphazoline HCl (Allerest)	A&C >12 y: 2 gtt or 0.05% spray in each nostril; q3–6h ≤ 5 d	C	Similar to phenylephrine	UK	UK	<10 min	UK	2–6 h
Oxymetazoline HCl (Afrin)	A&C >6 y: 0.05% gtt or spray; 2–3 gtt q nostril b.i.d. C 2–5 y (0.025% gtt only): 2–3 gtt b.i.d. (q10–12h)	C	Similar to phenylephrine	UK	UK	5–10 min	UK	5–6 h
Phenylephrine HCl (Neo-Synephrine, Sinex)	A: Sol (0.25–1%): 2–3 gtt or sprays in each nostril q3–4h C 6–12 y: Sol (0.25%): 2–3 gtt or sprays in each nostril q3–4h C 6 mo–5 y: Sol (0.125–0.16%): 1–2 gtt in each nostril q3h	C	*Increase* pressor effects with MAOIs, beta blockers	2.5 h	UK	15–30 min	UK	1–4 h

Drug	Dosage		Interactions/Comments	Half-life		Onset		Duration
Phenylpropanolamine HCl (Propadrine, Dimetapp)	A: PO: 25–50 mg t.i.d./q.i.d.; max: 150 mg/d C 6–12 y: 12.5 mg q4h; max: 75 mg/d C 2–5 y: 6.25 mg q4h	B	Similar to phenylephrine	3–4 h	UK	UK	PO: 15–30 min SR: 60 min	UK	3 h 12–14 h
Pseudoephedrine (Actifed, Novafed, Sudafed)	A: PO: 60 mg q4–6h; 120 mg SR q12h; max: 240 mg/d C 6–12 y: 30 mg q4–6h; max: 120 mg/d C 2–5 y: 15 mg q4–6h; max: 60 mg/d C 1–2 y: 7 gtt (0.2 mL)/kg q4–6h; max: 4 doses/d C 3–12 mo: 3 gtt/kg q4–6h; max: 4 doses/d	C	Similar to phenylephrine	9–15 h	UK	UK	PO: 15–30 min SR: 60 min	UK	4–6 h 12 h
Tetrahydrozoline HCl (Tyzine)	A&C >6 y: 2–4 gtt (0.1%) or spray q4–6h PRN C 2–6 y: 2–3 gtt (0.05%) q4–6h PRN Direct medical supervision for use >3–4 d	C	Hypotension with reserpine, methyldopa; may cause hypertensive crises with MAOIs	UK	UK	UK	UK		4–8 h
Xylometazoline HCl (Otrivin)	A&C >12 y: 2–3 gtt (0.1%) or spray q8–10h C <12 y: 2–3 gtt (0.5%) or spray q8–10h	C	Similar to tetrahydrozoline	UK	UK	<5–10 min	UK		5–10 h

KEY: For complete abbreviation key, see inside front cover.

Bronchodilator: Adrenergic

Metaproterenol SO$_4$

Metaproterenol SO$_4$
  (Alupent, Metaprel)
Adrenergic bronchodilator
Pregnancy Category: C
Drug Forms:
Tab 10, 20 mg
Syrup 10 mg/mL
Sol neb 0.6%, 5%
Aerosol 0.65 mg/dose

Dosage

A&C >9 y and >27 kg: PO: 20 mg
  t.i.d./q.i.d.
C: 6–9 y or <27 kg: PO: 10 mg
  t.i.d./q.i.d.
A&C >12 y: MDI: 2–3 inhalations as
  single dose; wait 2 min before
  second dose, if necessary; use only
  q3–4h to maximum of 12
  inhalations/d

Contraindications

Hypersensitivity, dysrhythmias
Caution: Narrow-angle glaucoma,
  cardiac disease, hypertension

Drug-Lab-Food Interactions

Increase action of both with
  sympathomimetics
Decrease with beta blockers
Lab: Decreased serum potassium

Pharmacokinetics

Absorption: PO: Well absorbed
Distribution: PB: UK
Metabolism: t 1/2: UK
Excretion: In urine as metabolites

Pharmacodynamics

PO: Onset: 15–30 min
    Peak: 1 h
    Duration: 4 h
MDI: Onset: 1–5 min
    Peak: 1 h
    Duration: 3–4 h

Therapeutic Effects/Uses: To treat bronchospasm, asthma; to promote bronchodilation.

Mode of Action: Relaxation of smooth muscle of bronchi.

Side Effects

Nervousness, tremors, restlessness,
  insomnia, headache, nausea,
  vomiting, hyperglycemia, muscle
  cramping in extremities

Adverse Reactions

Tachycardia, palpitations,
  hypertension
Life threatening: Cardiac
  dysrhythmias, cardiac arrest,
  paradoxical bronchoconstriction

KEY: For complete abbreviation key, see inside front cover.

■ NURSING PROCESS: Bronchodilator: Adrenergic

ASSESSMENT

- Obtain a medical and drug history; report probable drug-drug interactions.
- Obtain baseline VS for abnormalities and for future comparisons.
- Assess for wheezing, decreased breath sounds, cough, and sputum production.
- Assess sensorium levels for confusion and restlessness due to hypoxia and hypercapnia.
- Assess hydration; diuresis may result in dehydration in the elderly and children.

POTENTIAL NURSING DIAGNOSES
Airway clearance, ineffective
Noncompliance with drug therapy

PLANNING
• Client will be free of wheezing and lung fields will be clear within 2–5 d.
• Client is taking oral drug(s) and using inhaler as prescribed.

NURSING INTERVENTIONS
• Monitor VS. Blood pressure and heart rate can increase greatly. Check for cardiac dysrhythmias.
• Provide adequate hydration. Fluids aid in loosening secretions. Monitor drug therapy. Observe for side effects.
• Administer medication after meals to decrease GI distress.

CLIENT TEACHING
Skill
• Instruct to correctly use the inhaler or nebulizer. Caution against overuse since side effects and tolerance may result.
Correct use of metered-dose inhaler to deliver beta$_2$ agonist:
1. Insert the medication canister into the plastic holder.
2. Shake the inhaler well *before* using. Remove cap from mouthpiece.
3. Breathe *out* through the mouth. Open mouth wide and hold mouthpiece 1–2 inches from mouth. *Do not* put mouthpiece in mouth unless using a spacer. Discuss technique with health provider.
4. With mouth open, take *slow deep* breath through mouth and at same time push the top of the medication canister once.
5. Hold breath for a few seconds; then exhale slowly through pursed lips.
6. If a second dose is required, wait 2 min and repeat the procedure by first shaking the canister in the plastic holder with the cap on.
7. If the inhaler has not been used recently or when it is first used, "test spray" before administering the metered dose.
8. If a glucocorticoid inhalant is to be used with a bronchodilator, wait 5 min before using the inhaler containing the steroid for the bronchodilator effect.
• Teach client to monitor pulse rate.
• Teach client to monitor amount of medication remaining in the canister.
• Advise client not to take OTC preparations without first checking with the health care provider. Some OTC products may have an additive effect.
• Instruct the client to avoid smoking. Smoking increases drug elimination.
• Discuss ways to alleviate anxiety such as relaxation techniques and music.
• Advise client having asthma attacks to wear an ID bracelet or tags.

EVALUATION
• Evaluate the effectiveness of the bronchodilator. The client is breathing without wheezing and without side effects of the drug.

Sympathomimetics: Adrenergic Bronchodilators

Generic (Brand)	Route and Dosage	Preg Cat	Interaction	t1/2	PB	Onset	Peak	Duration
Alpha- and Beta-adrenergic Ephedrine SO$_4$	A: PO: 25–50 mg q3–4h; max: 400 mg/d PRN C >2 y: PO: 2–3 mg/kg/d in 4–6 divided doses C 6–12 y: PO: 6.25–12.5 mg q4h; max: 75 mg	C	*Increase* effects with tricyclic antidepressants, MAOIs, guanethidine, furazolidine	3–6 h	UK	15–60 min	15–60 min	2–4 h
Epinephrine (Adrenalin, Primatene Mist, Bronkaid Mist)	A: SC: 0.1–0.5 mg or mL of 1:1,000 sol; may repeat q10–15 min C: SC: 0.01 mg or mL of 1:1,000 sol; may repeat q20min–4h Inhal: 1–2 puffs of 1:100 q1–5 min	C	Hypertension with MAOIs; additive effect with other sympathomimetics	UK	UK	Inhal: 1 min SC: 3–5 min	20 min 20 min	1–3 h 20 min
Beta-Adrenergic Albuterol (Proventil, Ventolin)	A&C >6 y: Inhal: 1–2 puffs q4–6h or 2 puffs 15 min before exercise A: PO: 2–4 mg t.i.d. or q.i.d.; max: 8 mg q.i.d. SR: 4–8 mg q12h C 6–12 y: PO: 2 mg t.i.d/q.i.d. C 2–6 y: PO: 1 mg/kg t.i.d.	C	Similar to isoetharine	PO: 4–5 h Inhal: 2–3 h	UK	Inhal: 5–15 min PO: 30 min PO/SR: 30 min	30–90 min 2–3 h 2–3 h	4–6 h 4–6 h 8–12 h
Bitolterol mesylate (Tornalate)	A: Inhal: 2 (1–3 min apart) q6–8 h; max: 12 inhal/d	C	Similar to isoproterenol	3 h	UK	3–5 min	0.5–2 h	5–8 h

Drug	Preg. Cat.	Contraindications / Drug Interactions	Dosage			Onset	Peak	Duration
Isoetharine HCl (Bronkosol) Beta$_2$	C	Similar to isoproterenol; hypertensive crisis with MAOIs	Inhal: 1–2 puffs A: IPPB: 0.5–1.0 mL of 5% sol or 0.5 mL of 1% sol diluted in 3 mL of NSS	UK	UK	Inhal: Immediate	5–15 min	1–4 h
Isoproterenol (Isuprel) Beta$_1$ and beta$_2$	C	*Increase* effects with other sympathomimetics *Decrease* action with beta blockers	A&C: Inhal: 1–2 puffs q4–6h A: SL: 10–20 mg q6–8h C: SL: 5–10 mg q6–8h	2–5 min	UK	Inhal: Immediate SL: 15–30 min	UK	1 h / 2 h
Metaproterenol sulfate (Alupent, Metaprel) Beta$_1$ and beta$_2$			See Prototype Drug Chart				1–2 h	
Pirbuterol acetate (Maxair)	C	*Increase* toxicity with MAOIs, tricyclic antidepressants, beta agonists	*Prevention:* A&C >12 y: Inhal: 2 q4–6h *Bronchospasm:* A&C >12 y: Inhal: 2 (1–3 min apart) followed by 1	2–3 h	UK	<5 min	2–3 h	5 h
Anticholinergics Ipratropium bromide (Atrovent)	B	Avoid use with anticholinergics Forms precipitate with cromolyn sodium	*COPD:* A: Inhal: 2 q.i.d. >4 h intervals; max: 12 inhal/d	1.5–2 h	UK	5–15 min	1.5–2 h	4–6 h
Salmeterol (Serevent)	C	*Increase* effects of MAOIs, tricyclic antidepressants	*Maintenance bronchodilation:* A&C >12 y: Inhal: 2 q12h *Prevention exercise-induced bronchospasm:* A&C >12 y: Inhal: 2 ≥30–60 min before exercise	5.5 h	94–98%	10–20 min	3 h	12 h

continued

Sympathomimetics: Adrenergic Bronchodilators *Continued*

Generic (Brand)	Route and Dosage	Preg Cat	Interaction	t 1/2	PB	Action		
						Onset	Peak	Duration
Terbutaline SO$_4$ (Brethine, Bricanyl) Beta$_2$	Inhal: 1–2 puffs q4–6h A: PO: 2.5–5 mg t.i.d. A: SC: 0.25–0.5 mg q8h IV: 10 μg/min, gradually increase; max: 80 μg/min C >12 y: PO: 2.5 mg t.i.d.	B	Similar to isoetharine	3–11 h	25%	Inhal: 5–30 min PO: 30 min SC: 6–15 min	1–2 h 1–2 h 30–60 min	3–6 h 4–8 h 1.5–4 h

KEY: For complete abbreviation key, see inside front cover.

NOTES:

Bronchodilator: Methylxanthine

Theophylline

Theophylline
  (Theo-Dur, Theophyllin KI,
  Elixophyllin-KI, Somophyllin, Slo-
  phyllin, Slo-bid, Quibron)
Methylxanthine, respiratory smooth
  muscle relaxant

Pregnancy Category: C

Drug Forms:
Cap 50, 100, 200, 250 mg
Cap SR 50, 65, 100, 125, 130, 200, 250,
  260, 300, 400, 500 mg
Tab 100, 125, 200, 225, 250, 300 mg
Tab SR 100, 200, 250, 300, 400, 500 mg
Susp 300 mg/15 mL
Elix 80, 11.25 mg/15 mL
Liq 80, 150, 160 mg/15 mL
Sol 80 mg/15 mL, with/without
  alcohol

Dosage

Bronchospasm, Bronchial Asthma:
A: PO: 250–500 mg q8–12h
C: PO: 50–100 mg q6h; max:
  12 mg/kg/d
Dosing is highly individualized and
  is based on titration to serum levels
  between 10 and 20 μg/mL.
  Monitor levels and client response.

Contraindications

Severe cardiac dysrhythmias,
  hyperthyroidism, hypersensitivity
  to xanthines, peptic ulcer disease,
  uncontrolled seizure disorder
Caution: With young children and
  elderly

Drug-Lab-Food Interactions

Increase effect with allopurinol, oral
  contraceptives, clindamycin
Decrease effects of neuromuscular
  blockers, phenytoin, lithium;
  decrease effect with smoking,
  rifampin, phenobarbital,
  corticosteroids, and others
Food: Increase metabolism with low-
  carbohydrate, high-protein diet
Decrease elimination with high-
  carbohydrate diet (*increase* t 1/2)
Lab: Interaction with laboratory result
  is not common; however, check
  with each laboratory

Pharmacokinetics

Absorption: PO: Well absorbed; SR:
  slowly absorbed
Distribution: PB: Approx 60%
Metabolism: t 1/2: 7–9 h nonsmokers;
  4–5 h smokers
Excretion: In urine

Pharmacodynamics

PO: Onset: 30 min
  Peak: 1–2 h
  Duration: 6 h
PO/SR: Onset: 1–3 h
  Peak: 4–8 h
  Duration: 8–24 h
IV: Onset: Rapid
  Peak: UK
  Duration: 6–8 h

Bronchodilator: Methylxanthine

Therapeutic Effects/Uses: To promote bronchodilation; to treat asthma and chronic obstructive pulmonary disease.

Mode of Action: Increased cyclic AMP results in bronchodilation, diuresis; cardiac, CNS, and gastric acid stimulation.

Side Effects	Adverse Reactions
Anorexia, nausea, vomiting, restlessness, dizziness, insomnia, flushing, rash, headache	Irritability, tremors, tachycardia, palpitations, urticaria *Life threatening:* Seizures, cardiac dysrhythmias, convulsions

KEY: For complete abbreviation key, see inside front cover.

■ NURSING PROCESS: Bronchodilator

ASSESSMENT

• Obtain a medical and drug history; report probable drug-drug interaction.
• Obtain baseline VS for identifying abnormalities and for future comparisons.
• Assess for wheezing, decreased breath sounds, cough, and sputum production.
• Assess sensorium levels for confusion and restlessness due to hypoxia and hypercapnia.
• Assess theophylline blood levels. Toxicity occurs at a higher frequency with levels of >20 μg/mL.
• Assess hydration; diuresis may result in dehydration in the elderly and children.

POTENTIAL NURSING DIAGNOSES

Airway clearance, ineffective
Activity intolerance
Knowledge deficit related to OTC drugs

PLANNING

• Client will be free of wheezing or significantly improved and lung fields will be clear within 2–5 d.
• Client is taking oral drug(s) and using inhaler as prescribed.

NURSING INTERVENTIONS

• Monitor VS. Blood pressure may decrease and heart rate may increase. Check for cardiac dysrhythmias.
• Provide adequate hydration. Fluids aid in loosening secretions. Monitor drug therapy. Observe for side effects.
• Check serum and plasma theophylline levels (normal level is 10–20 μg/mL).
• Administer medication at regular intervals around the clock to have a sustained therapeutic level.
• Administer medication after meals to decrease GI distress.
• Do *not* crush enteric-coated or SR tablets or capsules.

CLIENT TEACHING

General

- Advise the client that if allergic reaction occurs (rash, urticaria), drug should be discontinued and health care provider notified.
- Advise the client not to take OTC preparations without first checking with the health care provider. Some OTC products may have an additive effect.
- Encourage the client to stop smoking under medical supervision. Avoid changing smoking amounts acutely since levels are titrated to $10-20$ µg/mL. Smoking increases drug elimination.
- Discuss ways to alleviate anxiety such as relaxation techniques and music.
- Advise the client having frequent or severe asthma attacks to wear an ID bracelet or tags.
- Encourage the client contemplating pregnancy to seek medical advice before taking a theophylline preparation.
- Advise the client to keep drug stored out of reach of small children; request child safety caps.

Skill

- Instruct the client to correctly use the nebulizer in conjunction with theophylline.
- Teach the client to monitor pulse rate and report any irregularities in comparison to baseline to health care provider.

Diet

- Advise the client that a high-protein, low-carbohydrate diet increases theophylline elimination. Conversely, a low-protein, high-carbohydrate diet prolongs the half-life; dosage may need adjustment.

EVALUATION

- Evaluate the effectiveness of the bronchodilators. The client is breathing without wheezing and without side effects of the drug.
- Evaluate serum theophylline levels to make sure they are within the accepted range.
- Evaluate tolerance to activity.

Generic (Brand)	Route and Dosage	Preg Cat	Interaction	t1/2	PB	Onset	Action Peak	Action Duration
Aminophylline (theophylline ethylenediamine)	A: PO: LD 500 mg; then 250–500 mg q6–8h IV: LD 6 mg/kg over 30 min; then 0.2–0.9 mg/kg/h C: PO: LD: 7.5 mg/kg; then 3–6 mg/kg q6–8h IV: LD 5.6 mg/kg then 1 mg/kg/h *Caution:* Need to stress that individual titration is based on levels, not specific doses	C	Similar to prototype theophylline	A: 9 h Smokers: 4 h C: 4–16 h	UK	PO: 15–60 min PO SR: UK IV: Rapid Rect: Rapid	1–2 h 4–7 h End of infusion 1–2 h	6–8 h 8–12 h 6–8 h 6–8 h
Dyphylline (dihydroxypropyl theophylline) (Dyline, Dilor, Lufyllin)	A: PO: 200–800 mg q.i.d. or q6h A: IM: 250–500 mg q6h C >6 y: PO: 4–7 mg/kg/d in 4 divided doses *Caution:* Titration to 10–20 µg/mL is indicated ¹⁄₁₀ bronchodilator effect of theophylline	C	Not hepatically metabolized, thus theophylline-like interactions do not apply. Caution with probenicid *Lab:* Use specific assay for drug; theophylline assay will give zero concentration	2 h	UK	UK	1 h	6 h
Oxtriphylline (choline theophyllinate) (Choledyl)	A: PO: 200 mg q.i.d. or q6h C: 2–12 y: PO: 4 mg/kg q6h *Caution:* Titration to 10–20 µg/mL is indicated	C	Similar to prototype theophylline	3–13 h	UK	PO: Liq: UK PO: Tab: 15–60 min PO SR: UK	1 h 5 h 4–7 h	UK 6–8 h 12 h
Theophylline	See Prototype Drug Chart							

KEY: For complete abbreviation key, see inside front cover.

CARDIOVASCULAR AGENTS

Cardiac Glycosides

Antianginals

Antidysrhythmics

Diuretics
Thiazides
Loop (High Ceiling), Osmotic, and
Carbonic Anhydrase Inhibitors
Potassium Sparing

Antihypertensives
Beta Blockers and Central Alpha$_2$
Agonist

Adrenergic Blockers
(Sympatholytics):
Alpha Blockers, Alpha-Beta
Blockers, Peripherally Acting
Blockers, and Direct-Acting
Vasodilators
Angiotensin Antagonists and
Calcium Blockers

**Anticoagulants, Antiplatelets, and
Anticoagulant Antagonists**

Thrombolytics

Antilipemics

Vasodilators (Peripheral)

Cardiac Glycosides (Cardiotonics)

Digoxin	Dosage
Digoxin (Lanoxin) Cardiac glycoside *Pregnancy Category:* C *Drug Forms:* Tab 0.125, 0.25, 0.5 mg Cap 0.1, 0.2 mg Elix 0.05 mg/mL (50 μg/mL) Inj 0.1, 0.25 mg/mL	A: PO: 0.5–1 mg initially in 2 divided doses (digitalization); maint: 0.125–0.5 mg/d; elderly: 0.125 mg/d IV: Same as PO dose given over 5 min C : PO: 1 mo–2 y: 0.01–0.02 mg/kg in 3 divided doses 2–10 y: 0.012–0.04 mg/kg in divided doses; maint: 0.012 mg/kg/d in 2 divided doses IV: Dosage varies

Contraindications	Drug-Lab-Food Interactions
Ventricular dysrhythmias, 2nd- or 3rd-degree heart block *Caution:* AMI, renal disease, hypothyroidism, hypokalemia	*Increase* digoxin serum level with quinidine, flecainide, verapamil *Decrease* digoxin absorption with antacids, colestipol *Increase* risk for digoxin toxicity with thiazide diuretics, loop diuretics *Lab:* hypokalemia, hypomagnesemia, hypercalcemia

Pharmacokinetics	Pharmacodynamics

Absorption: PO: 60–76%; liq PO: 90%
Distribution: PB: 25%
Metabolism: t 1/2: 30–45 h
Excretion: 70% in urine; 30% by liver metabolism
	PO: Onset: 1–5 h
	  Peak: 6–8 h
	  Duration: 2–4 d
	IV: Onset: 5–30 min
	  Peak: 1–5 h
	  Duration: 2–4 d

Therapeutic Effects/Uses: To treat CHF, atrial tachycardia, flutter, or fibrillation.

Mode of Action: It inhibits the sodium-potassium ATPase, thus promoting increased force of cardiac contraction, cardiac output, and tissue perfusion; decreases ventricular rate.

Side Effects	Adverse Reactions
Anorexia, nausea, vomiting, headache, blurred vision (yellow-green halos), diplopia, photophobia, drowsiness, fatigue, confusion	Bradycardia, visual disturbances *Life threatening:* Atrioventricular block, cardiac dysrhythmias

KEY: For complete abbreviation key, see inside front cover.

■ NURSING PROCESS: Cardiac Glycosides

ASSESSMENT

• Obtain a drug history. Report if a drug-drug interaction is probable. If the client is taking digoxin and a potassium-wasting diuretic or cortisone drug, hypokalemia might result, causing digitalis toxicity. A low serum potassium level enhances the action of digoxin. A client taking a thiazide and/or cortisone along with digoxin should be taking a potassium supplement.

Cardiac Glycosides (Cardiotonics)

- Obtain a baseline pulse rate for future comparisons. Apical pulse should be taken for a full minute and should be >60 bpm.
- Assess for signs and symptoms of digitalis toxicity. Common symptoms include anorexia, nausea, vomiting, bradycardia, cardiac dysrhythmias, and visual disturbances. Report symptoms immediately to the health care provider.

POTENTIAL NURSING DIAGNOSES
Decreased cardiac output
Altered tissue perfusion (cardiopulmonary, cerebral)
Anxiety related to cardiac problem

PLANNING
- Client checks pulse rate daily before taking digoxin. Client will report pulse rate of <60 bpm or a marked decline in pulse rate.
- Client eats foods rich in potassium to maintain a desired serum potassium level (see Client Teaching, Diet).

NURSING INTERVENTIONS
- Do *not* confuse **digoxin** with **digitoxin**. Read the drug labels carefully. Digoxin has a long half-life but has a shorter half-life than digitoxin.
- Check the apical pulse rate before administering digoxin. Do *not* administer if pulse rate is <60 bpm.
- Check for signs of peripheral and pulmonary edema, which indicate CHF.
- Check the serum digoxin level. The normal therapeutic drug range for digoxin is 0.5–2.0 ng/mL. A serum digoxin level of >2.0 ng/mL is indicative of digitalis toxicity. Check serum potassium level (normal range, 3.5–5.3 mEq/L) and report if hypokalemia (<3.5 mEq/L) is present.

CLIENT TEACHING
General
- Explain to the client the importance of compliance with the drug therapy. A visiting nurse may ensure that the medications are properly taken.
- Advise the client not to take OTC drugs without first consulting the health care provider to avoid adverse drug interactions.
- Keep drugs out of reach of small children. Request child safety cap bottle.
Skill
- Instruct the client how to check the pulse rate before taking digoxin and to call the health care provider for pulse rate <60 bpm or irregular pulse.
Diet
- Advise the client to eat foods rich in potassium such as fresh and dried fruits, fruit juices, and vegetables, including potatoes.
Side Effects
- Instruct the client to report side effects such as a pulse rate of <60 bpm, nausea, vomiting, headache, and visual disturbances, including diplopia.

EVALUATION
- Evaluate the effectiveness of digoxin by noting the client's response to the drug and the absence of side effects. Continue monitoring the pulse rate.

Cardiac Glycosides

Generic (Brand)	Route and Dosage	Preg Cat	Interaction	t 1/2	PB	Action Onset	Action Peak	Action Duration
Rapid-Acting Digitalis Deslanoside (Cedilanid-D)	A: IV: 1.2–1.6 mg/d in 1–2 divided doses; max: 1.6–2.0 mg	C	Similar to digoxin	33–36 h	20–25%	10–30 min	1–3 h	2.5–4 h
Digoxin (Lanoxin)	See Prototype Drug Chart							
Long-Acting Digitalis Digitoxin (Crystodigin)	A: PO/IV: LD: 0.8–1.2 mg; maint: PO: 0.05–3 mg/d	C	*Decrease* effects with barbiturate, phenytoin, cholestyramine, colestipol; decrease digitoxin level with thyroid drugs	1–3 wk	97%	0.5–2 h	4–12 h	2–3 wk
Positive Inotropic Bipyridines Amrinone lactate (Inocor)	A: IV: LD: 0.75 mg/kg within 2–3 min; maint: 5–10 µg/kg/min; max: 10 mg/kg/d	C	*Increase* hypotensive effect with disopyramide *Lab:* May *increase* serum liver enzyme	3.6–7 h	10–50%	2–5 min	10 min	0.5–2 h
Milrinone lactate (Primacor)	A: IV: Initially: 50 µg/kg/over 10 min *Continuous infusion:* 0.375–0.75 µg/kg/min with 0.45–0.9% saline	C	Do *not* mix with furosemide	1.5–2.5 h	70%	UK	2 min	3–6 h

KEY: For complete abbreviation key, see inside front cover.

NOTES:

Antianginals

Nitroglycerin

Nitroglycerin
  (Nitrostat, Nitro-Bid, Transderm-Nitro patch, NTG)
Nitrate
Pregnancy Category: C
Drug Forms:
Tab SL 0.15, 0.3, 0.4, 0.6 mg
Cap SR 2.5, 6.5, 9 mg
Oint 2% topical
Patch transderm 2.5, 5.0, 7.5, 10, 15 mg
Inj 0.5, 0.8, 5 mg/mL

Dosage

A: PO/SL: 0.3, 0.4, 0.6 mg; repeat q5min ×3 as needed.
  Cap: 2.5–9 mg q8–12 h
IV: Initially: 5 µg/min; dose may be increased
Oint 2%: 1–2 in
Patch: 2.5–15 mg/d

Contraindications

Marked hypotension, AMI, increased intracranial pressure (ICP), severe anemia
Caution: Severe renal or hepatic disease, early MI

Drug-Lab-Food Interactions

Increase effect with alcohol, beta blockers, calcium blockers, antihypertensives
Decrease effect of heparin

Pharmacokinetics

Absorption: SL: >75% absorbed; oint and patch: slow absorption
Distribution: PB: 60%
Metabolism: t 1/2: 1–4 min
Excretion: Liver and urine

Pharmacodynamics

SL: Onset: 1–3 min
         Peak: 4 min
         Duration: 20–30 min
SR: Cap: Onset: 20–45 min
         Duration: 3–8 h
Oint: Onset: 20–60 min
         Peak: 1–2 h
         Duration: 3–8 h
Patch: Onset: 30–60 min
         Peak: 1–2 h
         Duration: 20–24 h
IV: Onset: 1–3 min
         Duration: 0.5–2 h

Therapeutic Effects/Uses: To control anginal pectoris (pain).

Mode of Action: Decrease myocardial demand for oxygen; decrease preload by dilating veins, thus indirectly decreasing afterload.

Side Effects

Nausea, vomiting, headache, dizziness, syncope, weakness, flushing, confusion, pallor, rash, dry mouth

Adverse Reactions

Hypotension, reflex tachycardia, paradoxical bradycardia
Life threatening: Circulatory collapse

KEY: For complete abbreviation key, see inside front cover.

■ NURSING PROCESS: Antianginals: Nitroglycerin (Nitrostat, NTG)

ASSESSMENT

• Obtain baseline VS for future comparisons.
• Obtain medical and drug histories. Nitroglycerin is contraindicated for marked hypotension or AMI.

POTENTIAL NURSING DIAGNOSES

Decreased cardiac output
Anxiety related to cardiac problem(s)

PLANNING

• Client takes nitroglycerin or other antianginals and angina pain is controlled.

NURSING INTERVENTIONS

• Monitor VS. Hypotension is associated with most antianginal drugs.
• Have the client sit or lie down when taking a nitrate for the first time. After administration, check the VS while the client is lying down and then sitting up. Have the client rise slowly to a standing position.
• Offer sips of water before giving SL nitrates; dryness may inhibit drug absorption.
• Monitor effects of IV nitroglycerin. Report angina that persists.
• Apply Nitro-Bid ointment to the designated mark on paper. Do *not* use fingers because the drug can be absorbed; use a tongue blade or gloves. For the Transderm-Nitro patch, do not touch the medication portion.
• Do *not* apply the Nitro-Bid ointment or the Transderm-Nitro patch in any area on the chest in the vicinity of defibrillator-cardioverter paddle placement. Explosion and skin burns may result.

CLIENT TEACHING
General

• A nitroglycerin SL tablet is used if chest pain occurs. Repeat in 5 min if the pain has not subsided and again in another 5 min if it persists. Do *not* give more than 3 tablets. If the chest pain persists >15 min, immediate medical help is necessary.
• Instruct the client not to ingest alcohol while taking nitroglycerin to avoid hypotension, weakness, and faintness.
• Tolerance to nitroglycerin can occur. If the client's chest pain is not completely alleviated, the client should notify the physician.
Skill

• Instruct the client about SL nitroglycerin tablets. The tablet is placed under the tongue for quick absorption. A stinging or biting sensation may indicate the tablet is fresh. With the newer SL nitroglycerin, the biting sensation may not be present. The bottle is stored away from light and kept dry.
• Instruct the client about the Transderm-Nitro patch. Apply once a day, usually in the morning. Rotation of skin sites is necessary. Usually the patch is applied to the chest wall; however, the thighs and arms are used. Avoid hairy areas.
Side Effects

• Headaches commonly occur when first taking nitroglycerin products and last about 30 min. Acetaminophen is suggested for relief.
• If hypotension results from SL nitroglycerin, place the client in supine position with legs elevated.

EVALUATION

• Evaluate the nitrate product for relieving anginal pain. Note headache, dizziness, or faintness.

Generic (Brand)	Route and Dosage	Preg Cat	Interaction	t 1/2	PB	Onset	Action Peak	Duration
							(Peak)	
Nitrates								
Amyl nitrite	A: Inhal: 0.18–0.3 mL amp PRN	C	*Increase* hypotensive effect with alcohol antihypertensives, beta blockers *Decrease* effects of epinephrine	1–4 min	UK	30 sec	UK	3–5 min
Isosorbide dinitrate (Isordil, Sorbitrate)	A: SL: 2.5–10 mg q.i.d. Chewable: 5–10 mg PRN PO: 2.5–30 mg q.i.d. a.c. and h.s.	C	*Increase* hypotensive effect with alcohol, phenothiazides, antihypertensives including beta blockers	1–4 h	UK	SL: 3–30 min Chewable tab: 3–20 min PO: 1 h	SL: 15 min–1 h Chewable tab: 15 min–1 h PO: 1–2 h	SL: 1–4 h Chewable tab: 1–3 h PO: 4–6 h
Nitroglycerin (Nitrostat, Nitro-Bid, Transderm-Nitro)	See Prototype Drug Chart							
Pentaerythritol tetranitrate (Peritrate)	A: PO: 10–40 mg t.i.d./q.i.d. SR: 20–80 mg q12h	C	Same as isosorbide	10 min	UK	PO: 20–60 min SR: 0.5 h	PO: UK SR: UK	PO: 4–5 h SR: 8–12 h

Beta-Adrenergic Blockers							
Atenolol (Tenormin)	A: PO: 50–100 mg/d; max: 200 mg/d	C	*Increase* hypotensive effects with diuretics, antihypertensives; *increase* absorption with anticholinergics; *Lab:* may *increase* lidocaine levels	6–7 h	5–15%	1 h	2–4 h	24 h
Metoprolol tartrate (Lopressor)	A: PO: Initially: 50–100 mg/d in 1–2 divided doses; maint: 100–400 mg/d	C	*Increase* bradycardia with digoxin; *increase* hypotensive effects with alcohol, antihypertensives, anesthetics	3–7 h	12%	15 min–1 h	1.5–4 h	6–12 h
Propranolol HCl (Inderal)	A: PO: Initially: 10–20 mg t.i.d./ q.i.d.; maint: 20–60 mg t.i.d./q.i.d.; max: 320 mg/d SR: 80–160 mg/d IV: See Antidysrhythmics	C	Same as atenolol	3–6 h	90%	0.5–1 h	1–1.5 h SR: 6 h	12 h
Calcium Channel Blockers							
Amlodipine (Norvasc)	A: PO: Initially: 10 mg; maint: 2.5–10 mg/d	C	*May increase* hypotension with beta blockers, anesthetics *Decrease* effect with NSAIDs, adrenergics	30–50 h	95%	UK	6–12 h	24 h

continued

Antianginals *Continued*

Generic (Brand)	Route and Dosage	Preg Cat	Interaction	t 1/2	PB	Action Onset	Action Peak	Action Duration
Bepridal HCl (Vascor)	A: PO: Initially 200 mg/d ×10d; maint: 300 mg/d; max: 400 mg/d	C	*Increase* hypotensive effect with anesthesia; may *increase* effect of beta blockers *Lab:* May *increase* ALP, AST, ALT, CPK, LDH, liver enzymes	2–24 h	99%	1 h	2–3 h	UK
Diltiazem HCl (Cardizem)	A: PO: 30–60 mg q.i.d.; may increase to 360 mg/d in 4 divided doses SR: 60–120 mg q12h	C	Similar to nifedipine	3.5–9 h	70–85%	PO: 30 min SR: UK	PO: 2–3 h SR: 6–11 h	PO: 6–8 h SR: 12–24 h
Isradipine (DynaCirc)	A: PO: 2.5–7.5 mg t.i.d.	C	*Increase* effect of digoxin; *increase* effect with cimetidine, carbamazepine	5–11 h	99%	1–2 h	2–3 h	12 h

Drug	Dosage	Preg	Drug interactions			Onset	Peak	Duration
Nicardipine HCl (Cardene, Cardene SR)	A: PO: 20 mg t.i.d.; maint: 20–40 mg t.i.d. SR: 30 mg b.i.d.; maint: 30–60 mg b.i.d.	C	*Increase* effect with cimetidine, propranolol, theophylline *Decrease* effect with barbiturates, phenytoin *Lab:* Increase ALP, AST, ALT, creatine phosphokinase, LDH	5 h	95%	20 min	1–2 h	PO: 6–8 h
Nifedipine (Procardia, Adalat)	A: PO: 10–30 mg q6–8h; max: 180 mg/d	C	*Increase* effect with cimetidine; *increase* effects of theophylline, beta blockers, antihypertensives	2–5 h	92–98 h	PO: 20 min SR: UK	PO:1–4 h SR: UK	PO: 6–8 h SR: 24 h
Verapamil HCl (Calan, Isoptin, Verelan)	A: PO: 40–120 mg t.i.d.; max: 480 mg/d IV: 5–10 mg over 2 min	C	*Increase* effect with cimetidine; *increase* effects of theophylline, beta blockers, antihypertensives *Decrease* effect of lithium	3–8 h	90%	PO: 1–2 h SR: UK	PO: 0.5–1.5 h SR: 4–8 h	PO: 3–7 h SR: 24 h

KEY: For complete abbreviation key, see inside front cover.

Antidysrhythmics

Procainamide HCl
  (Procan, Pronestyl)
Fast channel (sodium) blocker
(type I)
Pregnancy Category: C
Drug Forms:
Tab and Cap 250, 375, 500 mg

Dosage

A: PO: 250–500 mg q3–4h
  SR: 250 mg–1 g q6h or
  50 mg/kg/d in 4 divided doses
  IV: 20–30 mg/min; maint:
  1–4 mg/min; max: 17 mg/kg
C: PO: 40–60 mg/kg/d in 4 divided
  doses
  IV: 3–6 mg/kg q10–30 min; max:
  100 mg/dose
TDM: 4–8 µg/mL

Contraindications

Hypersensitivity to procaine, blood
  dyscrasias, heart block, cardiogenic
  shock, myasthenia gravis
Caution: Hypotension, CHF, MI, renal
  or hepatic insufficiency

Drug-Lab-Food Interactions

Increase effects with histamine$_2$
  blockers; *increase* hypotensive
  effects with antihypertensives,
  nitrates
Decrease effects with barbiturates
Lab: May *increase* ALP, AST, LDH,
  bilirubin

Pharmacokinetics

Absorption: PO: 75–95%
Distribution: PB: 20%
Metabolism: t 1/2: 3–4 h
Excretion: 60% unchanged in urine
  (half as an active metabolite)

Pharmacodynamics

PO: Onset: 30 min
  Peak: 1–1.5 h
  Duration: 3–4 h (SR: 8 h)
IV: Onset: Minutes
  Peak: 25–60 min
  Duration: 3–4 h

Therapeutic Effects/Uses: To control cardiac dysrhythmias (premature ventricular
contractions [PVCs], ventricular tachycardia)

Mode of Action: Depression of myocardial excitability by slowing conduction of cardiac tissue through the atrium, bundle of His, and ventricle to decrease cardiac dysrhythmias.

Side Effects

Anorexia, nausea, vomiting,
  diarrhea, headache, dizziness,
  weakness, flushing, rash, pruritus,
  lupus-like syndrome with rash

Adverse Reactions

Life threatening: Atrioventricular
  block, pleural effusion, ventricular
  tachycardia/fibrillation,
  thrombocytopenia,
  agranulocytosis, cardiovascular
  collapse, torsade des pointes

KEY: For complete abbreviation key, see inside front cover.

■ NURSING PROCESS: Antidysrhythmics

ASSESSMENT
- Obtain health and drug histories. The history may include heart palpitations, coughing, chest pain (type, duration, and severity), previous angina or cardiac dysrhythmias, and drugs that the client is currently taking.
- Obtain baseline VS and ECG for future comparisons.
- Check early cardiac enzyme results (AST, LDH, CPK) to compare with future laboratory results.

POTENTIAL NURSING DIAGNOSES
Decreased cardiac output
Anxiety related to irregular heartbeat
High risk for activity intolerance

PLANNING
- Client will no longer experience abnormal sinus rhythm.
- Client will comply with the antidysrhythmic drug regimen.

NURSING INTERVENTIONS
- Monitor VS. Hypotension can occur.
- When the drug is ordered IV push or bolus, administer it over a period of 2–3 min or as prescribed.
- Monitor ECG for abnormal patterns and report findings, such as PVCs, increased PR and QT intervals, and/or widening of the QRS complex. Increased QT interval is a risk factor for torsade des pointes.

CLIENT TEACHING
General
- Instruct the client to take the prescribed drug as ordered. Drug compliance is essential.
- Provide specific instructions for each drug, such as photosensitivity for amiodarone.

Side Effects
- Instruct the client to report side effects and adverse reactions to the health care provider. These can include dizziness, faintness, nausea, and vomiting.
- Advise the client to avoid alcohol, caffeine, and cigarettes. Alcohol can intensify the hypotensive reaction; caffeine increases the catecholamine level; and cigarette smoking promotes vasoconstriction.

EVALUATION
- Evaluate the effectiveness of the prescribed antidysrhythmic by comparing heart rates with the baseline heart rate and assessing the client's response to the drug. Report side effects and adverse reactions. The drug regimen may need to be adjusted. A proarrhythmic effect may occur, which may require discontinuation of the drug.

Generic (Brand)	Route and Dosage	Preg Cat	Interaction	t 1/2	PB	Onset	Peak	Duration
							Action	
Fast (Sodium) Channel Blockers I								
Disopyramide phosphate (Norpace, Napamide)	A: PO: 100–200 mg q6h CR: 300 mg q12h C 4–12 y: PO: 10–15 mg/kg/d in divided doses 13–18 y: PO: 6–15 mg/kg/d in divided doses	C	*Increase* effect with other antidysrhythmics, beta blockers, lidocaine *Decrease* effect with phenytoin, rifampin *Lab:* May *increase* serum liver enzymes	4–10 h	50–65%	0.5–3.5 h	1–2 h	1.5–8 h
Procainamide (Pronestyl, Procan)	See Prototype Drug Chart							
Quinidine sulfate, polygalactorate, gluconate (Quinidex, Duraquin)	A: PO: 200–400 mg t.i.d./q.i.d. C: PO: 30 mg/kg or 900 mg/m² in 5 divided doses	C	*Increase* effect with beta blockers, thiazides, histamine₂ blockers, verapamil, sodium bicarbonate; *increase* effects of digoxin, warfarin *Decrease* effect with barbiturates, nifedipine, phenytoin, rifampin	6–7 h	80%	1–3 h	1–2 h	6–8 h

	A: Dosage	Pregnancy Category	Interactions	t½	%	Onset	Peak	Duration
Fast (Sodium) Channel Blockers II Encainide HCl (Enkaid) **Available for compassionate use only**	A: PO: 25 mg q8h; may increase to 50–75 mg q8h	B	*Increase* effect with histamine$_2$ blockers	3–12 h	75–85%	1–3 h	UK	8–12 h
Lidocaine (Xylocaine)	A: IV: 50–100 mg bolus in 2–3 min; then 20–50 µg/kg/min	B	*Increase* effect with beta blockers, histamine$_2$ blockers, other antihypertensives	1.5–2 h	60–80%	1–2 min	1–2 min	10–12 min
Mexiletine HCL (Mexitil)	A: PO: 200–400 mg q8h	C	*Increase* effect with H$_2$ blockers *Decrease* effect with barbiturates, phenytoin, antitubercular drugs, smoking	10–12 h	50–60%	0.5–2 h	2–3 h	8–12 h
Phenytoin (Dilantin)	A: IV: 100 mg q5–10 min until dysrhythmia ceases; max: 1000 mg	D	*Decrease* effects of steroids, oral contraceptives; decrease effect with barbiturate, theophylline, folic acid, antacids, CNS depressants *Food: Decrease* with calcium, vitamin D, folic acid	22 h	95%	UK	1.5–3 h	5 h
Tocainide HCL (Tonocard)	A: PO: LD: 600 mg PO: 400 mg q8h; max: 2.4 g/d	C	*Increase* effect with beta blockers, quinidine, other antihypertensives	10–17 h	70–80%	0.5–1 h	1–2 h	8–12 h

continued

| | | | | | | | Action | | |
Generic (Brand)	Route and Dosage	Preg Cat	Interaction	t 1/2	PB	Onset	Peak	Duration
Beta-Adrenergic Blockers *(Type II)*								
Acebutolol HCl (Sectral)	A: PO: 200 mg b.i.d.; may increase dose	B	*Increase* hypotensive effect with diuretics, other antihypertensives	3–13 h	26%	1 h	4–6 h	10 h
Propranolol HCl (Inderal)	A: PO: 10–30 mg t.i.d./q.i.d. A: IV bolus: 0.5–3 mg at 1 mg/min	C	Same as acebutolol	3–6 h	90%	0.5–1 h	1.5–4 h	UK
Sotalol HCl (Betapace)	A: PO: 80 mg b.i.d.; max: 240–320 mg/d Increase dose interval with renal dysfunction	B	May *increase* bradycardia with amiodarone; may *increase* hypoglycemic effect with oral antidiabetics *Food: Decrease* effect with milk and milk products	12 h	0%	UK	2–3 h	24 h
Calcium Channel Blockers *(Type IV)*								
Verapamil HCl (Calan)	A: PO: 240–480 mg/d in 3–4 divided doses IV: 5–10 mg IV push	C	*Increase* effect with cimetidine; *increase* effects of theophylline, beta blockers, antihypertensives *Decrease* effect of lithium	3–8 h	90%	PO: 0.5–1.5 h	PO: 1–2 h	PO: 3–7 h

Prolong Repolarization (Type III)							
Adenosine (Adenocard)	A: IV: 6 mg (bolus: 1–2 s); repeat if necessary, 12 mg bolus	C	<10 s	UK	<10 s	20–30 s	UK	May *increase* effect with dipyridamole *Decrease* effect with theophylline
Amiodarone HCl (Cordarone)	A: PO: LD: 400–1,600 mg/d in divided doses; maint: 200–600 mg/d	C	5–100 d	1–3 wk	2–3 d	UK	Weeks, months	*Increase* effects of digoxin, other antidysrhythmics, phenytoin *Lab:* May *increase* liver enzymes AST, ALT, ALP
Bretylium tosylate (Bretylol)	A: IM: 5–10 mg/kg q6–8h; IV: 5–10 mg/kg; repeat in 15–30 min, IV drip or IV bolus	C	4–17 h	UK	IM: 1–6 h IV: 5 min	IM: 6–9 h IV: End of infusion	IM/IV: 6–24 h	May *increase* hypotensive effect with beta blockers, other antidysrhythmics
Propafenone HCl (Rythmol)	A: PO: 150–300 mg q8h; max: 900 mg/d	C	5–8 h	97%	UK	1–3.5 h	UK	*Increase* digoxin effect May *prolong* clotting: Warfarin *Increase* effect with: cimetidine *Increase* effect of: Metoprolol, propranolol

KEY: For complete abbreviation key, see inside front cover.

Diuretic: Thiazides

Hydrochlorothiazide

Hydrochlorothiazide
  (HydroDIURIL, HCTZ, Esidrix,
  Oretic)
Thiazide diuretic
Pregnancy Category: B
Drug Forms:
Tab 25, 50, 100 mg
Oral sol 10, 100 mg/mL

Dosage

A: PO: Hypertension: 12.5–100 mg/d
    Edema: Initially: 25–200 mg in
    divided doses; maint:
    25–100 mg/d
C: PO: 1–2 mg/kg/d in divided
    doses
C: <6 mo: PO: 2–3 mg/kg/d in
    divided doses

Contraindications

Renal failure with anuria, electrolyte
  depletion
Caution: Hepatic cirrhosis, renal
  dysfunction, diabetes mellitus,
  gout, systemic lupus
  erythematosus (SLE)

Drug-Lab-Food Interactions

Increase digitalis toxicity with
  digitalis and hypokalemia; *increase*
  potassium loss with steroids;
  potassium loss
Decrease antidiabetic effect; decrease
  thiazide effect with cholestyramine
  and colestipol
Lab: *Increase* serum calcium, glucose,
  uric acid
Decrease serum potassium, sodium,
  magnesium

Pharmacokinetics

Absorption: Readily absorbed from
  the GI tract
Distribution: PB: 65%
Metabolism: t 1/2: 6–15 h
Excretion: In urine

Pharmacodynamics

PO: Onset: 2 h
     Peak: 3–6 h
     Duration: 6–12 h

Therapeutic Effects/Uses: To increase urine output. To treat hypertension, edema from CHF, hepatic cirrhosis, renal dysfunction.

Mode of Action: Action is on the renal distal tubules by promoting sodium, potassium, and water excretion. Acts on arterioles, causing vasodilation, thus decreasing blood pressure.

Side Effects

Dizziness, vertigo, weakness, nausea,
  vomiting, diarrhea, hyperglycemia,
  constipation, rash, photosensitivity

Adverse Reactions

Severe dehydration, hypotension
Life threatening: Severe potassium
  depletion, marked hypotension,
  uremia, aplastic anemia, hemolytic
  anemia, thrombocytopenia,
  agranulocytosis

KEY: For complete abbreviation key, see inside front cover.

■ NURSING PROCESS: Diuretics: Thiazides

ASSESSMENT
• Assess VS, weight, urine output, and serum chemistry values (electrolytes, glucose, uric acid) for baseline levels.
• Check peripheral extremities for presence of edema. Note pitting edema.
• Obtain a history of drugs that are taken daily. Review for drugs that may cause drug interaction, including digoxin, corticosteroids, antidiabetics.

POTENTIAL NURSING DIAGNOSIS
High risk for fluid volume deficit

PLANNING
• Client's blood pressure will be decreased and/or return to normal value.
• Client's edema will be decreased.
• Client's serum chemistry levels remain within normal ranges.

NURSING INTERVENTIONS
• Monitor VS and serum electrolytes, especially potassium and glucose levels. Report changes. If client is taking digoxin and hypokalemia occurs, digitalis toxicity frequently results.
• Observe for signs and symptoms of hypokalemia, such as muscle weakness, leg cramps, and cardiac dysrhythmias.
• Check the client's weight daily at a specified time. A weight gain of 2.2–2.5 lb is equivalent to an excess liter of body fluids.
• Monitor urine output to determine fluid loss or retention.

CLIENT TEACHING
General
• Suggest that the client take hydrochlorothiazide in early morning to avoid sleep disturbance due to nocturia.
• Keep drugs out of reach of small children. Request child safety cap bottle.

Skill
• Instruct the client or family member how to take and record his or her blood pressure. Record daily results.

Diet
• Instruct the client to eat foods rich in potassium, such as fruits, fruit juices, and vegetables. Potassium supplements may be ordered.
• Advise the client to take drugs with food to avoid GI upset.

Side Effects
• Instruct the client to change positions from lying to standing slowly because dizziness may occur due to orthostatic (postural) hypotension.
• Advise the client who may be prediabetic to have blood sugar checked periodically because large doses of hydrochlorothiazide increase blood glucose levels.
• Advise the client to use sunscreen when in direct sunlight.

EVALUATION
• Evaluate the effectiveness of drug therapy. Client's blood pressure and edema will be reduced and blood chemistry will remain within normal range.
• Determine the absence of side effects and adverse reactions to therapy.

Generic (Brand)	Route and Dosage	Interaction	Preg Cat	t1/2	PB	Action Onset	Action Peak	Action Duration
						Action		
						Onset	Peak	Duration
Short Acting								
Chlorothiazide (Diuril, Diachlor)	*Hypertension:* A: PO: 250–500 mg q.d. or b.i.d. *Edema:* A: PO: 500–2,000 mg q.d. or b.i.d. C >1 y: PO: 20 mg/kg/d C <6 mon: PO: 30 mg/kg/d in divided doses	May *increase* potassium and magnesium loss with digitalis, corticosteroids; *increase* toxicity with lithium *Decrease* effects of antidiabetics; *decrease* chlorothiazide absorption with colestipol	D	1–2 h	20–80%	1–2 h	4 h	6–12 h
Hydrochlorothiazide	See Prototype Drug Chart							
Intermediate Acting								
Bendroflumethiazide (Naturetin)	A: PO: 2.5–20 mg/d C: PO: maint: 0.05–0.1 mg/kg/d or 1.5–3 mg/m²	Same as chlorothiazide	UK	3–4 h	94%	1–2 h	6–12 h	18–24 h
Benzthiazide (Aquatag, Hydrex)	*Hypertension:* A: PO: 25–100 mg/q.d. or 25–100 mg in divided doses *Edema:* A: PO: 25–200 mg q.d. C: PO: 1–4 mg/kg/d in 3 divided doses	Same as chlorothiazide	D	UK	UK	2 h	4–6 h	12–18 h
Hydroflumethiazide (Saluron, Diucardin)	*Hypertension:* A: PO: 50–100 mg/d *Edema:* A: PO: 25–200 mg/d C: PO: 1 mg/kg/d	Same as chlorothiazide	C	17 h	74%	1–2 h	3–4 h	18–24 h

Long Acting

Drug	Dose	Preg. Cat.	Drug Interactions	Half-life	Protein Binding	Onset	Peak	Duration
Methyclothiazide (Aquatensen, Enduron)	*Hypertension/edema*: A: PO: 2.5–10 mg/d C: PO: 0.05–0.1 mg/kg/d	C	*Increase* hypokalemic effect with digitalis, glucocorticosteroids; *increase* hypoglycemic effect with antidiabetics (oral and insulin); *increase* toxicity with lithium; *may increase* risk of renal failure with NSAIDs	UK	UK	2h	6 h	>24 h
Polythiazide (Renese-R)	*Hypertension*: A: PO: 2–4 mg/d *Edema*: A: PO: 1–4 mg/d C: PO: 0.02–0.08 mg/kg/d	D	Similar to methyclothiazide	25 h	84%	2 h	6 h	24–48 h
Trichlormethiazide (Metahydrin, Naqua)	*Hypertension*: A: PO: 2–4 mg *Edema*: A: PO: 1–4 mg q.d. or b.i.d. C: PO: 0.07 mg/kg/d in divided doses	B	Similar to methyclothiazide	2.5–7 h	UK	2 h	6 h	24 h
Thiazide-Like Diuretics								
Chlorthalidone (Hygroton)	*Hypertension*: A: PO: 12.5–50 mg/d *Edema*: A: PO: 25–100 mg/d C: PO: 2 mg/kg 3×wk	C	Similar to methyclothiazide	40–54 h	75%	2 h	3–6 h	24–72 h
Indapamide (Lozol)	*Hypertension and edema*: A: PO: 2.5 mg/d; may increase to 5 mg/d	B	Similar to methyclothiazide	14–18 h	75%	1–2 h	<2 h	24–36 h
Metolazone (Zaroxolyn)	*Hypertension*: A: PO: 2.5–5.0 mg/d *Edema*: A: PO: 5–20 mg/d	D	Similar to methyclothiazide	8–14 h	33%	1 h	2–8 h	12–24 h
Quinethazone (Hydromox)	A: PO: 50–100 mg/d; max: 200 mg/d in divided doses	D	Similar to methyclothiazide	UK	UK	2 h	6 h	18–24 h

KEY: For complete abbreviation key, see inside front cover.

Diuretic: Loop (High Ceiling)

Furosemide

Furosemide
   (Lasix, Furomide)
High ceiling (loop) diuretic
Pregnancy Category: C
Drug Forms:
Tab 20, 40, 80 mg
Oral sol 10 mg/mL, 40 mg/5 mL
Inj 10 mg/mL

Dosage

A: PO: 20–80 mg single dose; repeat
   in 6–8 h max: 600 mg/d
   IM/IV: 20–100 mg single dose;
   over 1–2 min IV; repeat 20 mg in
   2 h
C: PO: 2 mg/kg single dose; repeat in
   6–8 h; max: 6 mg/kg/d
   IM/IV: 1 mg/kg single dose;
   repeat 1 mg/kg in 2 h

Contraindications

Presence of severe electrolyte
   imbalances, hypovolemia, anuria,
   hypersensitivity to sulfonamides,
   hepatic coma

Drug-Lab-Food Interactions

Increase orthostatic hypotension with
   alcohol; *increase* ototoxicity with
   aminoglycosides; *increase* bleeding
   with anticoagulants; *increase*
   potassium loss with steroids;
   increase digitalis toxicity and
   cardiac dysrhythmias with digitalis
   and hypokalemia
Lab: Increase BUN, blood/urine
   glucose, serum uric acid, ammonia
Decrease potassium, sodium, calcium,
   magnesium, chloride serum levels

Pharmacokinetics

Absorption: Readily absorbed from
   the GI tract
Distribution: PB: 95%
Metabolism: t 1/2: 30–50 min
Excretion: In urine, some in feces;
   crosses placenta

Pharmacodynamics

PO: Onset: <60 min
       Peak: 1–2 h
       Duration: 6–8 h
IV: Onset: 5 min
       Peak: 20–30 min
       Duration: 2 h

Therapeutic Effects/Uses: To treat fluid retention/fluid overload due to CHF, renal
dysfunction, cirrhosis; hypertension; acute pulmonary edema.

Mode of Action: Inhibition of sodium and water reabsorption from the loop of Henle
and distal renal tubules. Potassium, magnesium, and calcium also may be excreted.

Side Effects

Nausea, diarrhea, electrolyte
   imbalances, vertigo, cramping,
   rash, headache, weakness, ECG
   changes, blurred vision,
   photosensitivity

Adverse Reactions

Severe dehydration; marked
   hypotension
Life threatening: Renal failure,
   thrombocytopenia, agranulocytosis

KEY: For complete abbreviation key, see inside front cover.

■ NURSING PROCESS: Diuretics: Loop (High Ceiling)

ASSESSMENT

- Obtain a history of drugs that are taken daily. Note if client is taking a drug(s) that may cause an interaction, such as alcohol, aminoglycosides, anticoagulants, corticosteroids, or digitalis. Recognize that furosemide is highly protein-bound and can displace other protein-bound drugs such as Coumadin.
- Assess VS, serum electrolytes, weight, and urine output for baseline levels.
- Compare client's drug dose with recommended dose and report discrepancy.

POTENTIAL NURSING DIAGNOSIS

High risk for fluid volume deficit

PLANNING

- Client's edema and/or hypertension will be decreased.
- Client's serum chemistry levels will remain within normal ranges.

NURSING INTERVENTIONS

- Check the half-life of furosemide. With a short half-life, the drug can be repeated or given more than once a day.
- Check onset of action for furosemide, orally and intravenously. If the drug is given intravenously, the urine output should increase in 5–20 min. If urine output does not increase, notify the health care provider. Severe renal disorder may be present.
- Monitor urinary output to determine body fluid gain or loss. Urinary output should be at least 25 mL/h or 600 mL/24 h.
- Check the client's weight to determine fluid loss or gain. A loss of 2.2–2.5 lb is equivalent to a fluid loss of 1 liter.
- Monitor VS. Be alert for marked decrease in blood pressure.
- Administer IV furosemide slowly; hearing loss may occur if rapidly injected.
- Observe for signs and symptoms of hypokalemia (<3.5 mEq/L), such as muscle weakness, abdominal distention, and/or cardiac dysrhythmias.
- Check serum potassium levels, especially when a client is taking digoxin. Hypokalemia enhances the action of digitalis, causing digitalis toxicity.

CLIENT TEACHING

General

- Instruct the client to take furosemide early in the morning and *not* in the evening, to prevent sleep disturbance and nocturia.

Diet

- Suggest taking furosemide at mealtime or with food to avoid nausea.

Side Effects

- Instruct the client to arise slowly to prevent dizziness due to fluid loss.

EVALUATION

- Evaluate the effectiveness of drug action: decreased fluid retention or fluid overload, decreased respiratory distress, and increased cardiac output.
- Check for side effects and increase in urine output.

Diuretics: Loop (High Ceiling), Osmotics, Carbonic Anhydrase Inhibitors

Generic (Brand)	Route and Dosage	Preg Cat	Interaction	t 1/2	PB	Action Onset	Action Peak	Action Duration
Loop (High Ceiling) Bumetanide (Bumex)	A: PO: 0.5–2.0 mg/d, max: 10 mg/d IV: 0.5–1.0 mg/dose; repeat in 2–4 h C: PO: 0.015 mg/kg/d	C	*Increase* risk of ototoxicity with aminoglycosides, vancomycin, cisplatin; *increase* risk of toxicity with digoxin, lithium; *increase* drug effect with antihypertensives *Decrease* effects of antidiabetics (oral and insulin)	1–1.5 h	95%	PO: 0.5–1 h IV: 5–10 min	1–2 h 15–45 min	4–6 h 3–4 h
Ethacrynic acid (Edecrin)	A: PO: 50–200 mg/d IV: 0.5–1.0 mg/kg/dose C: PO: 25 mg/d	B	Similar to bumetanide	1–1.5 h	95%	PO: 30 min IV: 5–10 min	1–2 h 15–30 min	6–8 h 2–3 h
Furosemide	See Prototype Drug Chart							
Torsemide (Demadox)	*Hypertension* A: PO/IV: Initially: 5 mg/d; maint: PO: 5–10 mg/d IV: In 2 min *CHF:* A: PO/IV: 10–20 mg/d	C	Similar to furosemide	2–4 h	97–99%	30–60 min	1–4 h	6 h

Drug / Dose	C	Interactions				
Osmotics Mannitol *ICP, IOP:* A: IV: 1.5–2.0 g/kg; 15–25% sol infused over 30–60 min *Oliguria:* A: IV: 100 g; 15–20% sol infused over 90 min	C	*Incompatible* with whole blood *Decrease* effect of lithium	1.5 h	UK	IV: 1–3h	UK	4–6 h
Carbonic Anhydrase Inhibitors Acetazolamide (Diamox) A: PO/IV: 250 mg q12h; dose may vary C: PO: 10–15 mg/kg/d in divided doses C: IV: 5–10 mg/kg q6h	C	*Increase* effects of amphetamines, antidysrhythmics, tricyclic antidepressants; *increase* toxicity with salicylates; *increase* hypokalemia with other diuretics, corticosteroids, amphotericin B	2.5–5.5 h	90%	PO: 1–1.5 h PO/SR: 2 h IV 2 min	2–4 h 8–12 h 15 min	6–12 h 18–24 h 4–5 h
Dichlorphenamide (Daranide, Oratrol) A: PO: 100 mg q12h; maint: 25–50 mg q.d./t.i.d.	C	Similar to acetazolamide *Decrease* effect of lithium	UK	UK	PO 0.5–1 h	2–4 h	6–12 h
Methazolamide (Neptazane) A: PO: 50–100 mg b.i.d./t.i.d.	C	Same as dichlorphenamide	14 h	50–60%	2–4 h	6–8 h	10–18 h

KEY: For complete abbreviation key, see inside front cover.

Diuretic: Potassium Sparing

Triamterene

Triamterene
  (Dyrenium)
Potassium-sparing diuretic
Pregnancy Category: B
Drug Forms:
Cap 50, 100 mg

Dosage

A: PO: Edema: 100 mg q.d., b.i.d.; not
  to exceed 300 mg/d
C: PO: 2–4 mg/kg/d in divided
  doses

Contraindications

Severe kidney or hepatic disease,
  severe hyperkalemia
Caution: Renal or hepatic
  dysfunction, diabetes mellitus

Drug-Lab-Food Interactions

Increase serum potassium level with
  potassium supplements; *increase*
  effects of antihypertensives and
  lithium
Lab: Increase serum potassium level;
  may *increase* BUN, AST, alkaline
  phosphatase levels
  Decrease serum sodium, chloride

Pharmacokinetics

Absorption: Rapidly absorbed from GI
  tract
Distribution: PB: 67%
Metabolism: t 1/2: 1.5–2.5 h
Excretion: In urine, mostly as
  metabolites and bile

Pharmacodynamics

PO: Onset: 2–4 h
  Peak: 6–8 h
  Duration: 12–16 h

Therapeutic Effects/Use: To increase urine output; to treat fluid retention/overload
associated with CHF, hepatic cirrhosis, or nephrotic syndrome.

Mode of Action: Action on the distal renal tubules to promote sodium and water excretion and potassium retention.

Side Effects

Nausea, vomiting, diarrhea, rash,
  dizziness, headache, weakness, dry
  mouth, photosensitivity

Adverse Reactions

Life threatening: Severe hyperkalemia,
  thrombocytopenia, megaloblastic
  anemia

KEY: For complete abbreviation key, see inside front cover.

■ NURSING PROCESS: Diuretic: Potassium Sparing

ASSESSMENT

• Obtain a history of drugs that are taken daily. Note if the client is taking a potassium supplement or using a salt substitute.
• Assess VS, serum electrolytes, weight, and urinary output for baseline levels.
• Compare the client's drug dose with the recommended dose and report any discrepancy.

POTENTIAL NURSING DIAGNOSIS

High risk for fluid volume deficit

PLANNING

• Client's fluid retention and blood pressure will be decreased.
• Client's serum electrolytes remain within their normal values.

NURSING INTERVENTIONS

• Check the half-life of triamterene. With a long half-life, drug dose is usually administered once a day and sometimes twice a day.
• Monitor urinary output. Urine output should increase. Report if urine output is <30 mL/h, or 600 mL/day.
• Monitor VS. Report abnormal changes.
• Observe for signs and symptoms of hyperkalemia (increased serum potassium level: >5.3 mEq/L), such as nausea, diarrhea, abdominal cramps, tachycardia and later bradycardia, peaked narrow T wave (ECG), or oliguria.
• Administer triamterene in the early morning and not in the evening, to avoid nocturia.

CLIENT TEACHING

General

• Instruct the client to take triamterene with or after meals to avoid nausea.

Diet

• Advise clients with high average serum potassium levels to avoid foods rich in potassium when taking potassium-sparing diuretics.

Side Effects

• Instruct the client to avoid exposure to direct sunlight because the drug can cause photosensitivity.
• Advise the client to report possible side effects of the drug, such as rash, dizziness, or weakness.

EVALUATION

• Evaluate the effectiveness of the potassium-sparing diuretic such as triamterene. The presence of fluid retention (edema) is decreased or absent.
• Determine if urine output has increased and the serum potassium level is within normal range.

Diuretic: Potassium Sparing

Generic (Brand)	Route and Dosage	Preg Cat	Interaction	t 1/2	PB	Action Onset	Peak	Duration
Single Agents Amiloride HCl (Midamor)	A: PO: 5 mg/d; may increase to 10–20 mg/d in 1–2 divided doses	B	*Increase* hyperkalemia with potassium supplements, ACE inhibitors, salt substitutes; *increase* effect of lithium, antihypertensives	6–9 h	23%	PO: 2 h	6–10 h	24 h
Spironolactone (Aldactone)	*Hypertension:* A: PO: 25–100 mg/d *Edema:* A: PO: 25–200 mg/d in divided doses C: PO: 3.3 mg/kg/d in divided doses	C	Similar to amiloride *Decrease* drug effect with aspirin	1.5–2 h	98%	PO: 24–48 h	48–72 h	48–72 h
Triamterene	See Prototype Drug Chart							

Combinations:

Amiloride HCl and hydrochlorothiazide (Moduretic)	A: PO: 1–2 tab (amiloride 5 mg/hydrochlorothiazide 50 mg)	B	UK	UK	UK	UK	UK	UK
Spironolactone and hydrochlorothiazide (Aldactazide)	A: PO: 25/25 and 50/50 mg tab	B, C	UK	UK	UK	UK	UK	UK
Triamterene and hydrochlorothiazide (Dyazide, Maxzide)	A: PO: 1–2 cap b.i.d., p.c. (triamterene 50 mg/hydrochlorothiazide 25 mg)	B	UK	UK	UK	UK	UK	UK

KEY: For complete abbreviation key, see inside front cover.

Antihypertensives: Beta Blockers

Metoprolol tartrate	Dosage
Metoprolol tartrate (Lopressor, Betaloc, Apo- Metoprolol) Adrenergic blocker, sympatholytic, beta$_2$ blocker *Pregnancy Category:* C *Drug Forms:* Tab 50, 100 mg Inj 1 mg/mL	*Hypertension:* A: PO: 50–100 mg/d in 1–2 divided doses; maint: 100–450 mg in divided doses; max: 450 mg/d in divided doses *Myocardial Infarcton:* A: PO: 100 mg b.i.d. IV: 5 mg q2min × 3 doses

Contraindications	Drug-Lab-Food Interactions
Second- and third-degree heart block, cardiogenic shock, CHF, sinus bradycardia *Caution:* Hepatic, renal, or thyroid dysfunction; asthma; peripheral vascular disease	*Increase* bradycardia with digitalis; *increase* hypotensive effect with other antihypertensives, alcohol, anesthetics

Pharmacokinetics	Pharmacodynamics

Absorption: PO: 95%
Distribution: PB: 12%
Metabolism: t 1/2: 3–4 h
Excretion: In urine
	PO: Onset: 15 min
	    Peak: 1.5 h
	    Duration: 10–19 h
	IV: Onset: Immediate
	    Peak: 20 min
	    Duration: 5–10 h

Therapeutic Uses/Effects: To control hypertension.

Mode of Action: Promotion of blood pressure reduction via beta$_1$-blocking effect.

Side Effects	Adverse Reactions
Fatigue, weakness, dizziness, nausea, vomiting, diarrhea, mental changes, nasal stuffiness	Bradycardia, thrombocytopenia *Life threatening:* Complete heart block, bronchospasm, agranulocytosis

KEY: For complete abbreviation key, see inside front cover.

■ NURSING PROCESS: Antihypertensives: Beta Blockers

ASSESSMENT

● Obtain a medication history from the client. Report if a drug-drug interaction is probable.

● Obtain VS. Report abnormal blood pressure. Compare VS with baseline finding.

● Check laboratory values related to renal and liver function. An elevated BUN and serum creatinine may be caused by metoprolol or cardiac disorder. Elevated cardiac enzymes, such as AST and LDH, could result from use of metoprolol or from a cardiac disorder.

POTENTIAL NURSING DIAGNOSES
Decreased cardiac output
Noncompliance with drug regimen

PLANNING
- Client's blood pressure will be decreased and/or return to normal value.
- Client takes the medication as prescribed.

NURSING INTERVENTIONS
- Monitor VS, especially blood pressure and pulse.
- Monitor laboratory results, especially BUN, serum creatinine, AST, and LDH.

CLIENT TEACHING
General
- Instruct the client to comply with drug regimen: *abrupt discontinuation of the antihypertensive drug may cause rebound hypertension.*
- Suggest that the client avoid OTC drugs without first checking with the health care provider. Many OTC drugs carry warning against use in the presence of hypertension.
- Suggest that the client wear a Medic Alert bracelet or carry a card indicating the health problem and prescribed drugs.
- Instruct the client in a trauma situation to inform the physician of drugs taken daily, such as a beta blocker. Beta blockers block the compensatory effects of the body to the shock state. Glucagon may be needed to reverse the effects so that the client can be resuscitated.

Skill
- Instruct the client or family member how to take a radial pulse and blood pressure. Advise the client to report abnormal findings to the health care provider.

Diet
- Teach the client and family members nonpharmacologic methods to decrease blood pressure, such as a low-fat and low-salt diet, weight control, relaxation techniques, exercise, smoking cessation, and decreased alcohol ingestion (1–2 oz/d).
- Advise the client to report constipation. Foods high in fiber, a stool softener, and increased water intake (except in clients with CHF) are usually indicated.

Side Effects
- Advise the client that antihypertensives may cause dizziness due to orthostatic hypotension. Instruct the client to remain in a sitting position for several minutes before standing.
- Instruct the client to report dizziness, slow pulse rate, changes in blood pressure, heart palpitation, confusion, or GI upset to the health care provider.

EVALUATION
- Evaluate the effectiveness of the drug therapy, i.e, decreased blood pressure and the absence of side effects.
- Determine that the client is adhering to the drug regimen.

Antihypertensives: Beta Blockers and Central Alpha$_2$ Agonists

Generic (Brand)	Route and Dosage	Preg Cat	Interaction	t 1/2	PB	Onset	Peak	Duration
Beta-Adrenergic Blockers								
Acebutolol HCl (Sectral) Cardioselective beta$_1$	A: PO: 400–800 mg/d in 1 or 2 divided doses; max: 1,200 mg/d	B	*Increase* hypotensive effect with other antihypertensives and diuretics	3–13 h	26%	1 h	3–4 h	12–24 h
Atenolol (Tenormin) Cardioselective beta$_1$	A: PO: 25–100 mg/d	C	See acebutolol *Increase* absorption with anticholinergics; may *increase* lidocaine levels *Decrease* hypotensive effect with NSAIDs	6–7h	6–16%	1 h	2–4 h	24 h
Betaxolol HCl (Kerlone) Cardioselective beta$_1$	A: PO: 10–20 mg/d Also for ophthalmic use: glaucoma	C	May *increase* hypotension with calcium channel blockers	14–22 h	UK	30 min	2 h	12h
Bisoprolol fumarate (Zebeta) Beta$_1$ blocker	A: PO: Initially: 5 mg/d; maint: 2.5–20 mg/d	C	Similar to atenolol	9–12 h	<30%	UK	UK	UK
Carteolol HCl (Cartrol) Nonselective beta$_1$ and beta$_2$	A: PO: 2.5–5.0 mg/d	C	May *increase* hypoglycemia with insulin May *decrease* effect of theophylline; *decrease* blood pressure with aspirin and NSAIDs	4–6 h	23–30%	1 h	2–4 h	24–48 h

Drug	Dosage	Pregnancy Category	Uses and Considerations	t½	PB	Onset	Peak	Duration
Metoprolol (Lopressor) Cardioselective beta$_1$	See Prototype Drug Chart							
Nadolol (Corgard) Nonselective beta$_1$ and beta$_2$	A: PO: 40–80 mg/d; max: 320 mg/d	C	Similar to acebutolol and atenolol	10–24 h	30%	1 h	2–4 h	18–24 h
Penbutolol SO$_4$ (Levatol)	A: PO: 10–20 mg/d; max: 80 mg/d	C	Similar to acebutolol *Decrease* hypoglycemic effect of glyburide	5 h	80–98%	1 h	2–3 h	20–24 h
Pindolol (Visken) Nonselective beta$_1$ and beta$_2$	A: PO: 5 mg b.i.d., t.i.d.; maint: 10–30 mg in divided doses; max: 60 mg/d in divided doses	B	Similar to acebutolol and atenolol	3–4 h	50%	3 h	1–2 h	24 h
Propranolol (Inderal) Nonselective beta$_1$ and beta$_2$	A: PO: Initially: 40 mg b.i.d. SR: 80 mg/d; maint: 120–240 mg/d in divided doses C: PO: Initially 1 mg/kg/d in 2 divided doses; maint: 2 mg/kg/d	C	Similar to acebutolol and atenolol *Increase* effect with calcium channel blockers, phenothiazides *Decrease* absorption with antacid *Lab:* May *increase* AST, ALT, ALP, LDH, BUN	3–6 h	90%	0.5–1 h	1–1.5 h SR: 6 h	6–12 h
Timolol maleate (Blocadren) Nonselective beta$_1$ and beta$_2$	A: PO: Initially: 10 mg b.i.d.; maint: 20–40 mg/d in 2 divided doses; max: 60 mg/d Also for ophthalmic use: glaucoma	C	Similar to acebutolol	3–4 h	60%	1 h	2–4 h	12–24 h

continued

Generic (Brand)	Route and Dosage	Preg Cat	Interaction	t 1/2	PB	Action Onset	Action Peak	Action Duration
Central Alpha₂ Agonists								
Clonidine HCl (Catapres)	A: PO: Initially: 0.1 mg b.i.d.; maint: 0.2–1.2 mg/d in divided doses; max: 2.4 mg/d A: Transdermal patch: 100 μg (0.1 mg) b.i.d. or 200 μg (0.2 mg) q.d.	C	*Increase* hypotensive effect with diuretics, other antihypertensives; *increase* CNS depression with alcohol, CNS depressants *Decrease* hypotensive effects with tricyclic antidepressants, MAOIs	6–20 h	20–40%	PO: 0.5–1 h Transdermal: 1–3 d	2–4 h 2–3 d	8 h 7 d
Guanabenz acetate (Wytensin)	A: PO: 4 mg b.i.d.; may increase to 4–8 mg/d q 1–2 wk; max: 32 mg b.i.d.	C	*Increase* CNS depression with alcohol, CNS depressants *Decrease* hypotensive effect with tricyclic antidepressants	4–14 h	90%	1 h	2–5 h	6–12 h
Guanfacine HCl (Tenex)	A: PO: 1 mg h.s.; may increase to 2–3 mg/d	B	Similar to guanabenz	>17 h	70%	1–2 h	2–6 h	24 h
Methyldopa (Aldomet)	A: PO: 250–500 mg b.i.d.; max: 3 g/d IV: 250 mg–1 g q6h C: PO: 10 mg/kg/d in 2–4 divided doses	C	May *increase* effect with tricyclic antidepressants, phenothiazides; *increase* hypotension with levodopa; *increase* risk of lithium toxicity *Decrease* effects of ephedrine	1.7 h	<15%	12–24 h	2–6 h	12–24 h

KEY: For complete abbreviation key, see inside front cover.

NOTES:

Antihypertensives: Alpha-Adrenergic Blocker

Prazosin HCl	Dosage
Prazosin HCl (Minipress) Sympatholytic, selective alpha-adrenergic blocker *Pregnancy Category:* C *Drug Forms:* Cap 1, 2.5 mg	A: PO: 1 mg b.i.d./t.i.d.; maint: 3–15 mg/d; max: 20 mg/d in divided doses

Contraindications	Drug-Lab-Food Interactions
Renal disease	*Increase* hypotensive effect with other antihypertensives, nitrates, alcohol

Pharmacokinetics	Pharmacodynamics
Absorption: GI: 60% (5% to circulation) *Distribution:* PB: 95% *Metabolism:* t 1/2: 3 h *Excretion:* 10% in urine; in bile and feces	IV: Onset: 0.5–2 h Peak: 2–4 h Duration: 10 h

Therapeutic Uses/Effects: To control hypertension, refractory CHF.

Mode of Action: Dilation of peripheral blood vessels via blocking the alpha-adrenergic receptors.

Side Effects	Adverse Reactions
Dizziness, drowsiness, headache, nausea, vomiting, diarrhea, impotence, vertigo, urinary frequency, tinnitus, dry mouth, incontinence, abdominal discomfort	Orthostatic hypotension, palpitations, tachycardia, pancreatitis

KEY: For complete abbreviation key, see inside front cover.

■ **NURSING PROCESS: Antihypertensives: Adrenergic Blockers**

ASSESSMENT

- Obtain a medication history from the client, including current drugs. Report if a drug-drug interaction is probable. Prazosin is highly protein-bound and can displace other highly protein-bound drugs.
- Obtain baseline VS and weight for future comparisons.
- Check urinary output. Report if it is decreased (<600 mL/d), because drug is contraindicated if renal disease is present.

POTENTIAL NURSING DIAGNOSES
High risk for activity intolerance
Knowledge deficit related to drug regimen
Altered sexuality patterns

PLANNING
- Client's blood pressure will decrease.
- Client will follow proper drug regimen.

NURSING INTERVENTIONS
- Monitor VS. The desired therapeutic effect of prazosin may not fully occur for 4 wk. A sudden marked decrease in blood pressure should be reported.
- Check daily for fluid retention in the extremities. Prazosin may cause sodium and water retention.

CLIENT TEACHING

General
- Instruct the client to comply with drug regimen. *Abrupt discontinuation of the antihypertensive drug may cause rebound hypertension.*
- Inform the client that orthostatic hypotension may occur. Explain that before arising, the client should dangle his or her feet.

Skill
- Instruct the client or family member how to take a blood pressure reading. A record for daily blood pressures should be kept.

Diet
- Encourage the client to decrease salt intake unless otherwise indicated by the health care provider.

Side Effects
- Caution the client that dizziness, lightheadedness, and drowsiness may occur, especially when the drug is first prescribed. If these symptoms occur, the health care provider should be notified.
- Inform the male client that impotence may occur if high doses of the drug are prescribed. This problem should be reported to the health care provider.
- Instruct the client to report if edema is present in the morning.
- Instruct the client not to take cold, cough, or allergy OTC medications without first contacting the health care provider.

EVALUATION
- Evaluate the effectiveness of the drug in controlling blood pressure and the absence of side effects.
- Evaluate the client's adherence to medication schedule.

Antihypertensives: Sympatholytics: Alpha-Adrenergic, Alpha-Beta, and Peripherally Acting Blockers; and Direct-Acting Vasodilators

Generic (Brand)	Route and Dosage	Preg Cat	Interaction	t 1/2	PB	Onset	Peak	Duration
Selective Alpha-Adrenergic Blockers								
Doxazosin mesylate (Cardura)	A: PO: Initially: 1 mg/d; maint: 2–4 mg/d; max: 16 mg/d	C	Similar to terazosin	22 h	98%	1.5–2 h	2–6 h	6–12 h
Prazosin HCl (Minipress)	See Prototype Drug Chart							
Terazosin HCl (Hytrin)	A: PO: Initially 1 mg h.s.; maint: 1–5 mg/d; max: 20 mg/d	C	Increase hypotensive effect with diuretics, other antihypertensives, beta blockers, calcium channel blockers	9–12 h	95%	15 min	1–2 h	12–24 h
Alpha-Adrenergic Blockers								
Phenoxybenzamine HCl (Dibenzyline)	A: PO: Initially: 10 mg/d; maint: 20–40 mg/d C: PO: 0.2 mg/kg/d in 1–2 divided doses; may increase dose by 0.2 mg	C	Similar to phentolamine	24 h	UK	2 h	4–6 h	3–4 d
Phentolamine (Regitine)	A: IM/IV: 2.5–5 mg; repeat q5min until controlled; then q2–3h PRN C: IM/IV: 0.05–0.1 mg/kg; repeat if needed	C	Increase hypotensive effect with antihypertensives	20 min	UK	IM: 15–20 min IV: Immediate	IM: 20 min IV: 2 min	IM: 3–4 h IV: 15 min

Tolazoline HCl (Priscoline HCl)	NB: IV: Initially: 1–2 mg/kg; followed by 1–2 mg/kg/h for 24–48 h; expected effect within 30 min of initial dose A: IM/IV: 10–50 mg q.i.d.	C	Increase effect with alcohol, beta blockers, antihypertensives	3–10 h	UK	30 min	IM: 0.5–1 h	IM: 3–4 h
Peripherally Acting Sympatholytics								
Guanadrel sulfate (Hylorel)	A: PO: Initially: 5 mg b.i.d.; maint: 20–75 mg/d in divided doses	B	Same as guanethidine	10–12 h	20%	1–2 h	4–6 h	6–12 h
Guanethidine monosulfate (Ismelin sulfate)	A: PO: Initially: 10 mg /d; maint: 25–50 mg/d; max: 300 mg/d C: PO: 0.2 mg/kg/d; max: 1–1.6 mg/kg/d	C	Increase hypotensive effect with diuretics, alcohol, antihypertensives, levodopa Decrease hypotensive effects with decongestants, tricyclic antidepressants, phenothiazides	5 d	UK	0.5–2 h	6–8 h	1–3 wk
Reserpine (Serpasil)	A: PO: Initially: 0.25–5.0 mg daily for 1–2 wk; maint: 0.1–0.25 mg/d	D	Increase hypotensive effect with diuretics, beta blockers antihypertensives; increase CNS depression with alcohol, narcotics, barbiturates; increase cardiac depression with antidysrhythmics	11–50 h	96%	Days to 2 wk	Initially: 2–4 h Later: 3–6 wk	1–6 wk

continued

Generic (Brand)	Route and Dosage	Preg Cat	Interaction	t 1/2	PB	Action			
						Onset	Peak	Duration	

Generic (Brand)	Route and Dosage	Preg Cat	Interaction	t 1/2	PB	Onset	Peak	Duration
Direct-Acting Vasodilators								
Diazoxide (Hyperstat, Proglycem)	A & C: IV: 1–3 mg/kg in bolus (30 s); repeat in 5–15 min as needed; max: 150 mg	C	*Increase* hypotensive hyperglycemia, hyperuricemia effect with thiazide diuretics	20–45 h	90%	1–2 min	5 min	3–12 h
Hydralazine HCl (Apresoline HCl)	A: PO: Initially: 10 mg q.i.d.; maint: 25–50 mg q.i.d. Severe hypertension: IM-IV: 10–40 mg; repeat as needed C: PO: 3–7.5 mg/kg/d in 4 divided doses	C	*Increase* hypotensive effects with diuretics, beta blockers, antihypertensives	2–8 h	87%	PO: 20–30 min IM: 10–30 min IV: 5–20 min	PO: 1–2 h IM: 1 h IV: 2–6 h	PO: 2–5 h IM: 2–6 h IV: 2–6 h

Drug	Dosage		Contraindications–Caution	t½	PB	Onset	Peak	Duration
Minoxidil (Loniten, Rogaine, Minodyl)	A: PO: Initially: 5 mg/d; maint: 10–40 mg/d in single or divided doses; max: 100 mg/d C: PO: Initially: 0.2 mg/kg/d; max: 5 mg/d; maint: 0.25–1 mg/kg/d in divided doses; max: 50 mg/d *Topical for alopecia:* 2% sol b.i.d.	C	Similar to hydralazine *Lab:* May *increase* BUN, creatinine, ALP	3.5–4 h	0%	30 min	2–8 h	2–5 d
Sodium nitroprusside (Nipride, Nitropress)	A: IV: 1–3 μg/kg/min in D₅W; max: 10 μg/kg/min	C	None significant	2–7 d	UK	Immediate	2–5 min	10 min after infusion
Alpha- and Beta-Adrenergic Blocker								
Labetalol HCl (Trandate)	A: PO: Initially: 100 mg b.i.d.; maint: 200–800 mg/d in 2 divided doses A: IV: 2 mg/min in infusion; max: 300 mg as total dose	C	*Increase* hypotensive effect with diuretics, antihypertensives, nitrates, cimetidine, halothane; *increase* hypoglycemia with insulin, oral hypoglycemics *Decrease* effect with adrenergics, theophylline, lidocaine	4–8 h	50%	PO: 1–2 h IV: 2–5 min	PO: 2–4 h IV: 5–10 min	PO: 8–24 h IV: 2–4 h

KEY: For complete abbreviation key, see inside front cover.

305

Antihypertensives: Angiotensin Antagonist

Captopril	Dosage

Captopril
  (Capoten)
ACE inhibitor, angiotensin
  antagonist
Pregnancy Category: C
Drug Forms:
tab 12.5, 25, 50, 100 mg
	A: PO: 12.5–25 mg b.i.d./t.i.d.; max:
	  450 mg/d; maint: 25–50 mg t.i.d.

Contraindications	Drug-Lab-Food Interactions

Heart block
Caution: Leukemia, chronic
  obstructive pulmonary disease,
  renal or thyroid disease
	Increase hypotensive effect with
	  nitrates, diuretics, adrenergic
	  blockers, vasodilators, other
	  antihypertensives

Pharmacokinetics	Pharmacodynamics

Absorption: PO: 65% (food decreases
  absorption)
Distribution: PB: UK
Metabolism: t 1/2: 6–7 h
Excretion: In urine
	PO: Onset: 15 min
	     Peak: 1 h
	     Duration: 4–12 h

Therapeutic Uses/Effects: To reduce blood pressure; to control CHF.

Mode of Action: Suppression of the angiotensin-converting enzyme (ACE); inhibits angiotensin I conversion to angiotensin II.

Side Effects	Adverse Reactions

Dizziness, cough, nocturia,
  impotence, rash, polyuria,
  hyperkalemia, taste disturbance
	Oliguria, urticaria, severe
	  hypotension
	Life threatening: Acute renal failure,
	  bronchospasm, angioedema,
	  agranulocytosis

KEY: For complete abbreviation key, see inside front cover.

■ **NURSING PROCESS: Antihypertensives: Angiotensin Antagonist**

ASSESSMENT

• Obtain a drug history from the client of current drugs that are being taken. Report if a drug-drug interaction is probable.

• Obtain baseline VS for future comparisons.

• Check the laboratory values for serum protein, albumin, BUN, and creatinine, and compare with future serum levels.

POTENTIAL NURSING DIAGNOSES
Knowledge deficit related to drug regimen
Anxiety related to hypertensive state

PLANNING
• Client's blood pressure will be within desired range.
• Client is free of moderate to severe side effects

NURSING INTERVENTIONS
• Monitor laboratory tests related to renal function (BUN, creatinine, protein) and blood glucose levels. Caution: Watch for hypoglycemic reaction in a client with diabetes mellitus. Urine protein may be checked in the morning using a dipstick.
• Report to the health care provider occurrences of bruising, petechiae, and/or bleeding. These may indicate a severe adverse reaction to an angiotensin antagonist such as captopril.

CLIENT TEACHING
General
• Instruct the client not to abruptly discontinue use of captopril without notifying the health care provider. *Rebound hypertension could result.*
• Inform the client not to take OTC drugs (cold, allergy medications) without first contacting the health care provider.

Skill
• Teach the client how to take and record his or her blood pressure. Blood pressure chart should be established, and blood pressure changes should be reported.

Diet
• Instruct the client to take captopril 20 min–1 h before a meal. Food decreases 35% of captopril absorption.
• Inform the client that the taste of food may be diminished during the first month of drug therapy.

Side Effects
• Explain to the client that dizziness and/or lightheadedness may occur during the first week of captopril therapy. If dizziness persists, the health care provider should be notified.
• Instruct the client to report any occurrence of bleeding.

EVALUATION
• Evaluate the effectiveness of the drug therapy: in the absence of severe side effects and blood pressure return to desired range.

Antihypertensives: Angiotensin Antagonists and Calcium Blockers

Generic (Brand)	Route and Dosage	Preg Cat	Interaction	t 1/2	PB	Onset	Peak	Duration
Angiotensin Antagonists (ACE Inhibitors)								
Benazepril HCl (Lotensin)	A: PO: Initially: 10 mg/d; maint: 20–40 mg/d in 2 divided doses	D	Similar to ramipril	10 h	97%	UK	1–2 h	20 h
Captopril (Capoten)	See Prototype Drug Chart							
Enalapril maleate (Vasotec)	A: PO: Initially: 5 mg/d; maint: 10–40 mg/d in 1–2 divided doses IV: 1.25 mg q6h infuse in 5 min	C	*Increase* hypotensive effects with diuretics, antihypertensives; may *increase* lithium levels; *increase* potassium levels with potassium-sparing diuretics, potassium supplements *Decrease* effect with antacids, NSAIDs, aspirin	1.5–2 h	50–60%	PO: 1 h IV: 15 min	PO: 4–8 h IV: 1–4 h	PO: 24 h IV: 6 h
Lisinopril (Prinivil, Zestril)	A: PO: Initially: 10 mg/d; maint: 20–40 mg/d; max: 80 mg/d	C	Similar to enalapril	12 h	0%	1 h	6–8 h	24 h

Drug	Dosage	Pregnancy Category	Drug Interactions	$t_{1/2}$	Protein Binding	Onset	Peak	Duration
Ramipril (Altrace)	A: PO: 2.5–5 mg/d; max: 20 mg/d	D	May *increase* effect with lithium; *increase* hypotension with diuretics; *increase* risk of hyperkalemia with potassium supplements, potassium-sparing diuretics	2–3 h	97%	2 h	6–8 h	24 h
Calcium Channel Blockers								
Diltiazem HCl (Cardizem, Cardizem CD or SR)	A: PO SR: Initially: 60–120 mg b.i.d.; max: 240–360 mg/d	C	May *increase* effects of theophylline, beta blockers, digoxin; *increase* effect with cimetidine	3.5–9 h	70–85%	PO SR: UK	PO SR: 6–11 h	PO SR: >12 h
Felodipine (Plendil)	A: PO: Initially: 5 mg; maint: 5–10 mg/d; max: 20 mg/d	C	*Increase* effect of beta blockers, digoxin; *increase* effect with histamine₂ blockers. May *decrease* phenytoin, phenobarbital, carbamazepine. *Lab:* May *increase* ALP, AST, ALT, CPK, LDH	10–16 h	99%	1–2 h	2–5 h	20–24 h

continued

Antihypertensives: Angiotensin Antagonists and Calcium Blockers *Continued*

Generic (Brand)	Route and Dosage	Preg Cat	Interaction	t 1/2	PB	Onset	Peak	Duration
							Action	
Isradipine (DynaCirc)	*Hypertension:* A: PO: 1.25–10 mg b.i.d.; max: 20 mg/d	C	*Increase* effect of digoxin, cyclosporine	5–11 h	99%	1–2 h	2–3 h	12 h
Nifedipine (Procardia)	A: PO: 10–20 mg t.i.d. A: PO SR: 30–90 mg/d; max: 120 mg/d	C	*Increase* effect with cimetidine; *increase* effects of theophylline, beta blockers, antihypertensives	2–5 h	92–98%	PO: 20 min PO SR: UK	PO: 1–4 h PO SR: UK	PO: 6–8 h PO SR: 24 h
Verapamil (Calan SR, Isoptin SR)	A: PO SR: 120–240 mg/d in 2 divided doses; max: 480 mg/d	C	*Decrease* effect of lithium; other interactions similar to nifedipine	3–8 h	90%	PO SR: UK	PO SR: 4–8 h	PO SR: 24 h

KEY: For complete abbreviation key, see inside front cover.

NOTES:

_____

_____

_____

_____

_____

_____

_____

_____

_____

_____

Anticoagulants

Warfarin sodium

Warfarin sodium
  (Coumadin, Panwarfin)
Pregnancy Category: D
Drug Forms:
Tab 1, 2, 2.5, 5, 10 mg
Inj 50 mg/2 mL

Dosage

A: PO: LD: 10–15 mg/d for 2–3 d;
  maint: 2–10 mg/d
IM/IV: Dose is usually titrated
  according to PT—1.25 to 2.5 times
  control

Contraindications

Bleeding disorder, peptic ulcer,
  hepatic disease, blood dyscrasias,
  hemophilia, cerebral vascular
  accident (CVA), severe renal
  disease, eclampsia

Drug-Lab-Food Interactions

Increase effect with amiodarone,
  aspirin, NSAIDs, sulfonamides,
  thyroid drugs, allopurinol,
  histamine$_2$ blockers, oral
  hypoglycemics, metronidazole,
  miconazole, methyldopa, diuretics,
  oral antibiotics, vitamin E
Decrease effect with barbiturates,
  laxatives, phenytoin, estrogens,
  vitamins C and K, oral
  contraceptives, rifampin
Lab: May *increase* AST/ALT

Pharmacokinetics

Absorption: PO: Well absorbed
Distribution: PB: 99%
Metabolism: t 1/2: 0.5–3 d
Excretion: In urine and feces

Pharmacodynamics

PO: Onset: 12–24 h
  Peak: 1–3 d
  Duration: 2.5–5 d

Therapeutic Effects/Uses: To prevent blood clotting.

Mode of Action: Depression of hepatic synthesis of vitamin K–clotting factors (II, VII, IX, and X).

Side Effects

Anorexia, nausea, vomiting,
  diarrhea, abdominal cramps, rash,
  fever

Adverse Reactions

Bleeding, hematuria
Life threatening: Hemorrhage,
  thrombocytopenia, agranulocytosis

KEY: For complete abbreviation key, see inside front cover.

■ NURSING PROCESS: Anticoagulants: Warfarin (Coumadin)

ASSESSMENT

- Obtain a history of abnormal clotting or health problems that affect clotting, such as severe alcoholism or severe liver or renal disease. Warfarin is contraindicated for clients with blood dyscrasias, peptic ulcer, cerebral vascular accident (CVA), hemophilia, or severe hypertension. Caution its use in a client with acute traumatic injury.
- Obtain a drug history of current drugs the client is taking. Report if a drug-drug interaction is probable. Warfarin is highly protein-bound and can displace other highly protein-bound drugs, or warfarin could be displaced, which may result in bleeding.
- Develop a flow chart that lists PT and warfarin dosages. A baseline PT should be taken before warfarin is administered.

POTENTIAL NURSING DIAGNOSES

High risk for injury (bleeding)
Knowledge deficit

PLANNING

- Client's PT will be 1.25 to 2.5 times the control level. For a client receiving heparin, the aPTT should be checked.
- Abnormal bleeding will be rapidly addressed while the client is taking an anticoagulant. The PT level will be closely monitored.

NURSING INTERVENTIONS

- Monitor VS. An increased pulse rate followed by a decreased systolic pressure can indicate a fluid volume deficit due to external or internal bleeding.
- Check PT for warfarin (Coumadin) and aPTT for heparin before administering the anticoagulant. The PT should be 1.25 to 2.5 times the control level. The platelet count should be monitored, because anticoagulants can decrease platelet count.
- Check for bleeding from the mouth, nose (epistaxis), urine (hematuria), and skin (petechiae, purpura).
- Check stools periodically for occult blood.
- Monitor elderly clients receiving warfarin closely for bleeding. Their skin is thin and capillary beds are fragile. PT should be frequently checked.
- Keep anticoagulant antagonists (protamine, vitamin K_1, or vitamin K_3) available when drug dose is increased or there are indications of frank bleeding. Fresh or frozen plasma may be needed for transfusion.

CLIENT TEACHING

General

- Instruct the client to inform the dentist when taking an anticoagulant. Contacting the health care provider may be necessary.
- Instruct the client to use a soft toothbrush to avoid causing the gums to bleed.
- Instruct the client to shave with an electric razor. Bleeding from shaving cuts may be difficult to control.
- Advise the client to have laboratory tests such as PT performed as ordered by the health care provider. Warfarin dose is regulated according to the PT.

Anticoagulants

- Instruct the client to carry or wear a medical identification card or jewelry (Medic Alert) listing the person's name, telephone number, and drug name.
- Encourage the client *not* to smoke. Smoking increases metabolism; thus, the warfarin dose may need to be increased. If the person insists on smoking, notify the health care provider.
- Instruct the client to check with the health care provider before taking OTC drugs. Aspirin should *not* be taken with warfarin because aspirin intensifies its action and bleeding is apt to occur. Suggest that the client use acetaminophen.
- Teach the client to control external hemorrhage (bleeding) from accidents or injuries by applying firm, direct pressure for at least 5–10 min with a clean, dry absorbent material.

Diet

- Advise the client to avoid alcohol, which could contribute to increased bleeding, and large amounts of green leafy vegetables, fish, liver, coffee, or tea (caffeine), which are rich in vitamin K.

Side Effects

- Advise the client to report bleeding, such as petechiae, ecchymosis, purpura, tarry stools, bleeding gums, or expectoration of blood.

EVALUATION

- Evaluate the effectiveness of drug therapy. Client's PT values are within the desired range, and client is free of significant side effects.

Generic (Brand)	Route and Dosage	Preg Cat	Interaction	t 1/2	PB	Onset	Action Peak	Duration
Anticoagulants								
Dicumarol (Bishydroxycoumarin)	A: PO: LD: 200–300 mg/24 h; maint: 25–200 mg/d based on PT	D	*Increase* bleeding See warfarin	1–2 d	99%	Effect PT: 1–5 d	1–4 d	2–10 d
Enoxaparin sodium (Lovenox)	A: SC: 30 mg b.i.d.	B	*Increase* effect with other anticoagulants *Lab: Increase* AST, ALT	4.5 h	UK	UK	3 h	4–5 h
Heparin sodium (Lipo-Hepin, Pan-heprin)	A: SC: 5,000–7,500 U q6h or 8,000–10,000 U q8h A: IV: Bolus: 5,000 U Inf: 20,000–40,000 U over 24 h; dose varies according to APTT level C: IV: 50 U/kg bolus, 50–100 U/kg q4h or 20,000 U/m²/24 h	C	May *increase* bleeding with aspirin, NSAIDs *Decrease* effect with nitroglycerin, protamine *Lab: Increase* AST, ALT	1–1.5 h	95%	SC: 20–60 min IV: Rapid	SC: 5 min IV: 2 min	SC: 8–12 h IV: 2–6 h
Warfarin (Coumadin, Panwarfin)	See Prototype Drug Chart							

continued

Anticoagulants, Antiplatelets, and Anticoagulant Antagonists *Continued*

Generic (Brand)	Route and Dosage	Preg Cat	Interaction	$t\,1/2$	PB	Onset	Peak	Duration
						Action		
Antiplatelets								
Aspirin	A: PO: 325 mg/d or q.o.d.	D	*Increase* risk of bleeding with anticoagulant; *increase* risk of ulcer with glucocorticoids; *increase* risk of hypoglycemia with oral hypoglycemics *Lab: Decrease* potassium cholesterol, T_3, T_4	2–3 h	55%	15–30 min	1–2 h	4–6 h
Dipyridamole (Persantine)	A: PO: 50–100 mg t.i.d./q.i.d.	C	*Increase* effect with beta blockers, antidysrhythmics; *increase* antiplatelet effect with aspirin *Decrease* effect with phenytoin, rifampin	10–12 h	91–99%	0.5–1 h	1–2 h	6 h

Drug	Dosage	Pregnancy Category	Drug Interactions	3 h	95–99%	<1 h	1–2 h	4–6 h
Sulfinpyrazone (Anturane)	A: PO: 200–400 mg b.i.d.; max: 800 mg/d	C	*Increase* risk of hypoglycemia with oral hypoglycemics; *increase* PT with warfarin *Decrease* effect with aspirin, theophylline					
Anticoagulant Antagonists Protamine SO$_4$	A: IV: Initially: 1 mg/ 100 U heparin administered; 10–50 mg in 3–10 min slow push; max: 50 mg in any 10-min period	C	None significant	UK	UK	1–5 min	UK	2 h
Vitamin K$_1$, phytonadione (AquaMEPHYTON, Mephyton, Konakion)	A: PO/IM/IV: 2–10 mg q12–24 h as needed C: SC/IM: 5–10 mg	C	*Decrease* effects of warfarin, cholestyramine, colestipol	UK	UK	PO: 6–12 h SC/IM: 1–2 h IV: 15 min	SC/IM: 3–8 h Hemorrhage control	SC/IM: 12–14 h
Vitamin K$_3$, menadiol sodium diphosphate (Synkayvite)	A: PO/SC/IM/IV: 5–10 mg/d C: PO: 50–100 µg/d	C: preterm, term, X	*Decrease* effects of warfarin; *decrease* absorption by mineral oil, sucralfate	UK	UK	SC/IM: 1–2	UK	8–24 h

KEY: For complete abbreviation key, see inside front cover.

317

Thrombolytics

Streptokinase	Dosage
Streptokinase (Streptase, Kabikinase) Thrombolytic enzyme *Pregnancy Category:* C *Drug Forms:* Inj 250,000, 600,000, 750,000 IU	*Myocardial Infarction:* A: IV: 1,500,000 IU diluted in 45 mL; infuse over 60 min *Pulmonary Embolism (PE) and Deep Vein Thrombosis (DVT):* A: IV: LD: 250,000 IU Inf: 100,000 IU/h for 24–72 h (24 h for PE; 72 h for DVT)

Contraindications	Drug-Lab-Food Interactions
Recent CVA, cerebral neoplasm, active bleeding, severe hypertension, ulcerative colitis, anticoagulant therapy	*Increase* risk of bleeding with heparin, oral anticoagulants, aspirin, antiplatelets, NSAIDs

Pharmacokinetics	Pharmacodynamics
Absorption: IV: Directly administered *Distribution:* PB: UK *Metabolism:* t 1/2: 20–80 min *Excretion:* In urine and bile	PO: Onset: Immediate Peak: Rapid Duration: 4–12 h

Therapeutic Effects/Uses: To dissolve blood clots due to coronary artery thrombi, deep vein thrombosis, pulmonary embolism.

Mode of Action: Conversion of plasminogen to plasmin (fibrinolysin) for dissolving fibrin deposits.

Side Effects	Adverse Reactions
Headache, nausea, flushing, rash, fever	Bleeding, urticaria, unstable blood pressure *Life threatening:* Hemorrhage, bronchospasm, cardiac dysrhythmias, anaphylaxis

KEY: For complete abbreviation key, see inside front cover.

■ **NURSING PROCESS: Thrombolytics: Streptokinase**

ASSESSMENT

• Assess baseline VS and compare with future values.
• Check baseline PT value before administration of streptokinase.
• Obtain a medical and drug history. Contraindications for use of streptokinase include a recent CVA, active bleeding, severe hypertension, and anticoagulant therapy. It should be reported if the client is taking aspirin or NSAIDs. Thrombolytics are contraindicated for the client with a recent history of traumatic injury, especially head injury.

POTENTIAL NURSING DIAGNOSES
Decreased cardiac output
Anxiety related to severe health problem
Impaired tissue integrity

PLANNING
- The blood clot will be dissolved, and the client will be closely monitored for active bleeding.
- Client's VS will be monitored for stability during and after thrombolytic therapy.

NURSING INTERVENTIONS
- Monitor VS. Increased pulse rate followed by decreased blood pressure usually indicates blood loss and impending shock. Record VS and report changes.
- Observe for signs and symptoms of active bleeding from the mouth or rectum. Hemorrhage is a serious complication of thrombolytic treatment. Aminocaproic acid can be given as an intervention to stop the bleeding.
- Check for active bleeding for 24 h after thrombolytic therapy has been discontinued: q15min for the first hour, q30min until the eighth hour, and then hourly.
- Observe for signs of allergic reaction to streptokinase, such as itching, hives, flushing, fever, dyspnea, bronchospasm, hypotension, and/or cardiovascular collapse.
- Avoid administering aspirin or NSAIDs for pain or discomfort when the client is receiving a thrombolytic.
- Monitor the ECG for the presence of reperfusion dysrhythmias as the blood clot is dissolving; antidysrhythmic therapy may be indicated.

CLIENT TEACHING
General
- Explain the thrombolytic treatment to the client and family. Be supportive. If you cannot answer a question, refer the client or family to the health care provider.

Side Effects
- Instruct the client to report any side effects, such as lightheadedness, dizziness, palpitations, nausea, pruritus, or urticaria.

EVALUATION
- Determine the effectiveness of drug therapy. The client's clot has dissolved; VS are stable; there are no signs and symptoms of active bleeding; and the client is pain free.

Generic (Brand)	Route and Dosage	Preg Cat	Interaction	t 1/2	PB	Action		
						Onset	Peak	Duration
Thrombolytics								
Anistreplase (APSAC, Eminase)	A: IV: 30 U over 2–5 min	C	Similar to urokinase	1.5–2 h	UK	Immediate	45 min after injection	4–6 h
Streptokinase (Streptase, Kabikinase)	See Prototype Drug Chart							
Tissue-type plasminogen activator (t-PA, Alteplase)	*Acute Myocardial Infarction (AMI):* A: IV: Total: 100 mg over 3 h; bolus (1–2 min): 6–10 mg 1st hour: 60 mg; 2nd hour: 20 mg; 3rd hour: 20 mg *Pulmonary embolism:* A: IV: 100 mg over 2 h	C	*Increase* risk of bleeding with aspirin, heparin, dipyridamole	30 min	UK	Rapid	10–45 min	UK

Urokinase (Abbokinase)	B	A: IV: LD: 4,400 IU/kg diluted over 10 min Inf: 4,400 IU/kg over 12–24 h *Occluded coronary artery:* Dose may be increased	*Increase* risk of bleeding with aspirin, NSAIDs, anticoagulants	10–20 min	UK	Rapid	3–4 h	4–12 h
Plasminogen Inactivator Aminocaproic acid (Amicar)	C	A: PO/IV: LD: 5 g first hour Inf: 1–1.25 g/h for 8 h; max: 30 g/d	*Increase* coagulation with estrogens, oral contraceptives; may *increase* serum potassium level	1–2 h	0%	UK	<2 h	UK

KEY: For complete abbreviation key, see inside front cover.

Antilipemic

Lovastatin

Lovastatin
  (Mevacor)
Antilipemic, antihyperlipidemic
Pregnancy Category: X
Drug Forms:
Tab 20 mg

Dosage

A: PO: 20–80 mg/d in 1–2 divided
  doses with meals

Contraindications

Hepatic disease, pregnancy
Caution: Increase with alcohol
  consumption, seizure disorder,
  trauma

Drug-Lab-Food Interactions

Increase effect with other antilipemics;
  increase effect of Coumadin
Lab: May *increase* CPK, AST, ALT

Pharmacokinetics

Absorption: PO: 30%
Distribution: PB: 95%
Metabolism: t 1/2: 1–2 h
Excretion: 10% in urine, 80% in feces,
  bile

Pharmacodynamics

PO: Onset: 2–3 d
    Peak: UK
    Duration: UK

Therapeutic Effects/Uses: To control hypercholesterolemia; to decrease low-density
lipoprotein (LDL); and to increase high-density lipoprotein (HDL).

Mode of Action: Reduction of HMG-CoA reductase (enzyme), which inhibits cholesterol synthesis.

Side Effects

Nausea, diarrhea or constipation,
  abdominal pain or cramps,
  flatulence, dizziness, headache,
  blurred vision, rash, pruritus

Adverse Reactions

Hepatic dysfunction (elevated serum
  liver enzymes), myositis

KEY: For complete abbreviation key, see inside front cover.

■ NURSING PROCESS: Antilipemics: Lovastatin (Mevacor) and Others

ASSESSMENT
● Assess VS and serum chemistry values (cholesterol, triglycerides, AST, ALT, CPK) for baseline values.
● Obtain a medical history. Lovastatin is contraindicated for clients with a liver disorder. Pregnancy category is X.

POTENTIAL NURSING DIAGNOSES
Impaired tissue integrity
Anxiety related to elevated cholesterol level

PLANNING
● Client's cholesterol level will be <200 mg/dL in 6–8 wk.
● Client will be taught to choose foods low in fat, cholesterol, and complex sugars.

NURSING INTERVENTIONS
● Monitor the client's blood lipid levels (cholesterol, triglycerides, low-density lipoprotein [LDL], and high-density lipoprotein [HDL] every 6–8 wk for the first 6 mo after lovastatin therapy and then every 3–6 mo. For lipid level profile, the client should fast for 12–14 h. Desired cholesterol value is <200 mg/dL; triglyceride value is <150 mg/dL (can vary); LDL is <130 mg/dL; and HDL is >60 mg/dL. Cholesterol levels of >240 mg/dL, LDL levels of >160 mg/dL, and HDL levels of >35 mg/dL can lead to severe cardiovascular or cerebral vascular accident.
● Monitor laboratory tests for liver function, such as ALT, ALP, and GGTP. Antilipemic drugs may cause liver disorder.
● Observe for signs and symptoms of GI upset. Taking the drug with sufficient water or with meals may alleviate some of the GI discomfort.

CLIENT TEACHING
General
● Advise the client that if there is a family history of hyperlipidemia, his or her children should have a baseline blood lipid level obtained and monitored. Instruct the client that children should decrease fatty foods in the diet.
● Emphasize the need to comply with the drug regimen to lower the blood lipids. Side effects should be reported to the health care provider.
● Inform the client that it may take several weeks before blood lipid levels decline. Explain that laboratory tests for blood lipids (cholesterol, triglycerides, LDL, and HDL) are usually ordered every 3–6 mo.
● Advise the client to have serum liver enzymes monitored as indicated by the health care provider. Lovastatin is contraindicated in acute hepatic disease and pregnancy.
● Instruct the client to have an annual eye examination and to report changes in visual acuity.

Clofibrate, Gemfibrozil, Probucol
● Advise the client taking clofibrate and probucol that decreased libido and impotence may occur and should be reported. Drug dosage can be changed or another antilipemic may be ordered.

Antilipemic

- Instruct diabetic or prediabetic clients to monitor blood glucose levels if they are taking gemfibrozil. Dietary changes or insulin adjustment may be necessary.
- Advise the client with cardiac dysrhythmias to tell the health care provider before starting probucol. Dysrhythmias should be monitored and reported.

Skill

Cholestyramine and Cholestipol

- Instruct the client to mix the powder well in water or juice.

Diet

- Explain to the client that GI discomfort is a common problem with most antilipemics. Suggest increasing fluid intake when taking the medication.
- Instruct the client to maintain a low-fat diet by eating foods that are low in animal fat, cholesterol, and complex sugars. Lovastatin and other antilipemics are not a substitute for a diet that is low in fat.

Nicotinic Acid

- Advise the client to take the drug with meals to decrease GI discomfort.

Side Effects

Cholestyramine, Cholestipol, and Nicotinic Acid (Niacin)

- Advise the client that constipation may occur with cholestyramine and cholestipol. Increasing fluid intake and food bulk should help in alleviating the problem.
- Explain to the client that flushing is common and should decrease with continued use of the drug. Usually, the drug is started at a low dose.

EVALUATION

- Evaluate the effectiveness of the antilipemic drug. The client's cholesterol level is within desired range.
- Determine that the client is on a low-fat, low-cholesterol diet.

Generic (Brand)	Route and Dosage	Preg Cat	Interaction	t 1/2	PB	Action Onset	Action Peak	Action Duration
Cholestyramine resin (Questran)	A: PO: 4 g t.i.d. a.c. and hs; mix in 120–240 mL of fluid; max: 24 g/d	C	*Decrease* absorption of warfarin, digoxin, barbiturates, penicillins, tetracyclines, thyroid drugs, thiazides, iron, fat-soluble vitamins, folic acid *Lab: Increase* AST, ALT *Decrease* potassium and sodium levels	UK	UK	24–48 h	21 d	2–4 wk
Clofibrate (Atromid-S)	A: PO: 500 mg q.i.d.	C	*Increase* effects of insulin, oral hypoglycemics; *increase* risk of bleeding with warfarin; *increase* clofibrate effect with probenecid *Lab: Increase* AST, ALT, CPK	12–25 h	90–95%	UK	4–6 h	Weeks

continued

Antilipemics *Continued*

Generic (Brand)	Route and Dosage	Preg Cat	Interaction	t 1/2	PB	Onset	Peak	Duration
							Action	
						Onset	Peak	Duration
Colestipol HCl (Colestid)	A: PO: 10–30 g/d in divided doses before meals	C	Same as cholestyramine	UK	UK	24–48 h	Within 1 mo	4 wk
Fenofibrate (Lipidil)	A: PO: 100 mg/d	UK	None known	UK	UK	UK	UK	UK
Fluvastatin (Lescol)	A: PO: Initially: 20 mg h.s.; maint: 20–40 mg/d in 1 or 2 divided doses	B	*Decrease* effect with highly protein-bound drugs	UK	UK	UK	UK	UK
Gemfibrozil (Lopid)	A: PO: 600 mg b.i.d. before meals; max: 1,500 mg/d	B	*Increase* anticoagulant effect with warfarin *Lab:* May *increase* AST, ALT, ALP, LDH, bilirubin	1.5 h	90–95%	UK	1–2 h	UK
Lovastatin (Mevacor)	See Prototype Drug Chart							
Nicotinic acid (Niacin)	A: PO: Initially: 100 mg t.i.d.; maint: 1–3 g/d p.c. in 3 divided doses; max: 6 g/d	C	*Increase* hypotensive effect with antihypertensives	45 min	UK	Several days	0.5–1.2 h	UK
Pravastatin sodium (Pravachol)	A: PO: 10–40 mg/d	X	*Increase* effect of warfarin	1.5–2.5 h	55%	UK	1–1.5 h	UK

				20 d	UK	UK	1–3 mo	6–8 mo
Probucol (Lorelco)	A: PO: 500 mg b.i.d. with meals	B	*Increase* risk of ventricular arrhythmia with tricyclic antidepressants, beta blockers, phenothiazines, digoxin, quinidine *Lab: Increase* AST, ALT, ALP, BUN, blood glucose	20 d				6–8 mo
Simvastatin (Zocor)	A: PO: Initially: 5–10 mg/d in evening; maint: 20–40 mg/d in 1 or 2 divided doses; max 40 mg/d	X	May *increase* effect of digoxin; may *increase* bleeding with warfarin	UK	95%	Effect in 4 wk	1.3–2.4 h Max: 4 wk	UK

KEY: For complete abbreviation key, see inside front cover.

Vasodilators

Isoxsuprine HCl

Isoxsuprine HCl
  (Vasodilan, Voxsuprine)
Peripheral vasodilator,
  beta-adrenergic agonist
Pregnancy Category: C
Drug Forms:
Tab 10, 20 mg

Dosage

A: PO: 10–20 mg t.i.d./q.i.d.

Contraindications

Arterial bleeding, severe
  hypotension, postpartum,
  tachycardia
Caution: Bleeding disorders,
  tachycardia

Drug-Lab-Food Interactions

Decrease blood pressure with
  antihypertensives

Pharmacokinetics

Absorption: PO: Readily absorbed
Distribution: PB: UK
Metabolism: t 1/2: 1.25–1.5 h
Excretion: In urine

Pharmacodynamics

PO: Onset: 0.5 h
      Peak: 1 h
      Duration: 3 h

Therapeutic Effects/Uses: To increase circulation due to peripheral vascular disease (Raynaud's disease, arteriosclerosis obliterans) and cerebrovascular insufficiency.

Mode of Action: Action is directly on vascular smooth muscle.

Side Effects

Nausea, vomiting, dizziness,
  syncope, weakness, tremors, rash,
  flushing, abdominal distention,
  chest pain

Adverse Reactions

Hypotension, tachycardia,
  palpitations

KEY: For complete abbreviation key, see inside front cover.

■ NURSING PROCESS: Vasodilators: Isoxsuprine (Vasodilan)

ASSESSMENT
• Obtain baseline VS for future comparison.
• Assess for signs of inadequate blood flow to the extremities: pallor, coldness of extremity, and pain.

POTENTIAL NURSING DIAGNOSES
Impaired tissue integrity
Pain related to inadequate blood flow to extremity

PLANNING
• Client's blood flow to the extremities will improve, and the client's pain will be controlled.

NURSING INTERVENTIONS
• Monitor VS, especially blood pressure and heart rate. Tachycardia and orthostatic hypotension can be problematic with peripheral vasodilators.

CLIENT TEACHING
General
• Inform the client that a desired therapeutic response may take 1.5–3 mo.
• Advise the client not to smoke; smoking increases vasospasm.
• Instruct the client to use aspirin or aspirinlike compounds only with the health care provider approval. Salicylates help in preventing platelet aggregation.

Diet
• Advise the client with GI disturbances to take isoxsuprine with meals.
• Advise the client not to ingest alcohol with a vasodilator because it may cause a hypotensive reaction.

Side Effects
• Encourage the client to change position slowly but frequently to avoid orthostatic hypotension. Orthostatic hypotension is common when taking high doses of a vasodilator.
• Instruct the client to report side effects of isoxsuprine, such as flushing, headaches, and dizziness.

EVALUATION
• Evaluate the effectiveness of the isoxsuprine therapy; blood flow is increased in the extremities and pain has subsided.
• Client is experiencing no side effects from the prescribed drug.

Vasodilators (Peripheral)

Generic (Brand)	Route and Dosage	Preg Cat	Interaction	t 1/2	PB	Action Onset	Action Peak	Action Duration
Alpha-Adrenergic Blocker								
Tolazoline HCl (Priscoline HCl)	A: SC/IM/IV: 10–50 mg q.i.d. NB: IV: Initially: 1–2 mg/kg, followed by 1–2 mg/kg/h for 24–48 h; initial dose effect: 30 min	C	May first *decrease* blood pressure, then *increase* with epinephrine, norepinephrine	Neonate: 3–10 h May be longer in adult	UK	30 min	1–2 h	3–4 h
Beta₂-Adrenergic Agonists								
Isoxsuprine HCl (Vasodilan)	See Prototype Drug Chart							
Nylidrin HCl (Arlidin)	A: PO: 3–12 mg t.i.d./q.i.d.	C	*Increase* hypotensive effect with antihypertensives, phenothiazines, other vasodilators	UK	UK	10 min	30 min	2 h
Direct-Acting Peripheral Vasodilators								
Cyclandelate (Cyclospasmol)	A: PO: 20 mg q.i.d.; maint: 400–800 mg/d in 2–4 divided doses; dose may be reduced; max: 1,600 mg/d	C	May *increase* effects of alcohol, narcotics, tranquilizers (antipsychotics)	UK	UK	15 min	1–1.5 h	3–4 h

				t½	PB	Onset	Peak	Duration
Ergoloid mesylates (Hydergine)	A: PO/SL: 1 mg t.i.d.; dose may increase to 4–12 mg/d	C	UK	3–12 h	UK	UK	1–3 h	UK
Nicotinyl alcohol (Ronigen)	A: PO: 150–300 mg b.i.d. (Canada only)	UK	UK	UK	UK	UK	UK	UK
Papaverine (Pavabid)	A: PO: 100–300 mg, 3–5 ×d SR: 150 mg q12h; max: 300 mg q12h IV: 30–120 mg q3h PRN	C	*Increase* hypotensive effect with antihypertensives, vasodilators, alcohol *Decrease* effect of levodopa	1.5 h	90%	15 min	1–2 h	3–6 h
Hemorrheologic Pentoxifylline (Trental)	A: PO: 400 mg t.i.d. with meals	C	*Increase* effect with cimetidine, other histamine$_2$ antagonists, warfarin *Lab: Decrease* calcium magnesium levels; *increase* theophylline levels	0.5–1 h	UK	UK	1–4 h	UK

KEY: For complete abbreviation key, see inside front cover.

GASTROINTESTINAL AGENTS

Antiemetics
  Phenothiazines
  Cannabinoids and Miscellaneous
  Drugs for Motion Sickness

Emetics
  Emetics and Adsorbent

Antidiarrheals
  Opiates, Opiate-Related, and
    Adsorbents
  Miscellaneous and Combinations

Laxatives
  Osmotic and Contact
  Bulk Forming, Emollients, and
    Evacuant

Antiulcers
  Antacids
  Anticholinergics
  Histamine$_2$ Blockers
  Pepsin Inhibitor, Gastric Acid
      Secretion Inhibitor, and
      Prostaglandin Analog

Antiemetics: Phenothiazine

Perphenazine

Perphenazine
  (Trilafon)
Phenothiazine antiemetic
Pregnancy Category: C
Drug Forms:
Tab 2, 4, 6, 8, 16 mg
Tab SR 8 mg
Sol 16 mg/5 mL
Inj 5 mg/mL

Dosage

A: PO: 8–16 mg/d in divided doses;
  max: 24 mg
  IV: Max: 5 mg, diluted or slow IV
  drip
A&C >12 y: IM: 5–10 mg PRN; max:
  15 mg ambulatory care;
  max: 30 mg acute care

Contraindications

Narrow-angle glaucoma, severe liver
  disease, intestinal obstruction,
  blood dyscrasias, bone marrow
  depression
Caution: Children <12 y, seizures,
  cardiovascular disease

Drug-Lab-Food Interactions

Increase effects of alcohol, sedative-
  hypnotics, beta-adrenergic
  blockers
Decrease levodopa, lithium, other
  phenothiazines
Toxicity with epinephrine
Lab: Increase liver and cardiac
  enzymes, cholesterol, blood sugar
Decrease hormones; false pregnancy
  test

Pharmacokinetics

Absorption: PO: Erratic absorption;
  liquid: absorption is increased
Distribution: PB: UK
Metabolism: t 1/2: 8 h
Excretion: In urine and feces

Pharmacodynamics

PO: Onset: 2–6 h
  Peak: 2–4 h
  Duration: 6–12 h
IM: Onset: 10 min
  Peak: 1–2 h
  Duration: 6–12 h
IV: Onset: Rapid
  Peak: UK
  Duration: UK

Therapeutic Effects/Uses: To treat and prevent vomiting, especially from anticancer drug; to treat alcoholism.

Mode of Action: Effects of dopamine changed in CNS; inhibits medullary chemore-ceptor trigger zone as antiemetic; anticholinergic blocking agent.

Side Effects

Anorexia, dry mouth and eyes,
  constipation, blurred vision,
  extrapyramidal symptoms, rash,
  photosensitivity, orthostatic
  hypotension, impotence, weight
  gain, amenorrhea, gynecomastia,
  transient leukopenia, pain at IM
  injection site

Adverse Reactions

Extrapyramidal syndrome (tardive
  dyskinesia, akathesia), tachycardia
Life-threatening: Agranulocytosis,
  respiratory depression,
  laryngospasm, allergic reactions,
  cardiac arrest

KEY: For complete abbreviation key, see inside front cover.

■ NURSING PROCESS: Antiemetics: Phenothiazines

ASSESSMENT

- Obtain a history of the onset and frequency of vomiting and contents of the vomitus. If appropriate, elicit from the client possible causative factors such as food (seafood, mayonnaise).
- Obtain a history of present health problems. Clients with glaucoma should avoid many of the antiemetics.
- Assess VS for abnormalities and for future comparison.
- Assess urinalysis before and during therapy.

POTENTIAL NURSING DIAGNOSES

Altered nutrition: less than body requirements
High risk for fluid volume deficit related to vomiting

NURSING INTERVENTIONS

- Monitor VS. If vomiting is severe, dehydration may occur, and shocklike symptoms may be present.
- Monitor bowel sounds for hypoactivity or hyperactivity.
- Provide mouth care after vomiting. Encourage the client to maintain oral hygiene.

CLIENT TEACHING

General

- Instruct the client to store drug in tight, light-resistant container.
- Instruct the client to avoid OTC preparations.
- Instruct the client not to consume alcohol while taking antiemetics. Alcohol can intensify the sedative effect.
- Advise pregnant women to avoid antiemetics during the first trimester due to possible teratogenic effect on the fetus. Encourage them to seek medical advice about OTC or prescription antiemetics.

Side Effects

- Advise the client to report sore throat, fever, and mouth sores; notify health care provider and have blood drawn for a CBC.
- Instruct the client to avoid driving a motor vehicle or engage in dangerous activities because drowsiness is common with antiemetics. If drowsiness becomes a problem, a decrease in dosage may be indicated.
- Advise the client with a hepatic disorder to seek medical advice before taking phenothiazines. Instruct the client to report dizziness.
- Suggest to the client nonpharmacologic methods of alleviating nausea and vomiting such as flattened carbonated beverages, weak tea, crackers, and dry toast.

EVALUATION

- Evaluate the effectiveness of the nonpharmacologic methods or antiemetic by noting the absence of vomiting. Identify any side effects that may result from drug.

Generic (Brand)	Route and Dosage	Preg Cat	Interaction	t 1/2	PB	Action		
						Onset	Peak	Duration
Chlorpromazine (Thorazine)	See Prototype Drug Chart for Antipsychotics							
Perphenazine (Trilafon)	See Prototype Drug Chart							
Prochlorperazine maleate (Compazine)	A: PO: IM: 5–10 mg, t.i.d./ q.i.d., PRN SR: 10 mg q12h Rect: 5–25 mg PRN C: PO: Rect: 2.5 mg t.i.d.	C	Increase effect/toxicity with CNS depressants, anticonvulsants, epinephrine	23 h	≥90%	PO: 30–40 min SR: UK IM: 10–20 min Rect: 1h	UK UK UK UK	PO: 3–4 h SR: 12 h IM: 3–4 h Rect: 3–4 h
Thiethylperazine maleate (Torecan, Norzine)	A: PO/IM/PR: 10 mg q.d./t.i.d.	C	Increase anticholinergic effect with antidepressants Decrease absorption with antacids; decrease effects with barbiturates	UK	UK	PO: 30 min IM/PR: UK	UK UK	3–4 h UK
Triflupromazine (Vesprin)	A: PO: 20–30 mg/d A: IM: 5–15 mg q4–6h C: PO/IM: 0.2 mg/kg/d; max: 10 mg/d	C	Similar to chlorpromazine	UK	≥90%	20–40 min	UK	4 h

KEY: For complete abbreviation key, see inside front cover.

Antiemetics: Cannabinoids and Miscellaneous

Generic (Brand)	Route and Dosage	Preg Cat	Interaction	t 1/2	PB	Onset	Peak	Duration
Cannabinoids								
Dronabinol (Marinol) CSS II	*Chemotherapy-induced nausea:* A: PO: 5 mg/m² 1–3 h before chemotherapy; then q2–4h after; max: 15 mg/m²	B	*Increase* drowsiness with alcohol, sedatives, CNS depressants	20–24 h	98%	UK	2 h	6 h
Nabilone (Cesamet) CSS II	*Chemotherapy-induced nausea:* A: PO: 1–2 mg b.i.d. 1–3 h before chemotherapy, continue for 48 h after	B	*Increase* CNS depression with alcohol, other CNS depressants	2 h	UK	30–60 min	2 h	8 h
Miscellaneous								
Benzoquinamide HCl (Emete-con)	A&C >12 y: IM: 50 mg q3–4h PRN IV: 25 mg or 0.2–0.4 mg/kg diluted in D₅W as one dose	C	*Increase* CNS depression with alcohol, sedative-hypnotics, antihistamines	30–45 min	60%	IM: 15 min IV: 15 min	30 min UK	3–4 h 3–4 h
Dexamethasone	See Anti-inflammatory agents							
Diphenidol HCl (Vontrol)	*Nausea, vomiting, vertigo:* A: PO:25–50 mg q4h C >6 y: PO: 0.9 mg/kg	C	None significant known	4 h	UK	30–45 min	1.5–3 h	3–6 h
Droperidol (Inapsine)	A: IM/IV: 2.5–5 mg/dose q3–4h PRN C 2–12 y: IM/IV: 0.05–0.06 mg/kg/d q4–6h PRN C <2 y: Not recommended	C	*Increase* effect/toxicity with CNS depressants, analgesics, epinephrine, atropine, lithium	2.5 h	UK	5–10 min	30 min	2–12 h

continued

337

Generic (Brand)	Route and Dosage	Preg Cat	Interaction	t1/2	PB	Onset	Peak	Duration
							Action	
Granisetron (Kytril)	A: IV: 10 µg/kg 30 min before chemotherapy	B	None significant	4–11 h	65%	1–3 h	UK	18–24 h
Hydroxyzine (Atarax, Vistaril)	See Antihistamines							
Lorazepam (Ativan)	See Benzodiazepines							
Metoclopramide monohydrochloride monohydrate (Reglan)	A: PO: 10 mg a.c. and h.s. IV: 2 mg/kg 30 min before chemotherapy; then repeat q2h for 2 doses; then q3h for 3 doses; infuse diluted solution over not less than 15 min	B	*Increase* effect with opiate analgesics	4–7 h	30%	PO: 30–60 min IV: 1–3 min	1–2 h 1–2 h	1–3 h 1–3 h
Ondansetron HCl (Zofran)	A: IV: 0.15 mg/kg 30 min before chemotherapy; then 4 and 8 h after (total, 3 doses)	B	None significant	A: 4 h C: 2–3 h	70–75%	Rapid	15–30 min	4 h
Promethazine HCl (Phenergan)	See Antihistamines for Allergic Rhinitis							
Trimethobenzamide HCl (Tigan, Arrestin, Ticon)	A: PO: 250 mg t.i.d./q.i.d. IM/PR: 200 mg t.i.d./q.i.d. C: PO/PR: 15–20 mg/kg/d divided in 3–4 doses	C	Similar to benzquinamide	UK	UK	PO: 10–40 min IM: 15–30 min PR: 10–40 min	UK UK UK	3–4 h 3–4 h 3–4 h

KEY: For complete abbreviation key, see inside front cover.

Antiemetics: Drugs for Motion Sickness

Generic (Brand)	Route and Dosage	Preg Cat	Interaction	t 1/2	PB	Onset	Peak	Duration
Motion Sickness								
Buclizine HCl (Bucladin-S [Softab])	*Prophylaxis:* A: PO: 50 mg 0.5 h before travel; may repeat in 4–6 h	C	Increased toxicity with tricyclic antidepressants, MAOIs, CNS depressants	UK	UK	1 h	UK	4–6 h
Cyclizine HCl (Marezine)	A: PO: 50 mg 0.5 h before travel; may repeat in 4–6 h; max: 200 mg/d IM: 50 mg q4–6h PRN C 6–12 y: PO: 25 mg q.d./t.i.d. *Postoperative vomiting:* A: IM: 50 mg 0.5 h before surgery ends; may repeat q4–6h PRN	B	Increased toxicity with alcohol, CNS depressants	UK	UK	Rapid	UK	4–6 h
Dimenhydrinate (Calm-X, Dimetabs, Dramamine)	A: PO/IM/IV: 50–100 mg q4–6h; max: 400 mg/d C 6–12 y: PO: 25–50 mg q6–8h; max: 150 mg/d C <6 y: Not recommended	B	Increased effects/toxicity with anticholinergics, tricyclic antidepressants, MAOIs, CNS depressants	UK	UK	PO: 15–30 min IV: Immediate IM: 20–30 min	1–2 h UK 1–2 h	3–6 h 3–6 h 3–6 h
Meclizine HCl (Antivert, Antrizine)	A&C >12 y: PO: 25–50 mg 1 h before travel, after meal; may repeat q24h *Vertigo:* A: PO: 25–1,000 mg/d in divided doses	B	Increased toxicity with CNS depressants, anticholinergics, neuroleptics	6 h	UK	1–2 h	UK	8–24 h

KEY: For complete abbreviation key, see inside front cover.

339

Emetics

<table>
<tr><td>Ipecac Syrup</td><td>Dosage</td></tr>
<tr><td>

Ipecac Syrup
Emetic
Pregnancy Category: C
Drug Forms:
Liq
Fluid/extract is 14 times more
  concentrated than syrup

</td><td>

A: PO: 15–30 mL, followed by
  200–300 mL tepid water
C: >1–12 y: PO: 15 mL, followed by
  200–300 mL tepid water
C: <1 y: PO: 5–10 mL, followed by
  100–200 mL tepid water
Repeat initial dose if vomiting does
  not occur within 30 min.

</td></tr>
<tr><td>Contraindications</td><td>Drug-Lab-Food Interactions</td></tr>
<tr><td>

Hypersensitivity, depressed gag
  reflex, unconsciousness or
  semiconsciousness, poisoning with
  caustic or petroleum products,
  convulsions

</td><td>

Decrease effect with activated
  charcoal, carbonated beverages, or
  milk

</td></tr>
<tr><td>Pharmacokinetics</td><td>Pharmacodynamics</td></tr>
<tr><td>

Absorption: Minimal
Distribution: PB: UK
Metabolism: t 1/2: UK
Excretion: GI

</td><td>

PO: Onset: 15–30 min
    Peak: UK
    Duration: 20–25 min

</td></tr>
</table>

Therapeutic Effects/Uses: To induce vomiting after poisoning.

Mode of Action: Acts on chemoreceptor trigger zone (induces vomiting) and irritates gastric mucosa.

<table>
<tr><td>Side Effects</td><td>Adverse Reactions</td></tr>
<tr><td>

Diarrhea, sedation, lethargy,
  protracted vomiting

</td><td>

Life-threatening: Cardiotoxicity if
  ipecac is not vomited
  (hypotension, tachycardia, chest
  pain)

</td></tr>
</table>

KEY: For complete abbreviation key, see inside front cover.

■ NURSING PROCESS: Emetic: Ipecac Syrup

ASSESSMENT

- Determine the toxic substance ingested. Do *not* induce vomiting if caustics or petroleum products have been ingested.
- Determine the time elapsed since the ingestion; lavage may be indicated.
- Check the client's VS. Report abnormal findings.

POTENTIAL NURSING DIAGNOSES
Potential risk for absorption of toxic substance
Potential risk for infection

PLANNING
• Toxic substance will be expelled before absorption. There will be no bodily harm due to the toxic substance.
• Client will be closely monitored for adverse effects of the toxic substance for 24–48 h depending on the substance.

NURSING INTERVENTIONS
• Call the poison control center to report the toxic ingestion and for instructions.
• Monitor VS. Report changes.
• Offer sufficient fluids with ipecac syrup; warm clear liquids are best: *no* milk or milk products. Have client in high Fowler's position. Fluids dilute the toxic substance and are vehicles for expelling the substance; avoid carbonated beverages as they cause abdominal distention. If emetic is unsuccessful, gastric lavage may be performed or activated charcoal given to adsorb the toxic substances.
• Do not offer ipecac syrup or fluids to a semiconscious or unconscious person because of the danger of aspiration. Gastric lavage is usually performed in such cases.
• Do not induce vomiting if the toxic substance is a caustic or a petroleum distillate.
• Prepare for forceful vomiting; have large basin ready, and move clothing to protected area.

CLIENT TEACHING
General
• Instruct the parent or other family member to have ipecac syrup on hand. Explain that ipecac syrup is an OTC drug.
• Explain to the parent that ipecac should be given with sufficient fluids. Advise that ipecac syrup is *not* given if the toxic substance is a caustic or petroleum product.
• Advise the client or parents to *never* remove toxic substances from original labeled containers. Instruct parents on the use of child safety caps for future prevention.
• Advise the parent to keep readily available the telephone numbers of the poison control center and all emergency services.

EVALUATION
• Evaluate the effectiveness of ipecac syrup for inducing vomiting.
• Continue monitoring VS.
• Continue monitoring for signs and symptoms related to effect of ingested substance.

Emetics and Adsorbent

Generic (Brand)	Route and Dosage	Preg Cat	Interaction	t 1/2	PB	Action			
						Onset	Peak	Duration	
Emetics									
Apomorphine CSS II	A: SC: 4–10 mg C: SC: 0.07–0.1 mg/kg; 100–200 mL of water or evaporated milk before injection; do not repeat	C	Do not use with iodines, iron preparations, tannins, oxidizing agents	UK	UK	A: 10–15 min C: 1–2 min	UK	Sedation: 2 h 2 h	
Ipecac syrup (OTC preparation)	See Prototype Drug Chart								
Adsorbent									
Charcoal (Charcoaid, CharcoCaps)	A: PO: 520–1,000 mg after meals; repeat PRN; max: 4 g/d	C	Avoid sherbert, milk, ice cream Decrease absorption of all PO meds	NA	NA	UK	UK	UK	

KEY: For complete abbreviation key, see inside front cover.

NOTES:

_____

_____

_____

_____

_____

_____

_____

_____

_____

_____

Antidiarrheals

Diphenoxylate with atropine	Dosage
Diphenoxylate with atropine (Lomotil) *Pregnancy Category:* C CSS V *Drug Forms:* Tab 2.5 mg (2.5 mg of diphenoxylate/0.025 mg atropine)	A: PO: 2.5–5 mg b.i.d./q.i.d. C: >2 y: PO: 0.3–0.4 mg/kg daily in 4 divided doses or 2 mg 3–5×d

Contraindications	Drug-Lab-Food Interactions
Severe hepatic or renal disease, glaucoma, severe electrolyte imbalance, child <2 y	Alcohol, antihistamines, narcotics, sedative-hypnotics, MAOIs *Lab: Increase* serum liver enzymes, amylase

Pharmacokinetics	Pharmacodynamics
Absorption: PO: Well absorbed *Distribution:* PB: UK *Metabolism:* t 1/2: 2.5 h *Excretion:* In feces and urine	PO: Onset: 45–60 min Peak: 2 h Duration: 3–4 h

Therapeutic Effects/Uses: To treat diarrhea by slowing intestinal motility.

Mode of Action: Inhibition of gastric motility.

Side Effects	Adverse Reactions
Drowsiness, dizziness, constipation, dry mouth, weakness, flushing, rash, blurred vision, mydriasis, urine retention	Angioneurotic edema *Life-threatening:* Paralytic ileus, toxic megacolon, severe allergic reaction

KEY: For complete abbreviation key, see inside front cover.

■ **NURSING PROCESS: Antidiarrheals**

ASSESSMENT

• Obtain a history of any viral or bacterial infection, drugs taken, and foods ingested that could be contributing factors to diarrhea. Many of the antidiarrheals are contraindicated if the client has liver disease, narcotic dependence, ulcerative colitis, or glaucoma.

• Check VS to provide baseline for future comparison and to determine body fluid and electrolyte losses.

• Assess frequency and consistency of bowel movements.

• Assess bowel sounds. Hyperactive sounds can indicate increased intestinal motility.

• Report if the client has a narcotic drug history. If opiate or opiate-related antidiarrheals are given, drug misuse or abuse may occur.

POTENTIAL NURSING DIAGNOSES
Diarrhea
Altered nutrition
Alteration in fluid volume

PLANNING
- Client's bowel movements will no longer be diarrhea.
- Client's body fluids will be restored.

NURSING INTERVENTIONS
- Monitor VS. Report tachycardia or a systolic blood pressure decrease of 10–15 mm Hg. Monitor respirations. Opiates and opiate-related drugs can cause CNS depression.
- Monitor the frequency of bowel movements and bowel sounds. Notify the health care provider if intestinal hypoactivity occurs when taking drug.
- Check for signs and symptoms of dehydration due to persistent diarrhea. Fluid replacement may be necessary. With prolonged diarrhea, check serum electrolytes.
- Administer antidiarrheals cautiously to clients with glaucoma, liver disorders, or ulcerative colitis or who are pregnant.
- Recognize that drug may need to be withheld if diarrhea continues for more than 48 h or acute abdominal pain develops.

CLIENT TEACHING
General
- Instruct the client not to take sedatives, tranquilizers, or other narcotics with drug. CNS depression may occur.
- Advise the client to avoid OTC preparations; they may contain alcohol.
- Instruct the client to take the drug only as prescribed. Drug may be habit forming; do not exceed recommended dose.
- Encourage the client to drink clear liquids. Advise the client not to ingest fried foods or milk products until after the diarrhea has stopped.
- Advise the client that constipation can result from the overuse of this drug.

EVALUATION
- Evaluate the effectiveness of the drug; diarrhea has stopped.
- Monitor long-term use of opiates and opiate-related drugs for possible abuse and physical dependence.
- Continue to monitor VS. Report abnormal changes.

Antidiarrheals: Opiates, Opiate Related, and Adsorbents

Generic (Brand)	Route and Dosage	Preg Cat	Interaction	t1/2	PB	Onset	Peak	Duration
							Action	
						Onset	Peak	Duration
Opiates								
Deodorized opium tincture CSS II	A: PO: 0.6 mL or 10 gtt q.i.d. mixed with water; max: 6 mL/d C: PO: 0.005–0.01 mL/kg/dose q3–4 h; max: 6 doses/d	B (D, at term in high doses or prolonged time)	*Increase* effects of CNS depressants, MAOIs, tricyclic antidepressants daily *Lab: Increase* ALT, AST	2–3 h	UK	UK	UK	4 h
Camphorated opium tincture (Paregoric) CSS III	Camphorated: 5–10 mL b.i.d./q.i.d. C: PO: 0.25–0.5 mL/kg daily—q.i.d.							
Opiate Related								
Diphenoxylate with atropine (Lomotil) CSS V	A: PO: 2.5–5 mg b.i.d.–q.i.d. C >2 y: 0.3–0.4 mg/kg daily in 4 divided doses or 2 mg 3–5 × d	C B	*Increase* effects with: MAOIs, alcohol, CNS depressants *Increase* effects with CNS depressants	2.5 h	UK	45–60 min	2 h	3–4 h

Drug	Route and Dosage		Drug Interactions	t½	PB	Onset	Peak	Duration
Loperamide HCl (Imodium)	A: PO: Initially: 4 mg; then 2 mg after each loose stool; max: 16 mg/d C >2 y: PO: 0.4–0.8 mg/kg/d in divided doses q6–12 h			7–12 h	98%	30–60 min	2 h	4–5 h
Adsorbents Bismuth salts (Pepto-Bismol)	*Prevention of travelers' diarrhea:* A: PO: 2 tab q.i.d. a.c. and h.s. *Treatment:* A: PO: 2 tab or 30 mL q30–60 min PRN	UK	*Decrease effects of tetracycline, aspirin*	UK	UK	1 h	12 h	4 h
Kaolin-pectin (Kapectolin, Kaopectate)	A: 60–120 mL after each loose stool C 6–12 y: 30–60 mL after each loose stool	B	*Decrease absorption of chloroquine, digitalis, tetracyclines, penicillamine*	7–14 h	97%	30 min	UK	4 h

KEY: For complete abbreviation key, see inside front cover.

Antidiarrheals: Miscellaneous and Combinations

Generic (Brand)	Route and Dosage	Preg Cat	Interaction	t1/2	PB	Onset	Peak	Duration
							Action	
Miscellaneous								
Colistin sulfate (Coly-Mycin S)	Infants & children: PO: 5–15 mg/kg/d in 3 divided doses q8h	C	*Increase* nephrotoxicity with vancomycin; amphotericin B; *increase* respiratory depression with aminoglycosides	3–5 h	UK	UK	1–2 h	8–12 h
Difenoxin and atropine (Motofen) CSS IV	A: PO: Initially: 2 mg; then 1 mg after each loose stool; max: 8 mg/d for 2 d C <2 y: Not recommended	C	*Increase* CNS depression with barbiturates, narcotics, CNS depressants, tranquilizers; avoid use with MAOIs	12–24 h	UK	45–60 min	2 h	3–4 h
Furazolidine (Furoxone)	A: PO: 100 mg q.i.d. C >1 mo: PO: 5–8 mg/kg/d in 4 divided doses; max: 400 mg/d	C	*Increase* toxicity of levodopa; *increase* effects with tricyclic antidepressants, MAOIs, narcotics, anorexiants *Lab:* False-positive for glucose with Clinitest	UK	UK	UK	UK	UK
Lactobacillus acidophilus and Lactobacillus bulgaricus (one or both) (Bacid [plus carboxymethylcellulose sodium], Lactinix, More-Dophilus)	A&C >3 y: PO: 2 cap 2–9×/d Granules: 1 pkg with cereal, food, water t.i.d./q.i.d. Powder: 1 tsp daily with fluid C <3 y: Not recommended	NR	None significant known	UK	UK	UK	UK	UK

Drug	Route and Dosage	Pregnancy Category	Drug Interactions					
Octreotide acetate (Sandostatin)	*Diarrhea related to carcinoid tumors:* A: SC: Initially: 0.05 mg/d in divided doses for 2 wk; then increase according to response; max: 0.75 mg/d	B	*Decrease* effects with cyclosporines	1.5 h	65%	UK		9–12 h
Combinations								
Diphenoxylate with atropine (Lomotil)	See Prototype Drug Chart							
Kaolin, pectin, atropine SO$_4$, hyoscyamine SO$_4$, scopolamine hydrobromide (Donnagel)	A: PO: Initially: 30 mg; then 15–30 mg after each loose stool C: PO: 5–10 mg after each loose stool	C	Similar to diphenoxylate with atropine	UK	UK	UK	UK	UK
Powdered opium, kaolin, pectin, hyoscyamine SO$_4$, atropine SO$_4$, scopolamine hydrobromide, alcohol (Donnagel-PG) CSS V	A: PO: 15 mg q3h	C	Similar to diphenoxylate with atropine	UK	UK	UK	UK	UK
Parapectolin CSS V	A&C >12 y: 15–30 mL after each loose stool; max: 120 mL/d C 6–12 y: 5–10 mL after each loose stool; max:	C	*Increase* effect with depressants, MAOIs	UK	UK	UK	UK	UK

KEY: For complete abbreviation key, see inside front cover.

Laxatives: Contact

Bisacodyl	Dosage

Bisacodyl
  (Dulcolax)
Contact laxative
Pregnancy Category: C
Drug Forms:
Enteric-coated tab 5 mg
Rectal supp 10 mg
	A: PO: 10–15 mg in A.M./P.M.; max:
	  30 mg
	C: >3 y: PO: 5–10 mg; 0.3 mg/kg
	A&C >2 y: Rectal supp: 10 mg
	C <2 y & infants: 5 mg

Contraindications	Drug-Lab-Food Interactions

Hypersensitivity, fecal impaction,
  intestinal/biliary obstruction,
  appendicitis, abdominal pain,
  nausea, vomiting, rectal fissures
	Decrease effect with antacids,
	  histamine$_2$ blockers, milk

Pharmacokinetics	Pharmacodynamics

Absorption: Minimal absorption
Distribution: PB: UK
Metabolism: t 1/2: UK
Excretion: In bile and urine
	PO: Onset: 10–15 min; act: 6–12 h
	  Peak: UK
	  Duration: UK
	Rect: Onset: 15–25 min
	  Peak: UK
	  Duration: UK

Therapeutic Effects/Uses: Short-term treatment for constipation; bowel preparation for diagnostic tests.

Mode of Action: Increases peristalsis by direct effect on smooth muscle of intestine.

Side Effects	Adverse Reactions
Anorexia, nausea, vomiting, cramps, diarrhea	Dependence, hypokalemia *Life-threatening:* Tetany

KEY: For complete abbreviation key, see inside front cover.

■ NURSING PROCESS: Laxatives: Contact

ASSESSMENT

● Obtain a history of constipation and possible causes such as insufficient water/fluid intake, diet deficient in bulk or fiber, or inactivity; a history of the frequency and consistency of stools; and the general health status.

● Obtain baseline VS for identification of abnormalities and for future comparisons.

● Assess renal function.

● Assess electrolyte balance of clients with frequent laxative use.

POTENTIAL NURSING DIAGNOSES
Constipation
Altered nutrition
High risk for fluid deficit
Knowledge deficit related to overuse of laxatives
Altered health maintenance

PLANNING
• Client will be free of constipation.
• Client will exercise, eat foods high in fiber, and have adequate fluid intake to avoid constipation.

NURSING INTERVENTIONS
• Monitor fluid intake and output. Note signs and symptoms of fluid and electrolyte imbalances that may result from watery stools. Habitual use of laxatives can cause fluid volume deficit and electrolyte losses.

CLIENT TEACHING
General
• Instruct the client to increase water intake, if not contraindicated, which will decrease hard, dry stools.
• Advise the client to avoid overuse of laxatives, which can lead to fluid and electrolyte imbalances and drug dependence. Suggest exercise to help increase peristalsis.
• Instruct the client not to chew the tablets; swallow them whole.
• Advise the client to store suppositories at <86°F.
• Advise the client to take the drug only with water to increase absorption.
• Instruct the client not to take drug within 1 h of any other drug.
• Remind the client that drug is not for long-term use; tone of bowel may be lost.
• Instruct the client to time administration of drug so as to not interfere with activities or sleep.

Diet
• Advise the client to increase foods rich in fiber such as bran, grains, and fruits.

Side Effects
• Instruct the client to discontinue use if rectal bleeding, nausea, vomiting, or cramping occurs.

EVALUATION
• Evaluate the effectiveness of nonpharmacologic methods for alleviating constipation.
• Evaluate the client's use of laxatives in managing constipation; constipation will be alleviated. Identify laxative abuse.

Laxatives: Osmotic and Contact

Generic (Brand)	Route and Dosage	Preg Cat	Interaction	t1/2	PB	Onset	Peak	Duration
Osmotics: Saline Glycerin	A: Supp: 3 g C <6 y: Supp: 1–1.5 g	C	None significant	30–45 min	UK	15–30 min	NA	NA
Lactulose (Cephulac, Cholac, Constilec, Enulose)	*Chronic Constipation:* A: PO: 30–60 mL/d PRN C: PO: 7.5 mL/d after breakfast	C	Do not give with other laxatives	UK	UK	24–48 h	UK	UK
Magnesium citrate (Citroma, Citro-Nesia, Evac-Q-Mag)	A: PO: 120–240 mL C: PO: 4 mL/kg/dose	UK	*Increase* effects of neuromuscular blockers *Lab: Increase* magnesium level *Decrease* protein, calcium, potassium	UK	UK	0.5–3 h	UK	UK
Magnesium hydroxide (milk of magnesia)	A: PO: 20–60 mL C: PO: 0.5 mL/kg/dose	B	*Increase* effects of neuromuscular blockers *Decrease* absorption of digoxin, isoniazid, tetracyclines	UK	UK	4–8 h	UK	UK
Magnesium oxide (Maox)	A: PO: 2–4 g h.s. with 8 oz water Do not use in client with renal failure	B	*Decrease* effects of iron salts, digoxin, tetracyclines *Lab: Decrease* protein, calcium, potassium levels *Increase* magnesium level	UK	UK	4–8 h	UK	UK

Generic (Brand)	Route and Dosage	Pregnancy Category	Drug-Lab-Food Interactions	PB	t½	Onset	Peak	Duration
Magnesium SO₄ (Epsom salts)	A: PO: 10–30 g in 8 oz water C: PO: 0.3 g/kg in water	B	*Increase* CNS depression with barbiturates, anesthetics, CNS depressants	UK	UK	1–2 h	UK	UK
Sodium biphosphate (Fleet Phospho-Soda)	A: PO: 15–30 mL mixed in water	UK	None significant	UK	UK	PO: 0.5–3 h	UK	UK
Sodium phosphate with sodium biphosphate (Fleet enema)	*Enema:* A: 60–120 mL C: 30–60 mL	UK	None significant	UK	UK	Enema: 3–5 min	UK	UK
Contact Bisacodyl (Dulcolax)	See Prototype Drug Chart							
Cascara sagrada	A: PO: Tab: 325 mg/d Fluid extract: 1 mL/d Aromatic fluid extract: 5 mL/d	C	*Decrease* absorption of other oral medications	UK	UK	6–10 h	UK	UK
Castor oil (Emulsoil, Neoloid, Purge)	A: PO: 15–60 mL C 6–12 y: 5–15 mL	X	Similar to cascara sagrada	UK	UK	2–6 h	UK	UK
Phenolphthalein (Ex-Lax, Feen-A-Mint, Correctol)	A&C >12 y: 60–240 mg/d C 6–12 y: 30–60 mg	C	*Decrease* absorption of other oral medication	UK	UK	6–8 h	UK	2–3 d
Senna (Senokot)	A: PO: 1–4 tab or 1–4 tsp (granules) diluted in water	C	Similar to cascara sagrada	UK	UK	6–24 h	UK	UK

KEY: For complete abbreviation key, see inside front cover.

Laxatives: Bulk Forming

Psyllium Hydrophilic Muciloid	Dosage
Psyllium hydrophilic muciloid (Metamucil, Naturacil) Bulk-forming laxative *Pregnancy Category:* C *Drug Forms:* Chewable 1.7 g/piece Powder 500, 600, 950 mg/g, 1 g/g	A: PO: 1–3 tsp in 8 oz water, followed by 8 oz water C: >6 y: PO: 0.5–1 tsp in 4 oz water, followed by 4 oz water

Contraindications	Drug-Lab-Food Interactions
Hypersensitivity, fecal impaction, intestinal obstruction, abdominal pain	*Decrease* absorption of oral anticoagulants, aspirin, digoxin, nitrofurantoin

Pharmacokinetics	Pharmacodynamics
Absorption: Not absorbed *Distribution:* PB: UK *Metabolism:* t 1/2: UK *Excretion:* In feces	PO: Onset: 10–24 h Peak: 1–3 d Duration: UK

Therapeutic Effects/Uses: To control chronic constipation.
Mode of Action: Bulk-forming laxative by drawing in water.

Side Effects	Adverse Reactions
Anorexia, nausea, vomiting, cramps, diarrhea	Esophageal and/or intestinal obstruction if not taken with adequate water *Life-threatening:* Bronchospasm, anaphylaxis

KEY: For complete abbreviation key, see inside front cover.

■ **NURSING PROCESS: Laxatives: Bulk Forming**

ASSESSMENT

• Obtain a history of constipation and possible causes such as insufficient water/fluid intake, diet deficient in bulk or fiber, or inactivity; a history of the frequency and consistency of stools; and the general health status.
• Obtain baseline VS for identification of abnormalities and for future comparisons.
• Assess renal function, urine output, BUN, and serum creatinine.

POTENTIAL NURSING DIAGNOSES
Constipation
High risk for fluid deficit

PLANNING
- Client will be free of constipation.
- Client will exercise, eat foods high in fiber, and have adequate fluid intake to avoid constipation.

NURSING INTERVENTIONS
- Monitor fluid intake and output. Note signs and symptoms of fluid and electrolyte imbalances that may result from watery stools. Habitual use of laxatives can cause fluid volume deficit and electrolyte losses.
- Monitor bowel sounds.
- Identify the cause of constipation.
- Avoid inhalation of psyllium dust.

CLIENT TEACHING
General
- Instruct the client to mix drug with water immediately before use.
- Instruct the client to *not* swallow the drug in dry form.
- Advise the client to avoid overuse of laxatives, which can lead to fluid and electrolyte imbalances and drug dependence. Suggest exercise to help increase peristalsis.
- Advise the client to avoid inhaling psyllium dust; it may cause watery eyes, runny nose, and wheezing.

Diet
- Instruct the client to increase water intake, which will decrease hard, dry stools. Drink at least eight 8 oz glasses of fluids per day.
- Instruct the client to mix the drug in 8–10 oz of water, stir, and drink immediately. At least one glass of extra water should follow. Insufficient water can cause the drug to solidify and cause fecal impaction.
- Advise the client to increase foods rich in fiber such as bran, grains, and fruits.

Side Effects
- Instruct client to discontinue use if nausea, vomiting, cramping, or rectal bleeding occurs.

EVALUATION
- Evaluate the effectiveness of nonpharmacologic methods for alleviating constipation.
- Evaluate the client's use of laxatives in managing constipation. Identify laxative abuse.

Laxatives: Bulk Forming, Emollients, and Evacuants

Generic (Brand)	Route and Dosage	Preg Cat	Interaction	t1/2	PB	Onset	Peak	Duration
Bulk Forming								
Calcium polycarbophil (FiberCon, Fiberall, Mitrolan)	A: PO: 1 g, q.i.d. max: 6 g/d C 6–12 y: PO: 500 mg/d t.i.d.; max: 3 g C 2–5 y: PO: 500 mg/d b.i.d.; max: 1.5 g/d	C	*Decrease* absorption of tetracycline, digoxin, oral anticoagulants, potassium-sparing diuretics *Lab: Decrease* potassium	NA	NA	12–48 h	UK	UK
Methylcellulose (Cologel, Citrucel)	A: PO: 5–20 mL t.i.d. in 8–10 oz water C: 5–10 mL b.i.d. with 8 oz water	UK	*Decrease* absorption of salicylates, digitalis, antibiotics, oral anticoagulants	NA	NA	12–24 h	1–3 d	UK
Psyllium hydrophilic muciloid (Metamucil)	See Prototype Drug Chart							
Emollient: Stool Softeners								
Docusate calcium (Surfak)	A: PO: 240 mg/d C: PO: 60–120 mg/d	C	Similar to docusate sodium	NA	NA	12–72 h	UK	UK
Docusate potassium (Dialose)	A: PO: 100–300 mg/d	C	Similar to docusate sodium	NA	NA	12–72 h	UK	UK

356

Drug	Route and Dosage	Pregnancy Category	Uses and Considerations	Onset	Peak	Duration		
Docusate sodium (Colace)	A: PO: 50–300 mg/d C >6 y: 40–120 mg/d	C	*Decrease* effect of aspirin, warfarin sodium *Increase* toxicity with mineral oil, phenolphthalein	NA	NA	12–72 h	UK	UK
Docusate sodium with casanthranol (Peri-Colace)	A: PO: 1–2 cap/d C: PO: 1 cap/d	C	*Increase* absorption of mineral oil	NA	NA	8–12 h	UK	UK
Emollient: Lubricant Mineral oil	A: PO: 15–45 mL/h.s. C 6–12 y: PO: 5–20 mL	UK	*Decrease* absorption of vitamins A, D, E, K	NA	NA	6–8 h	UK	UK
Evacuant/Bowel Prep Polyethylene glycol–electrolyte solution (CoLyte, GoLYTELY)	Prep for GI exam requires 4 h; fasting for 3–4 h: A: PO: 240 mL q10–15 min for total of 4 L C: PO: 25–40 mL/kg/h for 4–10 h Administer via NGT to those unable or unwilling to drink solution (prepared with tap water and refrigerated)	C	Do not administer PO meds within 1 h of beginning drug	NA	NA	30–60 min	UK	4 h

KEY: For complete abbreviation key, see inside front cover.

Antiulcer: Antacids

Aluminum hydroxide

Aluminum hydroxide
   (Amphojel, ALternaGEL, Alu-Tab)
Antacid
Pregnancy Category: C
Drug Forms:
Cap 475, 500 mg
Tab 300, 500 mg
Tab chewable 600 mg
Liq 320 mg/5 mL, 600 mg/5 mL
Susp (4%) 600 mg/5 mL

Dosage

Antacid:
A: PO: 600 mg 1 h p.c. and h.s.;
   chewed with water or milk
Susp: 5–10 mL 1 h p.c. and h.s.
Hyperphosphatemia:
A: PO: 2 cap of 12.5 mL t.i.d./q.i.d.
   with meals

Contraindications

Hypersensitivity to aluminum
   products, hypophosphatemia
Caution: In elderly

Drug-Lab-Food Interactions

Decrease effects with tetracycline,
   phenothiazine, isoniazid,
   phenytoin, digitalis, quinidine,
   amphetamines
Lab: Increase urine pH

Pharmacokinetics

Absorption: PO: Small amount
   absorbed
Distribution: PB: UK
Metabolism: t 1/2: UK
Excretion: In feces; small amount in
   urine

Pharmacodynamics

PO: Onset: 15–30 min
   Peak: 0.5 h
   Duration: 1–3 h

Therapeutic Effects/Uses: To treat hyperacidity, peptic ulcer, and reflux esophagitis;
to reduce hyperphosphatemia.

Mode of Action: Neutralization of gastric acidity.

Side Effects

Constipation

Adverse Reactions

Hypophosphatemia, long term: GI
   obstruction

KEY: For complete abbreviation key, see inside front cover.

■ NURSING PROCESS: Antiulcer: Antacids

ASSESSMENT

• Assess the client's pain, including the type, duration, severity, and frequency.

• Assess the client's renal function.

• Assess for fluid and electrolyte imbalances, especially serum phosphate and calcium levels.

• Obtain drug history; report probable drug-drug interactions.

POTENTIAL NURSING DIAGNOSES
Pain
Knowledge deficit related to (mis)use of antacids

PLANNING
• Client will be free of abdominal pain after 1–2 wk of antiulcer drug management.

NURSING INTERVENTIONS
• Avoid administering antacids with other oral drugs, since antacids can delay their absorption. An antacid should definitely not be given with tetracycline, digoxin, or quinidine because it binds with and inactivates most of the drug. Antacids are given 1–2 h after other medications.
• Shake suspension well before administering: follow with water.
• Monitor urinary pH, calcium, and phosphate levels, and electrolytes.

CLIENT TEACHING
General
• Instruct the client to report pain, coughing, or vomiting of blood.
• Encourage client to drink 1 oz of water after antacid to ensure that the drug reaches the stomach.
• Advise the client to take the antacid 1–3 h after meals and at bedtime. Do not take antacids at mealtime; they slow gastric emptying time, causing increased GI activity and gastric secretions.
• Advise the client to notify the health care provider if constipation or diarrhea occurs; the antacid may have to be changed. Self-treatment should be avoided.
• Stress that antacids are not candy and that an unlimited amount is contraindicated.
• Advise the client to avoid taking acids with milk or foods high in vitamin D.
• Instruct the client to avoid taking antacids within 1–2 h of other oral medications since there may be interference with absorption.
• Advise the client to check antacid labels for sodium content if on a sodium-restricted diet.
• Alert the client to consult with the health care provider before taking self-prescribed antacids for longer than 2 wk.
• Instruct the client on the use of relaxation techniques.

Skill
• Instruct the client how to take antacids correctly. Chewable tablets should be thoroughly chewed and followed with water. With liquid antacid, 2–4 oz of water should follow the antacid.

Side Effects
• Advise the client to avoid foods and liquids that can cause gastric irritation, such as caffeine-containing beverages, alcohol, and spices.
• Advise that stools may become speckled or white.

EVALUATION
• Determine the effectiveness of the antiulcer treatment and the presence of side effects. The client should be free of pain, and healing should be progressing.

Generic (Brand)	Route and Dosage	Preg Cat	Interaction	t 1/2	PB	Action Onset	Action Peak	Action Duration
Aluminum carbonate (Basaljel)	A: PO: 10–30 mL or 2 tab/cap q2h Extra strength 5–15 mL	C	Similar to aluminum hydroxide	NA	NA	Slow	UK	Short
Aluminum hydroxide (Amphojel, ALternaGEL)	A: PO: 30 mL, 1–3 h p.c. and h.s. *Peptic ulcer disease:* A: PO: 15–45 mL 1–3 h p.c. and h.s. C: PO: 5–15 mL 1–3 h p.c. and h.s. *Prophylaxis GI bleeding:* A: PO: 30–60 mL qh C: PO: 5–15 mL q1–2h; maintain gastric pH >5	C	*Decrease* effects of digoxin, tetracyclines, isoniazid, corticosteroids, phenothiazine, histamine$_2$ antagonists	NA	NA	Slow	UK	Prolonged
Calcium carbonate (Tums, Dicarbosil)	A: PO: 2 tab or 10 mL q2h; max: 12 doses/d	C	*Decrease* absorption of tetracyclines *Lab:* Increase calcium level	UK	UK	UK	UK	UK
Dihydroxyaluminum sodium carbonate (Rolaids Antacid)	A: PO: Chew 1–2 tab PRN	C	*Decrease* absorption of quinolones, tetracyclines	UK	UK	Fast	UK	Moderate

Drug	Dosage		Uses and Considerations					
Magaldrate (Riopan, Lowsium [plus simethicone])	A: PO: 5–15 mL PRN; max: 100 mL/d; or 1–2 tab PRN; max: 20 tab/d	C	Decrease absorption of phenothiazines, isoniazid, fluoroquinolones, tetracyclines	UK	UK	Immediate	UK	Prolonged
Magnesium hydroxide and aluminum hydroxide (Maalox)	A: PO: 2–4 tab PRN; max: 16 tab/d	UK	None significant known	UK	UK	Fast	UK	Short
Magnesium hydroxide, aluminum hydroxide, and calcium carbonate (Camalox)	A: PO: 10–20 mL PRN; max: 80 mL/d; or 2–4 tab PRN; max: 16 tab	UK	None significant known	UK	UK	Fast	UK	Prolonged
Magnesium hydroxide and aluminum hydroxide with simethicone (Aludrox, Mylanta, Mylanta III, Maalox Plus, Gelusil-I, Gelusil-II, Gelusil-M, Di-Gel)	A: PO: 10–20 mL PRN; max: 120 mL/d; or 2–4 tab PRN; max: 24 tab	UK	None significant known	UK	UK	UK	UK	UK
Magnesium trisilicate (Gaviscon)	A: PO: 1–2 tab PRN; max: 8 tab/d	UK	None significant known	UK	UK	Slow	UK	Prolonged
Sodium bicarbonate	A: PO: 0.5 tsp of powder in 8 oz water	C	Increase effects of amphetamines, quinidine, ephedrine Decrease effects of lithium, salicylates	UK	UK	Fast	UK	Short

KEY: For complete abbreviation key, see inside front cover.

Generic (Brand)	Route and Dosage	Preg Cat	Interaction	t 1/2	PB	Onset	Peak	Duration
							Action	
						Onset	Peak	Duration
Belladonna tincture	A: PO: 0.3–1 mL t.i.d/q.i.d.	C	*Increase* cholinergic effects with MAOIs, antidepressants	18–36 h	UK	1–2 h	UK	4–6 h
Clidinium bromide and chlordiazepoxide HCl (Librax)	A: PO: 1–2 cap t.i.d/q.i.d. a.c., h.s.	C	Similar to belladonna	UK	UK	1 h	UK	3 h
Glycopyrrolate (Robinul)	A: PO: 1 mg b.i.d./t.i.d. IM/IV: 0.1–0.2 mg (100–200 μg) t.i.d/q.i.d.	B	Similar to belladonna	UK	UK	PO: 50 min IM: 20–45 min IV: 10–15 min	1 h 45 min 10–15 min	6 h 7 h 4 h
Propantheline bromine (Pro-Banthine)	A: PO: 15 mg t.i.d. a.c. and 30 mg h.s.	C	*Increase* cholinergic effects with antidepressants, atropine, antihistamines, phenothiazines	UK	UK	30–45 min	2–6 h	4–6 h
Tridihexethyl chloride (Pathilon)	A: PO: 25–50 mg t.i.d/q.i.d. a.c. and h.s.	C	Similar to belladonna	UK	UK	UK	UK	UK

KEY: For complete abbreviation key, see inside front cover.

NOTES:

_____

_____

_____

_____

_____

_____

_____

_____

_____

_____

Antiulcer: Histamine₂ Blockers

Ranitidine	Dosage
Ranitidine (Zantac) Histamine₂ blocker *Pregnancy Category:* B *Drug Forms:* Tab 150, 300 mg Inj 25 mg/mL	A: PO: 150 mg q12h or 300 mg h.s.; maint: 300 mg h.s. IM: 50 mg q6–8 h IV: 50 mg q6–8 h diluted C: PO: 2–4 mg/kg/d divided q12h IV: 1–2 mg/kg/d divided q6–8 h

Contraindications	Drug-Lab-Food Interactions
Hypersensitivity, severe renal or liver disease *Caution:* Pregnancy, lactation	*Decrease* absorption with antacids; *decrease* absorption of ketoconazole; *toxicity* with metoprolol *Lab: Increase* serum alkaline phosphatase

Pharmacokinetics	Pharmacodynamics
Absorption: PO: Well absorbed, 50% *Distribution:* PB: 15% *Metabolism:* t 1/2: 2–3 h *Excretion:* In urine and feces	PO: Onset: 15 min Peak: 1–3 h Duration: 8–12 h IM/IV: Onset: 10–15 min Peak: 15 min Duration: 8–12 h

Therapeutic Effects/Uses: To prevent and treat peptic ulcers, gastroesophageal reflux, and stress ulcers.

Mode of Action: Inhibition of gastric acid secretion by inhibiting histamine at histamine₂ receptors in parietal cells.

Side Effects	Adverse Reactions
Headache, confusion, nausea, diarrhea or constipation, depression, rash, blurred vision	*Life-threatening:* Hepatotoxicity, cardiac dysrhythmias, blood dyscrasias

KEY: For complete abbreviation key, see inside front cover.

Antiulcer: Histamine₂ Blockers

■ NURSING PROCESS: Antiulcer: Histamine₂ Blockers

ASSESSMENT
- Assess the client's pain, including the type, duration, severity, frequency, and location.
- Assess GI complaints.
- Assess mental status.
- Assess fluid and electrolyte imbalances, including intake and output.
- Assess gastric pH (>5 is desired), BUN, and creatinine.
- Assess drug history; report probable drug-drug interactions.

POTENTIAL NURSING DIAGNOSES
Pain related to gastric dysfunction

PLANNING
- Client will no longer experience abdominal pain after 1–2 wk of drug therapy.

NURSING INTERVENTIONS
- Do not confuse drug with alprazolam (Xanax).
- Administer drug just before meals to decrease food-induced acid secretion.
- Be alert that reduced doses of drug are needed by the elderly, who have less gastric acid; need to prevent metabolic acidosis.
- Administer drug intravenously in 20–100 mL of IV solution.

CLIENT TEACHING

General
- Instruct the client to report pain, coughing, or vomiting of blood.
- Advise the client to avoid smoking because it can hamper the effectiveness of the drug.
- Remind the client that the drug must be taken exactly as prescribed to be effective.
- Instruct the client to separate ranitidine and antacid dosage by at least 1 h, if possible.
- Instruct the client not to drive a motor vehicle or engage in dangerous activities until stabilized on the drug.
- Tell the client that drug-induced impotence and gynecomastia are reversible.
- Instruct the client on the use of relaxation techniques to decrease anxiety.

Diet
- Advise the client to eat foods rich in vitamin B_{12} to avoid deficiency as a result of drug therapy.
- Advise the client to avoid foods and liquids that can cause gastric irritation, such as caffeine-containing beverages, alcohol, and spices.

EVALUATION
- Determine the effectiveness of the drug therapy and the presence of any side effects or adverse reactions. The client should be free of pain, and healing should be progressing.

Generic (Brand)	Route and Dosage	Preg Cat	Interaction	t 1/2	PB	Action			
						Onset	Peak	Duration	

Generic (Brand)	Route and Dosage	Preg Cat	Interaction	t 1/2	PB	Onset	Peak	Duration
Cimetidine (Tagamet)	A: PO: 300 mg q.i.d. with meals and h.s. or 800 mg h.s.; maint: 300 mg h.s. IV: 300 mg q6–8h diluted in 50 mL (administered over 15–30 min) C: PO/IV: 10–40 mg/kg/d divided q6h	B	*Increase* effects of lidocaine, phenytoin, oral anticoagulants, theophylline *Decrease* effects of drug with smoking, antacids	1–2 h	20%	PO: 30 min IM/IV: 10–15 min	60–90 min 30 min	4–5 h 4–5 h
Famotidine (Pepcid)	A: PO: 20 mg q12h or 40 mg h.s.; maint: 20 mg h.s. IV: 20 mg q12h diluted C: PO: 1 mg/kg/d divided q8–12h C: IV: 0.6–0.8 mg/kg/d divided q8–12h	B	*Decrease* absorption with antacids; *decrease* effects of ketoconazole	2.5–4 h	15–20%	PO: 30–60 min IV: <1 h	1–4 h 1–3 h	6–12 h 8–15 h
Nizatidine (Axid)	A: PO: 150 mg q12h or 300 mg h.s.; maint: 150 mg h.s.	B	*Increase* effects of salicylates *Decrease* effects with antacids	1.5 h	35%	UK	0.5–3 h	8–12 h
Ranitidine (Zantac)	See Prototype Drug Chart							

KEY: For complete abbreviation key, see inside front cover.

NOTES:

Antiulcer: Pepsin Inhibitor

Sucralfate

Sucralfate
  (Carafate)
Antiulcer agent, pepsin inhibitor
Pregnancy Category: B
Drug Forms:
Tab 1 g

Dosage

Active Disease:
A: PO: 1 g q.i.d. 1 h a.c. and h.s.
Maintenance:
A: PO: 1 g b.i.d.

Contraindications

Hypersensitivity
Caution: Renal failure

Drug-Lab-Food Interactions

Decrease effects with tetracycline,
  phenytoin, fat-soluble vitamins,
  digoxin; *altered absorption* with
  ciprofloxacin, norfloxacin, antacids

Pharmacokinetics

Absorption: PO: Minimal absorption
  (<5%)
Distribution: PB: UK
Metabolism: t 1/2: 6–20 h
Excretion: In urine

Pharmacodynamics

PO: Onset: 30 min
    Peak: UK
    Duration: 5 h

Therapeutic Effects/Uses: To prevent gastric mucosal injury from drug-induced ulcers (aspirin, NSAIDs); to manage duodenal ulcers.

Mode of Action: In combination with gastric acid forms a protective covering on the ulcer surface.

Side Effects

Dizziness, nausea, constipation, dry
  mouth, rash, pruritus, back pain,
  sleepiness

Adverse Reactions

None significant

KEY: For complete abbreviation key, see inside front cover.

Antiulcer: Pepsin Inhibitor

■ NURSING PROCESS: Antiulcer: Pepsin Inhibitor

ASSESSMENT
- Assess the client's pain, including the type, duration, severity, and frequency. Ulcer pain usually occurs after meals and during the night.
- Assess the client's renal function. Report urine output of <600 mL/d or <25 mL/h.
- Assess for fluid and electrolyte imbalances.
- Assess gastric pH (>5 is desired).

POTENTIAL NURSING DIAGNOSES
Pain related to GI dysfunction

PLANNING
- Client will be free of abdominal pain after 1−2 wk of antiulcer drug management.

NURSING INTERVENTIONS
- Administer drug on empty stomach.
- Administer an antacid 30 min before or after sucralfate. Allow 1 to 2 h to elapse between sucralfate and other prescribed drugs; sucralfate binds with certain drugs such as tetracycline and phenytoin, thus reducing the effect of the other drugs.

CLIENT TEACHING
General
- Advise client to take drug exactly as ordered. Therapy usually requires 4−8 wk for optimal ulcer healing. Advise the client to continue to take drug even if feeling better.
- Increase fluids and dietary bulk, and exercise to relieve constipation.
- Instruct the client on the use of relaxation techniques.
- Monitor for severe, persistent constipation.
- Stress need for follow-up medical care.
- Emphasize cessation of smoking, as indicated.

Diet
- Advise the client to avoid foods and liquids that can cause gastric irritation, such as caffeine-containing beverages, alcohol, and spices.

Side Effects
- Instruct the client to report pain, coughing, or vomiting of blood.

EVALUATION
- Determine the effectiveness of the antiulcer treatment and the presence of any side effects. The client should be free of pain, and healing should be progressing.

Antiulcer: Pepsin Inhibitor, Gastric Acid Secretion Inhibitor, and Prostaglandin Analog

Generic (Brand)	Route and Dosage	Preg Cat	Interaction	t 1/2	PB	Onset	Peak	Duration
						Action		
Pepsin Inhibitor Sucralfate (Carafate)	See Prototype Drug Chart							
Gastric Acid Secretion Inhibitor Omeprazole (Prilosec)	Gastroesophageal reflux disease (GERD) A: PO: 20 mg/d for 4–8 wk *Hypersecretory:* A: PO: Initially: 60 mg daily; may increase to 120 mg t.i.d. in divided doses up to 80 mg/d	C	*Increase* levels of diazepam, warfarin, phenytoin	30–90 min	95%	0.5–4 h	5 d	72–96 h
Prostaglandin Analog Misoprostol (Cytotec)	A: PO: 100–200 µg q.i.d. with food C <18 y: PO: Safety and efficacy not established	X	*Increase* diarrhea with magnesium antacids	1.5 h	85%	30 min	60–90 min	3–6 h

KEY: For complete abbreviation key, see inside front cover.

OPHTHALMIC AND OTIC AGENTS

Ophthalmic:
  Miotics: Cholinergics and
    Beta-Adrenergic Blockers
  Carbonic Anhydrase
    Inhibitors (CAIs)
  Osmotics

Mydriatics and Cycloplegics
Anti-Infectives
Anti-Inflammatories

Otic:
  Anti-Infectives

Miotics

Pilocarpine

Pilocarpine
  (Isopto Carpine, Pilopine HS,
  Ocusert Pilo-20 and -40)
Miotic
Pregnancy Category: C
Drug Forms:
Sol 0.25–10%
Ocusert Pilo-20 and -40 gel 4%

Dosage

A&C : sol: 1–2%, 1–2 gtt, up to 6 × d
Gel: Apply 0.5-in ribbon in lower eye-
  lid at bedtime

Contraindications

Retinal detachment, adhesions
  between iris and lens, acute ocular
  inflammation; must avoid systemic
  absorption of drug with coronary
  artery disease, obstruction of
  GI/GU tract, epilepsy, asthma

Drug-Lab-Food Interactions

Avoid use with carbachol and
  echothiophate
Decrease antiglaucoma effects with
  belladonna alkaloids; *decrease*
  dilation with phenylephrine

Pharmacokinetics

Absorption: Some systemic absorption
Distribution: PB: UK
Metabolism: t 1/2: UK; binds to ocular
  tissue
Excretion: UK

Pharmacodynamics

Miosis:
Ophthalmic: Onset: 10–30 min
              Peak: 20 min
              Duration: 4–8 h
Reduce IOP:
Ophthalmic: Onset: 45–60 min
              Peak: 75 min
              Duration: 4–14 h
Ocusert: Onset: 1 h
          Peak: 1.5–2 h
          Duration: 7 d
Gel: Onset: 1 h
      Peak: 3–12 h
      Duration: 18–24 h

Therapeutic Effects/Uses: To induce miosis; to decrease IOP in glaucoma.
Mode of Action: Stimulation of pupillary and ciliary sphincter muscles.

Side Effects

Blurred vision, eye pain, headache,
  eye irritation, brow ache, stinging
  and burning, nausea, vomiting,
  diarrhea, increased salivation and
  sweating, muscle tremors, contact
  allergy
Conjunctival irritation with Ocusert

Adverse Reactions

Dyspnea, hypertension, tachycardia,
  retinal detachment; long term:
  bronchospasm
Corneal abrasion and visual
  impairment potential with Ocusert

KEY: For complete abbreviation key, see inside front cover.

■ NURSING PROCESS: Miotics

ASSESSMENT
- Obtain medical and drug history. Miotics are contraindicated in clients with narrow-angle glaucoma, acute inflammation of the eye, heart block, coronary heart disease, obstruction of the GI and/or GU tracts, and asthma. Report probable drug-drug interactions.
- Assess VS. Baseline VS can be compared with future findings.
- Assess the client's level of anxiety. The possibility of diminished vision or blindness increases anxiety.
- Assess the client's eye pigment. Heavily pigmented eyes may benefit from pilocarpine concentration of <4%.

POTENTIAL NURSING DIAGNOSES
Altered visual perception
High risk for injury

PLANNING
- Client will take miotics as prescribed.
- Client's intraocular pressure will decrease and be within the accepted range.

NURSING INTERVENTIONS
- Apply gentle pressure to the inner canthus when administering eye drops to prevent or minimize systemic absorption.
- Monitor VS. Heart rate and blood pressure may decrease with large doses of cholinergics.
- Monitor for side effects, such as headache, eye pain, and decreased vision.
- Monitor for postural hypotension. Instruct the client to arise slowly from a recumbent position.
- Check breath sounds for rales and rhonchi; cholinergics can cause bronchospasm and increase bronchial secretions.
- Maintain oral hygiene with excessive salivation.
- Have atropine available for antidote for pilocarpine.

CLIENT TEACHING

General
- Instruct the client not to use discolored solution.
- Instruct the client not to rinse the dropper; do not touch tip of dropper to any surface.
- Encourage the client not to close eyes tightly or blink frequently.
- Instruct the client on need for regular and ongoing medical supervision.
- Instruct the client to increase light for reading; dim light reduces acuity.
- Advise the client to avoid driving motor vehicles or engaging in dangerous activities while vision is impaired.
- Alert the client that long-term drug therapy is a possibility.
- Instruct the client on the use of relaxation techniques for decreasing anxiety, if indicated.
- Instruct the client with glaucoma to avoid atropinelike-drugs because they increase intraocular pressure. Clients should check drug label on OTC preparations.

Miotics

• Instruct the client not to suddenly stop medication without prior approval of health care provider.

Skill

• Instruct the client or family on correct administration of eye drops; include return demonstration.

1. WASH HANDS.
2. Instruct the client to lie or sit down and to look up toward the ceiling.
3. Gently draw skin down below the affected eye to expose the conjunctival sac.
4. Administer the prescribed number of drops into the center or outer aspect of the sac. Medication placed directly on the cornea can cause discomfort and/or damage. Do not touch eyelids or eyelashes with dropper.
5. Gently press on lacrimal duct with sterile cotton ball or tissue for 1–2 min after instillation of drops to prevent systemic absorption through lacrimal canal.
6. Client should keep eyes gently closed for 1–2 min after instillation to promote absorption.

Side Effects

• Advise the client that blurred vision after drug administration decreases with repeated use of drug.

OCULAR THERAPEUTIC SYSTEMS (OCUSERT)

• Instruct the client to follow directions related to insertion and removal.
• Wash hands with soap and water thoroughly before insertion.
• Store drug in refrigerator.
• Instruct the client to check for presence of disc in conjunctival sac at bedtime and when arising. Discard damaged or contaminated discs.
• Explain that myopia is minimized by bedtime insertion of drug in the upper conjunctival sac.
• Explain that temporary stinging is expected; notify health care provider if blurred vision or brow pain occurs.

EVALUATION

• Evaluate the effectiveness of drug.
• Intraocular pressure will be within the desired range.

Miotics: Cholinergics and Beta-Adrenergic Blockers

Generic (Brand)	Route and Dosage	Preg Cat	Interaction	t 1/2	PB	Onset	Peak	Duration
Direct-Acting Cholinergics								
Acetylcholine Cl (Miochol)	A: Intraocular: 5–20 mg of 1% sol injected in anterior chamber before or after suturing	C	*Decrease* effects with suprofen, flurbiprofen	NA	NA	Miosis: Prompt	UK	10 min
Carbachol (Miostat [intraocular], Carbacel [topical])	A: Ophthalmic: 1–2 gtt 1–4 × d A: IO: 0.5 mL into anterior chamber before or after suturing	C	Similar to pilocarpine	NA	NA	Ophthalmic: 10–20 min IO: 2–5 min	UK	IOP: 4–8 h 24 h
Pilocarpine HCl (Isopto Carpine)	See Prototype Drug Chart							
Pilocarpine nitrate (Ocusert Pilo-20, Pilo-40)	See Prototype Drug Chart							
Echothiophate iodide (Phospholine Iodide)	A: 0.03–0.06% sol: 1 gtt q.d./b.i.d.	C	*Increase* toxicity with carbamate pesticides, succinylcholine	NA	NA	Miosis: 10–30 min IOP: 4–8 h	UK	1–4 wk
Indirect-Acting Cholinesterase Inhibitors: Short Acting								
Physostigmine salicylate (Isopto Eserine)	A&C: Oint 0.25%: 1/4 in up to 3 × d Sol 0.25–0.5%: 1–2 gtt q.d./q.i.d.	C	*Decrease* cholinergic effects with antidepressants, atropine, phenothiazines, antihistamines; atropine *decreases* optimal effects	NA	NA	Miosis: 20–30 min Decrease IOP: UK	UK 2–6 h	12–36 h 12–36 h

continued

Generic (Brand)	Route and Dosage	Preg Cat	Interaction	t1/2	PB	Action			
						Onset	Peak	Duration	

Generic (Brand)	Route and Dosage	Preg Cat	Interaction	t1/2	PB	Onset	Peak	Duration
Long-Acting Demecarium bromide (Humorsol)	A: Sol 0.125–0.25%: 1–2 gtt 2×wk or 1–2 gtt b.i.d.	X	Similar to physostigmine salicylate	NA	NA	Miosis: 15–60 min IOP: UK	2–4 h	3–10 d
Isoflurophate (Floropryl)	A&C: Oint 0.025%: 1/4 in q8–72h	X	Additive effects of anticholinesterase drugs	NA	NA	Miosis: 5–10 min Decrease IOP: UK	20–30 min 24 h	1–4 wk 1 wk
Beta-Adrenergic Blockers Betaxolol HCl (Betoptic)	Sol 0.25% (susp) or 5.0% (sol): Usual dose: 1 gt b.i.d.	C	Increase effects with other ocular hypotensives Lab: Alters GTT	15–20 h	UK	30 min	2 h	12 h
Levobunolol HCl (Betagan Liquifilm)	Sol: 1 gt q.d./b.i.d.	C	Similar to betaxolol	60–90 min	UK	45–60 min	2–6 h	12–24 h
Timolol maleate (Timoptic)	A: Sol 0.25% or 5.0%: Initially: 1 gt b.i.d.; maint: 1 gt q.d. once response occurs with initial dosage	C	Additive effects with systemic beta blockers Increase effect of quinidine, verapamil Decrease effects of theophylline, isoproterenol Lab: Increase liver function tests, BUN, serum potassium Decrease hemoglobin, hematocrit	4 h	10%	30 min	1–2 h	12–24 h

KEY: For complete abbreviation key, see inside front cover.

Carbonic Anhydrase Inhibitors (CAIs)

Generic (Brand)	Route and Dosage	Preg Cat	Interaction	t 1/2	PB	Onset	Peak	Duration
							Action	
						Onset	Peak	Duration
Acetazolamide (Diamox Sequals)	A: PO: Short term: 250 mg q4h or b.i.d.; acute: 500 mg, then 125–250 mg q4h IV: 250–500 mg; may repeat ×1 in 24 h C: PO: 10–15 mg/kg/24 h in divided doses q6–8h IV: 5–10 mg/kg/dose q6h	C	*Increase* toxicity of CAI with salicylates, cyclosporine *Decrease* effect with phenobarbital	2–6 h	UK	PO: SR 2 h IV: 2 min PO: 1–1.5 h	3–6 h 15 min 1–4 h	18–24 h 4–5 h 8–12 h
Dichlorphenamide (Daranide)	A: PO: Initially: 100–200 mg; then 100 mg q12h until desired results; maint: 25–50 mg q.d./t.i.d.; given with miotics	C	*Decrease* excretion of ephedrine, procainamide, tricyclic antidepressants *Increase* excretion of lithium, phenobarbital	UK	UK	1 h	2–4 h	6–12 h
Methazolamide (Neptazane)	A: PO: 50–100 mg b.i.d./t.i.d.	C	May induce digitalis and salicylate toxicities due to hypokalemia	14 h	UK	2–4 h	6–8 h	10–18 h

KEY: For complete abbreviation key, see inside front cover.

Generic (Brand)	Route and Dosage	Preg Cat	Interaction	t 1/2	PB	**Action**			
						Onset	Peak	Duration	
Glycerin (Glyrol)	A&C: 1–2 g/kg 1–1.5 h before surgery	C	None significant reported	30–45 min	UK	Decrease IOP: 10–30 min	1–1.5 h	4–8 h	
Isosorbide (Ismotic)	A: PO: 45% sol 1.5–3 g/kg b.i.d./q.i.d. IV: 15–25% sol 1.5–2 g/kg over 30–60 min	C	None significant reported	5–9.5 h	UK	Decrease ICP: 10–60 min 10–30 min	UK 1–1.5 h	2–3 h 5–6 h	
Mannitol (Osmitrol)	A: IV: 15–20% sol 1.5–2 g/kg over 30–60 min	C	Decrease effect with lithium	15–100 min	UK	30–60 min Decrease ICP: 15 min	1 h	6–8 h	
Urea (Ureaphil)	A: IV: 30% sol 1–1.5 g/kg; over 1-3 h; max: 4 mL/min C >2 y: IV: 0.5-1.5 g/kg; max: 4 mL/min C <2 y: IV: 0.1 g/kg; max: 4 mL/min	C	Decrease effect with lithium	<60 min	UK	30–45 min	1–2 h	5–6 h	

KEY: For complete abbreviation key, see inside front cover.

Generic (Brand)	Route and Dosage	Preg Cat	Interaction*	t 1/2	PB	Action Onset	Action Peak	Action Duration
Atropine sulfate (BufOpto-atropine)	A: Sol 1%: 1–2 gtt up to q.i.d. C: Sol 0.5% 1–2 gtt up to t.i.d. Oint: Apply in lower eyelid sac up to t.i.d.	C	May *decrease* effects with miotics	NA	NA	M: 30–60 min C: 1–2 h	30–60 min 1–2 h	5–12 d 5–6 d
Cyclopentolate HCl (Cyclogyl)	A: Sol 0.5–2%: 1–2 gtt; then 1 gtt in 5 min C: 1–2 gtt ×1; may repeat ×1 in 5–10 min with 0.5% or 1% sol	C	*Decrease* effect of cholinesterase inhibitors, carbachol	NA	NA	M&C: 10–15 min	25–60 min	6–24 h
Dipivefrin HCl (Propine)	A: Sol 0.1%; 1 gtt q12h	B	*Increase* effects with other agents to decrease IOP	NA	NA	M: 30 min C: <30 min	1 h 1 h	6 h 12+ h
Epinephrine HCl (Epifrin)	A&C: Sol 0.25–2%: 1–2 gtt q.d./b.i.d.	C	Inactivates chymotrypsin, ophthalmic beta blockers Use with MAOIs may lead to hypertensive crises	NA	NA	<5 min	30 min	12 h
Epinephrine borate (Epinal, Eppy/N)	*Surgery:* A: 0.1% sol: Instill 1–2 gtt ≤3× *Open angle glaucoma:* A: 0.5% or 1.0% sol: Instill 1 gtt in eye b.i.d.	C	*Increase* effect of lowering IOP with osmotics, carbonic anhydrase inhibitors	UK	UK	<1 h	4–8 h	24 h

continued

379

Mydriatics and Cycloplegics Continued

Generic (Brand)	Route and Dosage	Preg Cat	Interaction*	t1/2	PB	Onset	Peak	Duration
							Action	
Homatropine hydrobromide (Isopto Homatropine)	A&C: Sol 2% and 5%: 1–2 gtt q3–4h *C: Use only 2%	C	None significant known	NA	NA	M: 10–15 min C: 30–60 min	40–60 min 30–60 min	1–3 d 1–3 d
Phenylephrine HCl (AK-Dilate, AK-Nefrin Ophthalmic)	*Mydriasis:* A&C: 2.5% or 10% sol: Instill 1 gt in eye before examination *Mydriasis with vasoconstriction:* A&C >12 y: Instill 1 gt in eye; repeat ×1 in 1h PRN C: 2.5% sol: Instill 1 gt in eye; repeat ×1 in 1h PRN	C	*Increase* effect with adrenergic and oxytocic drugs *Decrease* effect with alpha and beta blockers	UK	UK	Several minutes	10–90 min	3–7 h
Scopolamine hydrobromide (Isopto Hyoscine)	A: Sol 0.25% 1–2 gtt 1 h before exam; 1–2 gtt for treatment up to q.i.d.	C	Similar to atropine sulfate	NA	NA	M&C: 15–30 min	30–60 min	3–7 d
Tropicamide (Mydriacyl Ophthalmic)	*Refraction:* 1%: 1–2 gtt; repeat in 5 min *Fundus exam:* 0.5: 1–2 gtt 15–20 min before exam	C	None significant known	NA	NA	M&C: 10–15 min	20–40 min	6 h

*KEY: *To minimize systemic absorption, apply gentle pressure to lacrimal duct. For complete abbreviation key, see inside front cover.*
M: Mydriatic; C: Cycloplegic.

Generic (Brand)	Route and Dosage	Preg Cat	Interaction*	t 1/2	PB	Onset	Peak	Duration
							Action	
Antibiotics								
Chloramphenicol (AK-Chlor, Chloromycetin Ophthalmic)	A&C: Ophthalmic: Instill 1–2 gtt or 1/2 in oint q3–4 h for 48 h; increase interval to b.i.d./t.i.d.	C	None significant reported	NA	NA	UK	UK	UK
Ciprofloxacin HCl (Ciloxan)	*Acute infections:* A&C: Instill 1–2 gtt q15–30 min; decrease frequency gradually as infection is controlled *Moderate infection:* A&C: Instill 1–2 gtt 4–6 ×d	C	None significant reported	NA	NA	UK	UK	UK
Erythromycin (Ilotycin)	Oint 0.5%: 0.5–1 cm q,d./q.i.d.	B	None significant reported	1.5 h	75–90%	UK	UK	UK
Gentamicin sulfate (Garamycin Ophthalmic)	A&C: Sol 0.3%: 1–2 gtt q4h; may increase to 2 gtt q1h Oint 0.3%: 1/2 in ribbon b.i.d./t.i.d.	C	None significant reported	NA	NA	UK	UK	UK
Norfloxacin (Chibroxin)	A&C >1 y: Instill 1–2 gtt in affected eye(s) q.i.d. for ≤7 d	C	None significant reported	NA	NA	UK	UK	UK
Polymyxin B sulfate (Neomycin Sulfate, Bacitracin, Aerosporin)	A&C: Sol: 1–2 gtt b.i.d./q.i.d. for 7–10 d	B	None significant reported	4–6 h	UK	UK	UK	UK

continued

Generic (Brand)	Route and Dosage	Preg Cat	Interaction*	t 1/2	PB	Onset	Peak	Duration
Antibiotics Silver nitrate 1% (Dey-Drop)	Neonate: Instill 2 gtt to each eye within 1 h of birth	C	None significant reported	NA	NA	UK	UK	UK
Tetracycline HCl (Achromycin Ophthalmic)	A: Instill 1–2 gtt b.i.d./q.i.d. A: Oint: 1/4–1/2 in q2–12h	D	None significant reported	NA	NA	UK	UK	UK
Antifungal Natamycin (Natacyn Ophthalmic)	A&C: Sol 5%: 1 gt q2h for 3–4 d; then 1 gt q3h for 14–21 d	C	Avoid ophthalmic glucocorticoids	NA	NA	2 d	2–4 wk	UK
Antiviral Idoxuridine (IDU, Herplex Liquifilm)	A&C: Sol: Initially: 1 gt q1h during the day and q2h at night; when definite improvement occurs, use 1 gt q2h during the day and q4h at night; continue 3–7 d after healing occurs	C	Topical corticosteroids may be used concomitantly; avoid boric acid–containing products and systemic glucocorticoids	NA	NA	5–7 d	UK	UK
Trifluridine (Viroptic)	A: 1% sol: Instill 1 gt into infected eye q2h while awake; max: 9 gtt/d until corneal ulcer re-epithelialized; then 1 gt q4h for 7 d; max: 21 d of treatment	C	Systemic absorption negligible	NA	NA	UK	UK	UK
Vidarabine (Vira-A Ophthalmic)	*Keratoconjunctivitis, herpes simplex keratitis:* A&C: Oint 3%: 1/2 in 5 ×/d at 3-h intervals	C	Allopurinol increases neurologic side effects	UK	UK	UK	UK	UK

KEY: *To minimize systemic absorption, apply gentle pressure to lacrimal duct. For complete abbreviation key, see inside front cover.

Generic (Brand)	Route and Dosage	Preg Cat	Interaction	t 1/2	PB	Action Onset	Action Peak	Action Duration
Dexamethasone (Ocu-Dex)	A&C: Oint: Apply into conjunctival sac t.i.d./q.i.d.; gradually decrease to discontinue Susp: Instill 2 gtt qh while awake and q2h during night; taper to q3–4h; then t.i.d./q.i.d.	C	None significant reported	NA	NA	UK	UK	UK
Diclofenac Na (Cataflam, Voltaren)	A: 1 gt to affected eye q.i.d. for 2 wk; start 24 h after cataract surgery	B	None significant reported	NA	NA	Rapid	UK	UK
Flurbiprofen Na (Ocufen)	A: Instill 1 gt q30 min 2 h before surgery	C	None significant reported	NA	NA	UK	UK	UK
Ketorolac tromethamine (Acular)	A: 0.5% sol: Instill 1 gt q.i.d.	B	None significant reported	NA	NA	UK	UK	UK
Medrysone (HMS Liquifilm)	A&C: 1% sol: Initially: Instill 1 gt in conjunctival sac q1–2h (1–2 d); then 1 gt b.i.d./q.i.d.	C	None significant reported	NA	NA	UK	UK	UK
Prednisolone acetate (AK-Tate, Econopred, Predforte [Pred Forte], Pred Mild Ophthamic)	A: Initially: Instill 1–2 gtt in conjunctival sac qh while awake, q2h during night until desired effect; maint: 1 gt q4h	C	None significant reported	NA	NA	UK	UK	UK
Prednisolone Na phosphate (AK-Pred Inflamase)	*Preoperative:* A: Instill 2 gtt in conjunctival sac at 3, 2, and 1 h before surgery	C	*Decrease effects of ophthalmic acetylcholine or carbachol*	NA	NA	UK	UK	UK

KEY: *To minimize systemic absorption, apply gentle pressure to lacrimal duct. For complete abbreviation key, see inside front cover.*

Generic (Brand)	Route and Dosage	Preg Cat	Interaction	t 1/2	PB	Onset	Peak	Duration
							Action	
						Onset	Peak	Duration
External								
Acetic acid and aluminum acetate (Otic Domeboro)	A&C: Sol 2%: Insert saturated wick, keep moist ×24h; instill 4–6 gtt q2–3h	UK	None significant reported	NA	NA	UK	UK	UK
Boric acid (Ear-Dry)	A&C >12 y: Instill 5–10 gtt b.i.d.; tilt head to unaffected side to keep	C	None significant reported	NA	NA	UK	UK	UK
Carbamide peroxide (Debrox)	gtt in ear or put cotton plug in outer ear	C	None significant reported	NA	NA	UK	UK	UK
Chloramphenicol (Chloromycetin Otic)	A&C: Otic sol: Instill 2–3 gtt into ear t.i.d.	C	None significant reported	NA	NA	UK	UK	UK
Polymyxin B	A&C: 3–4 gtt t.i.d./q.i.d. for 7–10 d	B	None significant reported	NA	NA	UK	UK	UK
Tetracycline (Achromycin)	A&C: 1–2 gtt b.i.d./q.i.d.	D	None significant reported	NA	NA	UK	UK	UK
Trolamine polypeptide oleate-condensate (Cerumenex)	A&C: Fill ear canal and insert cotton plug for 15–30 min; flush ear with lukewarm water; repeat ×1 if needed	C	None significant reported	NA	NA	24 h	UK	UK

Internal								
Amoxicillin (Amoxil, Augmentin)	B	Dose varies See Antibacterials: Penicillins	Similar to penicillin	1–1.5 h	20%	PO: 30 min	1–2 h	6–8 h
Ampicillin trihydrate (Polycillin)	B	Dose and route vary See Antibacterials: Penicillins	*Increase* risk for rash with allopurinol Similar to penicillin *Decrease* effect of oral contraceptives	1–2 h	15–25%	PO: Rapid IM: Rapid IV: Rapid	2 h 1 h 5 min	6–8 h 6–8 h 6–8 h
Cefaclor (Ceclor)	B	Usual dose: A: PO: 250 mg q8h C: PO: 20 mg/kg/d in divided doses q8h; max: 1g/d	Similar to penicillin	30–60 min; *increase* to 2–3 h with renal dysfunction	25%	PO: Rapid	30–60 min	UK

continued

Generic (Brand)	Route and Dosage	Preg Cat	Interaction	t1/2	PB	Onset	Peak	Duration
							Action	
Erythromycin (E-Mycin)	Dose and route vary	B	*Increase* effects of digitalis, theophylline; *increase* risk of toxicity with oral anticoagulants, carbamazepine	1–3 h; may *increase* to 5–6 h with renal dysfunction	70%	PO: 1 h IV: Rapid	1–4 h End of infusion	6 h UK
Penicillin (Pentids, Pen-V)	Dose varies by route Pen G: IM/IV/PO Pen V: PO only See Antibacterials: Penicillins	B	*Decrease* effects with erythromycin, tetracyclines; *decrease* effect of oral contraceptives	30–60 min	Pen V: 80% Pen G: 60%	PO: Rapid IM: Rapid IV: Rapid	1 h 15–30 min Rapid	6 h 6 h 6 h
Sulfonamides (Azulfidine [sulfasalazine], Gantrisin [sulfisoxazole], Bactrim [trimethoprim and sulfamethoxazole])	Dose and route vary See Antibacterials: Sulfonamides	Safety not established	*Increase* effect of anticoagulants, sulfonylureas; *increase* toxicity with methotrexate; may *increase* toxicity of cyclosporine *Decrease* effect of digoxin	6–10 h	68%	UK	UK	UK

KEY: For complete abbreviation key, see inside front cover.

ENDOCRINE AGENTS

Pituitary Hormones

Thyroid Hormone Replacements and Antithyroid Agents

Parathyroid Hormones: Replacements and Supplements

Adrenal Hormones: Glucocorticoids

Antidiabetics
  Insulin
  Sulfonylureas

Pituitary: Adrenocorticotropic Hormone (ACTH)

Corticotropin	Dosage
Corticotropin (Acthar, Acthar gel, Cortrophin-Zinc) Anterior pituitary hormone *Pregnancy Category:* C *Drug Forms:* Inj 25, 40 U per vial	A: SC/IM: 20 U q.i.d. IV: 10–25 U in 500 mL D_5W q8h C: SC/IM: 1.6 U/kg/d or $\quad$ 50 U/m^2/d in divided doses

Contraindications	Drug-Lab-Food Interactions
Severe fungal infection, CHF, peptic ulcer *Caution:* Hepatic disease, psychiatric disorder, myasthenia gravis	*Increase* ulcer formation with aspirin; may *increase* effect of diuretics *Decrease* effects of oral antidiabetics or insulin

Pharmacokinetics	Pharmacodynamics
Absorption: IM: Well absorbed *Distribution:* PB: UK *Metabolism:* t 1/2: 15–20 min *Excretion:* In urine	IM: Onset <6 h $\quad$ Peak: 6–18 h $\quad$ Duration: 12–24 h IV: Onset: UK $\quad$ Peak: 1 h $\quad$ Duration: UK

Therapeutic Effects/Uses: To diagnose adrenocortical disorders; acts as an anti-inflammatory agent; to treat acute multiple sclerosis (MS).

Mode of Action: Stimulation of the adrenal cortex to secrete cortisol.

Side Effects	Adverse Reactions
Nausea, vomiting, increased appetite, mood swing (euphoria to depression), petechiae, water and sodium retention, hypokalemia, hypocalcemia	Edema, ecchymosis, osteoporosis, muscle atrophy, growth retardation, decreased wound healing, cataracts, glaucoma, menstrual irregularities *Life-threatening:* Ulcer perforation, pancreatitis

KEY: For complete abbreviation key, see inside front cover.

■ NURSING PROCESS: Pituitary Hormones

ASSESSMENT
- Obtain baseline VS for future comparison. Report abnormal results.
- Assess the client's urinary output and weight.
- Assess the client for an infectious process. Corticotropin can suppress signs and symptoms of infection.
- Assess the client's physical growth. Compare child's growth with reported standards. Report findings.

POTENTIAL NURSING DIAGNOSES
- Altered health maintenance
- Altered growth and development

PLANNING

• Client will be free of pituitary disorder with appropriate drug regimen.

NURSING INTERVENTIONS

Antidiuretic Hormone (ADH)

• Monitor VS. Increased heart rate and decreased systolic pressure can indicate fluid volume loss due to decreased ADH production. With less ADH secretion, more water is excreted, decreasing vascular fluid (hypovolemia).
• Monitor urinary output. Increased output can indicate fluid loss due to a decrease in ADH.

Adrenocorticotropic Hormone (ACTH), Corticotropin

• Avoid administering corticotropin to clients with adrenocortical hyperfunction. Corticotropin stimulates the release of cortisol from the adrenal glands.
• Monitor the growth and development of a child receiving corticotropin.
• Monitor the client's weight. If a weight gain occurs, check for edema. A side effect of corticotropin (ACTH) is sodium and water retention.
• Monitor for adverse effects when corticotropin is discontinued. Dose should be tapered and not stopped abruptly because adrenal hypofunction may result.
• Check laboratory findings, especially electrolyte levels. Electrolyte replacement may be necessary.

Growth Hormone (GH)

• Monitor blood sugar and electrolyte levels in clients receiving GH. Hyperglycemia can occur with high doses.

Client Teaching
ACTH

• Advise the client to adhere to the drug regimen. Discontinuation of certain drugs, such as corticotropin, can cause hypofunction of the gland being stimulated.
• Advise the client to decrease salt intake to decrease or avoid edema. Potassium supplement may be needed.
• Instruct the client to report side effects, such as muscle weakness, edema, petechiae, ecchymosis, decrease in growth, decreased wound healing, and menstrual irregularities.

Growth Hormone

• Advise athletes not to take GH due to its side effects. GH can be effective for children whose height is markedly below the expected norm for their age. Because GH acts on the newly forming bone, it should be administered before the epiphyses are fused.
• Inform the diabetic client to closely monitor blood sugar levels. Insulin regulation may be necessary.
• Suggest that the client or family monitors the client's growth rate.

EVALUATION

• Evaluate the effectiveness of the drug therapy.

Generic (Brand)	Route and Dosage	Preg Cat	Interaction	t 1/2	PB	Action		
						Onset	Peak	Duration
Anterior: Growth Hormone (GH)								
Sermorelin acetate (Geref)	*Diagnostic:* A & C: IV: 0.3–1 µg/kg	C	*Increase* effects with clonidine, levodopa	UK	UK	UK	UK	UK
Somatrem (Protropin)	C: SC/IM: 100 µg/kg (0.1 mg/kg) 3×wk or 0.2 U/kg 3×wk; 48-h interval is recommended between doses	C	*Increase* epiphyseal closure with androgens, estrogens, thyroid drugs *Decrease* somatrem effect with ACTH, glucocorticoids	20–30 min	UK	UK	UK	18–20 h
Somatropin (Humatrope)	C: SC/IM: 60 µg/kg (0.06 mg/kg) 3×wk or 0.16 IU/kg 3×wk; 48-h interval is recommended between doses	D	Same as somatrem	15–50 min	UK	UK	UK	18–20 h
Thyroid-Stimulating Hormone (TSH)								
Thyrotropin (Thytropar)	*Hypothyroidism and treatment of thyroid cancer:* A: SC/IM: 10 IU/d for 1–3 d; cancer treatment: 3–8 d	C	None significant reported	35 min with normal thyroid	UK	8 h	UK	24–28 h

Drug	Route and Dosage	Pregnancy Category	Drug Interactions	$t_{1/2}$	PB	Onset	Peak	Duration
Adrenocorticotropic Hormone (ACTH) Corticotropin (Acthar)	See Prototype Drug Chart A: SC/IM: 40–80 U/q24–48h							
Corticotropin repository (Acthar gel)	See Corticotropin, Prototype Drug Chart							
Cosyntropin (Cortrosyn)	A: C >2 y: IM: 0.25–0.75 mg IV: 0.25 mg C <2 y: IM: 0.125 mg IV: 0.125 mg (0.04 mg/h)	C	May *increase* effect of spironolactone; may *increase* plasma cortisol level when taken with cortisone preparations	15 min (plasma)	UK	IM: 15–30 min IV: 5–15 min	1 h	2–4 h
Posterior: Antidiuretic Hormone (ADH) Desmopressin acetate (DDAVP)	A: Intranasal: 0.1–0.4 mL/d in divided doses C <12 y: Intranasal: 0.05–0.3 mL/d in divided doses	B	May *increase* ADH effect with carbamazepine, chlorpropamide May *decrease* ADH effect with other vasopressors, lithium	76 min	UK	0.5–1 h	1–5 h	5–20 h
Desmopressin (Stimate)	A: Inf: 0.3 μg/kg diluted in 50 mL of NSS admin over 20–30 min C <12 y: Inf: 0.3 μg/kg diluted in 10 mL of NSS	B	Same as DDAVP	76 min	UK	0.5–1 h	1–5 h	5–20 h
Lypressin (Diapid)	*Diabetes insipidus:* A&C: Intranasal: 1–2 sprays per nostril q.i.d.	B	May *decrease* ADH effect with other vasopressors, lithium	15 min	UK	0.5–2 h	0.5–2 h	3–8 h

continued

Generic (Brand)	Route and Dosage	Preg Cat	Interaction	t 1/2	PB	Action Onset	Action Peak	Action Duration
Vasopressin (aqueous) (Pitressin)	*Diabetes insipidus:* A: SC/IM: 5–10 U b.i.d./t.i.d. C: SC/IM: 2.5–10 U b.i.d./q.i.d.	X	May *increase* ADH effect with thiazides, carbamazepine, chlorpropamide May *decrease* ADH effect with alcohol, phenytoin, heparin, lithium	15 min	UK	UK	UK	2–8 h
Vasopressin tanate/oil (Pitressin Tannate)	A: IM: 1.5–5.0 U q2–3d C: IM: 1.25–2.5 U q2–3d	X	Same as aqueous vasopressin	10–20 min	UK	UK	UK	24–72 h

KEY: For complete abbreviation key, see inside front cover.

NOTES:

_____

_____

_____

_____

_____

_____

_____

_____

_____

_____

Thyroid Hormone: Replacement

Levothyroxine Na

Levothyroxine sodium
(Synthroid, Levothroid)
Thyroid synthetic hormone

Pregnancy Category: A

Drug Forms:
Tab 25, 50, 75, 100, 125, 150, 200,
300 μg
Inj 200, 500 μg per vial

Dosage

A: PO: Initially: 50 μg/d (0.05 mg/d);
maint: 50–200 μg/d (0.05–0.2
mg/d)
IV: 0.2–0.5 mg in sol
C : >3 y: PO: 50–100 μg/d
(0.05–0.1 mg/d)

Contraindications

Thyrotoxicosis, MI, severe renal
disease

Caution: Cardiovascular disease,
hypertension, angina pectoris

Drug-Lab-Food Interactions

Increase cardiac insufficiency with
epinephrine; *increase* effects of
anticoagulants, tricyclic
antidepressants, vasopressors,
decongestants

Decrease effects of antidiabetics (oral
and insulin), digitalis products;
decrease absorption with
cholestyramine, colestipol

Pharmacokinetics

Absorption: PO: 50–75%
Distribution: PB: 99%
Metabolism: t 1/2: 6–7 d
Excretion: In bile and feces

Pharmacodynamics

PO: Onset: UK
Peak: 24 h–1 wk
Duration: 1–3 wk
IV: Onset: 6–8 h
Peak: 24–48 h
Duration: UK

Therapeutic Effects/Uses: To treat hypothyroidism, myxedema, and cretinism.

Mode of Action: Increase metabolic rate, oxygen consumption, and body growth.

Side Effects

Nausea, vomiting, diarrhea, cramps,
tremors, nervousness, insomnia,
headache, weight loss

Adverse Reactions

Tachycardia, hypertension,
palpitations
Life-threatening: Thyroid crisis, angina
pectoris, cardiac dysrhythmias,
cardiovascular collapse

KEY: For complete abbreviation key, see inside front cover.

■ **NURSING PROCESS: Thyroid Hormone: Replacement and Antithyroids Drugs**

ASSESSMENT

- Obtain baseline VS to compare with future data. Report abnormal results.
- Check serum T_3, T_4, and TSH levels. Report abnormal results.

THYROID REPLACEMENT

- Obtain a history of drugs the client is currently taking. Be aware that thyroid drugs enhance the action of oral anticoagulants, sympathomimetics, and antidepressants and decrease the action of insulin, oral hypoglycemics, and digitalis preparation. Phenytoin and aspirin can enhance the action of thyroid hormone.

ANTITHYROID DRUGS

- Assess for signs and symptoms of a thyroid crisis (thyroid storm), which includes tachycardia, dysrhythmias, fever, heart failure, flushed skin, apathy, confusion, behavioral changes, and later hypotension and vascular collapse. Thyroid crisis can result from a thyroidectomy (excess thyroid hormones released), abrupt withdrawal of antithyroid drug, excess ingestion of thyroid hormone, or failure to give antithyroid medication before thyroid surgery.

POTENTIAL NURSING DIAGNOSES

Altered health maintenance
Altered tissue perfusion

PLANNING

- Client's signs and symptoms of hypothyroidism will be alleviated within 2–4 wk with prescribed thyroid drug replacement, and the client will not experience side effects.
- Client's signs and symptoms of hyperthyroidism will be alleviated in 1–3 wk with the prescribed antithyroid drug.

NURSING INTERVENTIONS

- Monitor VS. With hypothyroidism, the temperature, heart rate, and blood pressure are usually decreased. With hyperthyroidism, tachycardia and palpitations usually occur.
- Monitor the client's weight. Weight gain commonly occurs in clients with hypothyroidism.

Client Teaching

Thyroid Drug Replacement for Hypothyroidism

- Instruct the client to take the drug at the same time each day, preferably before breakfast. Food will hamper absorption rate.
- Advise the client to check cautions on labels of OTC drugs. Avoid OTC drugs that caution against use by persons with heart or thyroid disease.
- Advise the client to report symptoms of hyperthyroidism (tachycardia, chest pain, palpitations, excess sweating) due to drug accumulation or overdosing.
- Suggest that the client carry a medical alert card, tag, or bracelet with health condition and thyroid drug listed.

Diet

• Instruct the client to avoid foods that can inhibit thyroid secretion, such as strawberries, peaches, pears, cabbage, turnips, spinach, kale, Brussels sprouts, cauliflower, radishes, and peas.

Antithyroid Drugs for Hyperthyroidism

• Instruct the client to take the drug with meals to decrease GI symptoms.
• Advise the client about the effects of iodine and its presence in iodized salt, shellfish, and OTC cough medicines.
• Emphasize the importance of drug compliance; abruptly stopping the antithyroid drug could bring on a thyroid crisis.
• Teach the client the signs and symptoms of hypothyroidism: lethargy, puffy eyelids and face, thick tongue, slow speech with hoarseness, lack of perspiration, and slow pulse. Hypothyroidism can result from treatment of hyperthyroidism.
• Advise the client to avoid antithyroid drugs if pregnant or breast feeding. Antithyroid drugs taken during pregnancy can cause hypothyroidism in the fetus or infant.

Skill

• Demonstrate to the client how to take a pulse rate. Instruct the client to monitor the pulse rate and report increases or marked decreases in pulse rate.

Side Effects

• Teach the client the side effects of antithyroid drugs, such as skin rash, hives, nausea, alopecia, loss of hair pigment, petechiae or ecchymoses, and weakness.
• Advise the client to contact the health care provider if a sore throat and fever occur while taking antithyroid drugs. A serious adverse reaction of antithyroid drugs is agranulocytosis (loss of WBCs). CBC should be monitored for leukopenia.

EVALUATION

Thyroid Replacement

• Evaluate the effectiveness of the thyroid drug and drug compliance.
• Continue monitoring for side effects from drug accumulation or overdosing.

Antithyroid Drugs

• Evaluate the effectiveness of the antithyroid drug in decreasing signs and symptoms of hyperthyroidism. If signs and symptoms persist after 2–3 wk of therapy, other methods for correcting hyperthyroidism may be necessary.

Generic (Brand)	Route and Dosage	Preg Cat	Interaction	t 1/2	PB	Onset	Peak	Duration
						Action		
Thyroid Replacements: Hypothyroidism								
Levothyroxine Na (Synthroid)	See Prototype Drug Chart							
Liothyronine Na (Cytomel)	A: PO: Initially: 5–25 µg/d; maint: 25–100 µg/d C: PO: Initially: 5 µg/d > 3 y: 50–100 µg/d	A	Similar to thyroid	6–7 d	99%	UK	24–72 h	72 h
Liotrix (Euthroid, Thyrolar)	A: PO: Initially: 15–30 mg/d, increase q2–3wk; maint: 60–120 mg/d C: 6–12 y: 100–150 µg/d	A	Similar to thyroid	6–7 d	99%	UK	24–48 h	72 h
Thyroglobulin (Proloid)	A: PO: Initially: 32 mg/d; maint: 32–200 mg/d Elderly: Initially: 16 mg/d	A	Similar to thyroid	6–7 d	99%	UK	12–24 h	UK
Thyroid (Armour Thyroid, Thyrar)	A: PO: Initially: 15–65 mg/d, increase monthly as needed; maint: 65–195 mg/d C: PO: 15 mg/d, increase q2wk as needed	A	May increase effects of anticoagulants, tricyclic antidepressants, adrenergics May increase dose requirement for insulin, oral hypoglycemics Decrease thyroid effect with cholestyramine, colestipol, phenytoin	6–7 d	99%	UK	1–3 wk	UK

continued

Generic (Brand)	Route and Dosage	Preg Cat	Interaction	t 1/2	PB	Onset	Peak	Duration
							Action	
Antithyroid Drugs: Hyperthyroidism								
Methimazole (Tapazole)	A: PO: Initially: 15–60 mg/d in 3 divided doses; maint: 5–15 mg/d C: PO: Initially: 0.4 mg/kg/d in divided doses; maint: 0.2 mg/kg/d in divided doses	D	Similar to propylthiouracil	3–5 h	Not significant	0.5–1 h	1–2 h	2–4 h
Thioamide: Propylthiouracil (PTU)	A: PO: Initially: 300–400 mg/d in divided doses; maint: 100–300 mg/d C: 6–10 y: PO: 50–150 mg/d >10 y: PO: Same as adult or 150 mg/m²/d	D	May *increase* effect of oral anticoagulants	1–2 h	80%	UK	1–1.5 h	UK
Iodine: strong iodine solution (Lugol solution, potassium iodide solution)	A & C: PO: 0.1–0.3 mL (3–5 gtt) t.i.d. *Thyroid crisis:* A & C: PO: 1 mL in water p.c. t.i.d.	D	*Increase* antithyroid effect with other antithyroid drugs *Lab:* May *increase* serum potassium level	UK	UK	24 h	10–15 d	UK

KEY: For complete abbreviation key, see inside front cover.

NOTES:

_____

_____

_____

_____

_____

_____

_____

_____

_____

_____

Parathyroid Hormone

Calcitriol

Calcitriol
  (Rocaltrol)
Vitamin D analog
Pregnancy Category: C
Drug Forms:
Cap 0.25, 0.5 μg

Dosage

A: PO: 0.25 μg/d

Contraindications

Hypersensitivity, hypercalcemia,
  hyperphosphatemia,
  hypervitaminosis D,
  malabsorption syndrome
Caution: Cardiovascular disease,
  renal calculi

Drug-Lab-Food Interactions

Increase cardiac dysrhythmias with
  digoxin, verapamil
Decrease calcitriol absorption with
  cholestyramine
Lab: Increase serum calcium with
  thiazide diuretics, calcium
  supplements

Pharmacokinetics

Absorption: PO: Well absorbed
Distribution: PB: UK; crosses the
  placenta
Metabolism: t 1/2: 3–8 h
Excretion: Mostly in feces

Pharmacodynamics

PO: Onset: 2–6 h
     Peak: 10–12 h
     Duration: 3–5 d

Therapeutic Effects/Uses: To treat hypocalcemia in chronic renal failure.

Mode of Action: Enhancement of calcium deposits in bones.

Side Effects

Anorexia, nausea, vomiting,
  diarrhea, cramps, drowsiness,
  headache, dizziness, lethargy,
  photophobia

Adverse Reactions

Hypercalciuria, hyperphosphatemia,
  hematuria

KEY: For complete abbreviation key, see inside front cover.

■ **NURSING PROCESS: Parathyroid Hormone**

ASSESSMENT

• Assess serum calcium level. Report abnormal results.
• Assess for symptoms of tetany in hypocalcemia: twitching of the mouth, tingling and numbness of the fingers, carpopedal spasm, spasmodic contractions, and laryngeal spasm.

POTENTIAL NURSING DIAGNOSES

High risk for impaired tissue integrity
Altered health maintenance

PLANNING

• The client's serum calcium level will be within the normal range.

NURSING INTERVENTIONS

• Monitor the serum calcium level. Normal reference value is 8.5–10.5 mg/dL, or 4.5–5.5 mEq/L. A serum calcium level <8.5 mg/dL, or <4.5 mEq/L, indicates hypocalcemia, and a serum calcium level >10.5 mg/dL, or >5.5 mEq/L, indicates hypercalcemia. Serum ionized calcium levels are usually used because much of the calcium is protein-bound and is nonionized and nonactive.

Client Teaching
Hypoparathyroidism

• Advise the client to report symptoms of tetany (see Assessment).

Hyperparathyroidism

• Advise the client to report signs and symptoms of hypercalcemia: bone pain, anorexia, nausea, vomiting, thirst, constipation, lethargy, bradycardia, and polyuria.
• Instruct women to inform their health care provider about pregnancy status before taking calcitonin preparation.
• Advise the client to check OTC drugs for possible calcium content, especially if the client has an elevated serum calcium level. Some vitamins and antacids contain calcium. Tell the client to contact the health care provider before taking drugs with calcium.

EVALUATION

• Monitor the effectiveness of drug therapy.
• Continue monitoring for signs and symptoms of hypocalcemia (tetany) when commercially prepared calcitonin has been given.

Parathyroid Hormones: Replacements and Supplements

Generic (Brand)	Route and Dosage	Preg Cat	Interaction	t 1/2	PB	Onset	Peak	Duration
							Action	
						Onset	Peak	Duration
Hypoparathyroidism and Hypocalcemia: Vitamin D Analogs								
Calcifediol (Calderol)	A: PO: 50–100 µg/d or 100–200 µg q.o.d.	C	*Increase* cardiac dysrhythmias with digoxin; may *increase* hypercalcemia with thiazide diuretics *Decrease* absorption with cholestyramine, colestipol; *decrease* effect with glucocorticoids	12–22 d	Bound to specific alpha globulins for transport	UK	4 h	15–20 d
Calcitriol (Rocaltrol)	A: PO: 0.25 µg/d; may increase 0.25 µg q4wk; max: 1.0 µg/d IV: 0.5 µg 3×wk at end of dialysis C: PO: 0.014–0.041 µg/kd/d	C	Similar to calcifediol	3–6 h	Alpha globulins	2–6 h	7–12 h	1–5 d

		C	Similar to calcifediol	12–24 h	Alpha globulins	12–24 h	4 wk	2–6 mo
Ergocalciferol (Drisdol Drops)	A & C: PO: 50,000–200,000 U/d or 1.25–5.0 µg/d	C	Similar to calcifediol	12–24 h	Alpha globulins	12–24 h	4 wk	2–6 mo
Hyperparathyroidism and Hypercalcemia								
Calcitonin (human) (Cibacalcin)	A: SC: Initially: 0.5 mg/d; maint: 0.25 mg q.d.–0.5 mg b.i.d.	C	None significant reported	1 h	UK	15 min	4 h	8–24 h
Calcitonin (salmon) (Calcimar)	A: SC/IM: Initially: 4 IU/kg/d; maint: 4–8 IU/kg q12h	C	None significant reported	1–1.5 h	UK	15 min	4 h	8–24 h

KEY: For complete abbreviation key, see inside front cover.

Adrenal Hormone

Prednisone

Prednisone
  (Deltasone, Meticorten, Orasone,
  Panasol-S)
Glucocorticoid
Pregnancy Category: C
Drug Forms:
Tab 2.5, 5, 10, 25, 50 mg
Liq 5 mg/5 mL
Syrup 5 mg/5 mL

Dosage

A: PO: 5–60 mg/d in divided doses
C : PO: 0.1–0.15 mg/kg/d in 2–4
    divided doses or 4–5 mg/m^2/d in
    2 doses

Contraindications

Hypersensitivity, psychosis, fungal
  infection
Caution: Diabetes mellitus

Drug-Lab-Food Interactions

Increase effect with barbiturates,
  phenytoin, rifampin, ephedrine,
  theophylline
Decrease effects of aspirin,
  anticonvulsants, isoniazid (INH),
  antidiabetics, vaccines

Pharmacokinetics

Absorption: PO: Well absorbed
Distribution: PB: UK; crosses the
  placenta
Metabolism: t 1/2: 3–4 h
Excretion: In urine

Pharmacodynamics

PO: Onset: UK
     Peak: 1–2 h
     Duration: 24–36 h

Therapeutic Effects/Uses: To decrease inflammatory occurrence; as an immunosuppressant; to treat dermatologic disorders.

Mode of Action: Suppression of inflammation and adrenal function.

Side Effects

Nausea, diarrhea, abdominal
  distention, increased appetite,
  sweating, headache, depression,
  flushing, mood changes

Adverse Reactions

Petechiae, ecchymosis, hypertension,
  tachycardia, osteoporosis, muscle
  wasting
Life-threatening: GI hemorrhage,
  pancreatitis, circulatory collapse,
  thrombophlebitis, embolism

KEY: For complete abbreviation key, see inside front cover.

Adrenal Hormone

■ NURSING PROCESS: Adrenal Hormone: Glucocorticoids

ASSESSMENT
- Obtain baseline VS for future comparison.
- Assess laboratory test results, especially serum electrolytes and blood sugar. Serum potassium level usually decreases and blood sugar level increases when a glucocorticoid such as prednisone is taken over an extensive period of time.
- Obtain the client's weight and urine output to use for future comparison.
- Assess the client's medical history. Report if the client has glaucoma, cataracts, peptic ulcer, psychiatric problems, or diabetes mellitus. Glucocorticoid can intensify these health problems.

POTENTIAL NURSING DIAGNOSES
Fluid volume excess
High risk for impaired tissue integrity

PLANNING
- The client's inflammatory process will abate. Side effects of glucocorticoid will be minimal.

NURSING INTERVENTIONS
- Monitor VS. Glucocorticoids such as prednisone can increase blood pressure and sodium and water retention.
- Administer glucocorticoids only as ordered. Routes of administration include PO, IM (not in the deltoid muscle), IV, aerosol, and topical. Topical glucocorticoid drugs should be applied in thin layers. Rashes, infection, and purpura should be noted and reported.
- Monitor weight. Report weight gain of 5 lb in several days; this would most likely be due to water retention.
- Monitor laboratory values, especially serum electrolytes and blood sugar. Serum potassium level would probably decrease to <3.5 mEq/L, and blood sugar level would probably increase.
- Observe for signs and symptoms of hypokalemia, such as nausea, vomiting, muscular weakness, abdominal distention, paralytic ileus, and irregular heart rate.
- Observe for side effects from glucocorticoid drugs when therapy has lasted >10 d and the drug is taken in high dosages. The cortisone preparation should not be abruptly stopped because adrenal crisis can result.
- Monitor older adults for signs and symptoms of increased osteoporosis. Glucocorticoids promote calcium loss from the bone.
- Report changes in muscle strength. High doses of glucocorticoids promote loss of muscle tone.

CLIENT TEACHING
General
- Advise the client to take the drug as prescribed. Instruct the client *NOT* to abruptly stop the drug. When the drug is discontinued, the dose is tapered over 1–2 wk.
- For short-term use of glucocorticoids such as prednisone or other cortisone preparations (<10 d), the drug dose still needs to be tapered. Prepare a

schedule for the client to decrease the dose over a period of 4–5 d. For example, take 1 tab q.i.d.; the next day take 1 tab t.i.d.; the next day, take 1 tab b.i.d.; and then take 1 tab q.d.

• Advise the client not to take cortisone preparations (PO or topical) during pregnancy unless necessary and prescribed by the health care provider. These drugs may be harmful to the fetus.

• Instruct the client to avoid persons with respiratory infections since these drugs suppress the immune system. This is especially important if the client is receiving a high dose of glucocorticoids.

• Advise the client receiving glucocorticoids to inform other health care providers of all drugs taken, especially before surgery.

• Advise the client to have a medical alert card, tag, or bracelet stating the glucocorticoid drug being taken.

Skill

• Teach the client how to use an aerosol nebulizer. Warn the client against overuse of the aerosol to avoid possible rebound effect.

Diet

• Instruct the client to take cortisone preparations at mealtime or with food. Glucocorticoid drugs can irritate the gastric mucosa and cause a peptic ulcer.

• Advise the client to eat foods rich in potassium, such as fresh and dried fruits, vegetables, meats, and nuts. Prednisone promotes potassium loss and, thus, hypokalemia.

Side Effects

• Teach the client to report signs and symptoms of drug overdose or Cushing's syndrome, including a moon face, puffy eyelids, edema in the feet, increased bruising, dizziness, bleeding, and menstrual irregularity.

EVALUATION

• Evaluate the effectiveness of glucocorticoid drug therapy. If the inflammation has improved, a change in drug therapy may be necessary.

• Continue monitoring for side effects, especially when the client is receiving high doses of glucocorticoids.

						Action		
Generic (Brand)	Route and Dosage	Preg Cat	Interaction	t 1/2	PB	Onset	Peak	Duration
Beclomethasone Dipropionate (Vanceril)	A: Inhal: 2 puffs b.i.d./q.i.d.	C	None significant reported	5–15 h	87%	UK	1–2 wk	UK
Betamethasone (Celestone, Celestone Phosphate)	A: PO: 0.6–7.2 mg/d in single or divided doses IM/IV: 1–9 mg/d; max: IM: 12 mg/d	C	*Increase* effect with aspirin, estrogens, oral contraceptives, erythromycin; *increase* risk of hypokalemia with diuretics, amphotercin B, ticarcillin; *increase* need of insulin, oral hypoglycemics *Decrease* effect with barbiturates, phenytoin, theophylline, rifampin, cholestyramine, ephedrine; *decrease* effects of anticoagulants, antidiabetics, aspirin	36–50 h (tissue)	80–90%	PO: 1 h IM/IV: Rapid	PO: 1–2 h IM/IV: 2–8 h	PO: 3 d IV: 1–3 d

continued

Adrenal Hormones: Glucocorticoids Continued

Generic (Brand)	Route and Dosage	Preg Cat	Interaction	t 1/2	PB	Onset	Peak	Duration
							Action	
Cortisone acetate (Cortone Acetate, Cortistan)	A: PO/IM: 25–300 mg/d; decrease dose periodically	C	Same as betamethasone	0.5–12 h	UK	PO: UK IM: UK	PO: 2 h IM: 24–48 h	PO: 1.5 d IM: 1.5 d
Dexamethasone (Decadron)	*Inflammation:* A: PO: 0.25–4 mg b.i.d./q.i.d. IM: 4–16 mg q1–3wk C: PO: 0.2 mg/kg/d in divided doses *Shock:* A: IV: 1–6 mg/kg as a single dose	C	Same as betamethasone	3–4 h	80–90%	PO: UK IM: UK	PO: 1–2 h IM: 8 h	PO: 2–2.5 d IM: Days to 1–3 wk
Fludrocortisone acetate (Florinef Acetate)	A & C: PO: 0.1–0.2 mg/d	C	*Increase* potassium loss with thiazides, loop diuretics	≥3.5 h	92%	UK	1.5–2 h	1–2 d
Hydrocortisone (Cortef, Hydrocortone)	A: PO: 20–240 mg/d in 2–4 divided doses IV: 15–240 mg (phosphate) q12h Rectal supp: 10–25 mg	C	Similar to betamethasone	2–12 h	79%	PO: 1–2 h IV: Rapid	PO: 1 h IV: UK	PO: 1–1.5 d IV: 1–1.5 d
Methylprednisolone (Medrol, Solu-Medrol [sodium succinate], Depo-Medrol [acetate])	A: PO: 4–48 mg/d in one or more divided doses IM/IV: Succinate: 10–250 mg q6h IM: Acetate: 40–80 mg/wk	C	Similar to betamethasone	Tissue: 18–36 h	UK	PO: UK IM: Acetate: 6–48 h IV: Rapid	PO: 1–2 h IM: Acetate: 4–8 d IV: UK	PO: 1.5 d IM: Acetate: 1–5 wk IV: UK

Paramethasone acetate (Haldrone)	A: PO: 0.5–6 mg t.i.d./q.i.d. C: PO: 58–800 µg/kg/d in 3–4 divided doses	C	Similar to fludrocortisone May *change* PT with warfarin *Increase* risk of GI distress with NSAIDs, other steroids; *Decrease* effect with barbiturates, phenytoin, rifampin; *decrease* antibody response with toxoids, vaccines	3–4.5 h Tissue: 36–54 h	95%	UK	1–2 h	2 d
Prednisolone (Delta-Cortef, Hydeltrasol [phosphate])	A: PO: 2.5–15 mg b.i.d./q.i.d. IV: Phosphate: 2–30 mg q12h C: PO: 0.14–2 mg/kg/d in a single or divided doses	C	Similar to betamethasone	Tissue: 18–36 h	80–90%	PO: UK	PO: 1–2 h	PO: 1.5–2 d
Prednisone	See Prototype Drug Chart							

KEY: For complete abbreviation key, see inside front cover.

Antidiabetic: Insulins

Regular Insulin	Dosage

Regular Insulin
  NPH Insulin
  Injectable insulins
Pregnancy Category: B
Drug Forms:
Inj 100 U/mL; 40 and 50 U/mL
	Varies according to client's blood sugar

Contraindications	Drug-Lab-Food Interactions
Hypersensitivity to beef, zinc, protamine insulins	*Increase* hypoglycemic effect with aspirin, oral anticoagulant, alcohol, oral hypoglycemics, beta blockers, tricyclic antidepressants, MAOIs, tetracycline *Decrease* hypoglycemic effect with thiazides, glucocorticoids, oral contraceptives, thyroid drugs, smoking

Pharmacokinetics	Pharmacodynamics

Absorption: SC: Well absorbed
Distribution: PB: UK
Metabolism: t 1/2: Regular IV insulin: 5–9 min; varies with type of insulin
Excretion: Mostly in urine
	Regular Insulin:
	SC: Onset: 0.5–1 h
	  Peak: 2–4 h
	  Duration: 4–8 h
	IV: Onset: 10–20 min
	  Peak: 15–30 min
	  Duration: 1–2 h
	NPH Insulin:
	SC: Onset: 1–2 h
	  Peak: 6–12 h
	  Duration: 18–24 h

Therapeutic Effects/Uses: To control diabetes mellitus; to lower blood sugar.

Mode of Action: Insulin promotes utilization of glucose by body cells.

Side Effects	Adverse Reactions
Hunger, tremors, weakness, headache, lethargy, fatigue, redness, irritation or swelling at insulin injection site, flushing, confusion, agitation	Urticaria, tachycardia, palpitations, hypoglycemic reaction, rebound hyperglycemia (Somogyi effect), lipodystrophy *Life-threatening:* Shock; anaphylaxis

KEY: For complete abbreviation key, see inside front cover.

■ NURSING PROCESS: Antidiabetics: Insulin

ASSESSMENT

• Assess the drugs the client is currently taking. Certain drugs, such as alcohol, aspirin, oral anticoagulants, oral hypoglycemics, beta blockers, tricyclic antidepressants, MAOIs, and tetracycline, increase the hypoglycemic effect when taken with insulin. Note that thiazides, glucocorticoids, oral contraceptives, thyroid drugs, and smoking can increase blood sugar.

Antidiabetic: Insulins

- Assess the type of insulin and dosage. Note if it is given once or twice a day.
- Check VS and blood sugar levels. Report abnormal findings.
- Assess the client's knowledge of diabetes mellitus and the use of insulins.
- Assess for signs and symptoms of a hypoglycemic reaction (insulin shock) and hyperglycemia or ketoacidosis.

POTENTIAL NURSING DIAGNOSES
High risk for impaired tissue integrity
Altered nutrition: more or less than body requirements
High risk for injury

PLANNING
- Client's blood sugar will be within the normal values (70–110 mg/dL).

NURSING INTERVENTIONS
- Monitor VS. Tachycardia can occur during an insulin reaction.
- Monitor blood glucose levels and report changes. The reference value is 60–100 mg/dL for blood glucose and 70–110 mg/dL for serum glucose.
- Prepare a teaching plan based on the client's knowledge of the health problem, diet, and drug therapy.

CLIENT TEACHING

General
- Instruct the client to report immediately symptoms of a hypoglycemic (insulin) reaction, such as headache, nervousness, sweating, tremors, and rapid pulse, and symptoms of a hyperglycemic reaction (diabetic acidosis), such as thirst, increased urine output, and sweet fruity breath odor.
- Advise the client that hypoglycemic reactions are more likely to occur during the peak action time. Most diabetics know if they are having a hypoglycemic reaction; however, some have a higher tolerance to low blood sugar and can have a severe hypoglycemic reaction without realizing it.
- Explain that orange juice, sugar-containing drinks, and hard candy may be used when a hypoglycemic reaction begins.
- Instruct family members in administering glucagon by injection if the client has a hypoglycemic reaction and cannot drink sugar-containing fluid.
- Instruct the client about the necessity for compliance to prescribed insulin and diet.
- Advise the client to obtain a medical alert card, tag, and/or bracelet indicating the health problem and insulin dosage.

Skill
- Instruct the client how to check the blood sugar using Chemstrip bG test.
- Instruct the client in the care of the insulin bottle and syringes. Inform the client taking NPH or lente insulin with regular insulin that the regular insulin should be drawn up before the NPH or lente insulin.

Diet
- Advise the client taking insulin to eat the prescribed diet on schedule. The diet may be from the American Diabetic Association (ADA).

EVALUATION
- Evaluate the effectiveness of the insulin therapy by noting whether blood sugar level is within the accepted range.
- Evaluate the client's knowledge of the signs and symptoms of hypoglycemic or hyperglycemic reaction.

Antidiabetic: Insulins									

Generic (Brand)	Route and Dosage	Preg Cat	Interaction	t 1/2	PB	Onset	Peak	Duration
							Action	
						Onset	Peak	Duration
Rapid-Acting Humulin R	Same as regular insulin							
Regular	A & C: SC/IV: 100 U/mL; dose is individualized according to blood sugar	B	May *increase* insulin effect with aspirin, beta blockers, tetracyclines, MAOIs, tricyclic antidepressants, oral anticoagulants May *decrease* insulin effect with thiazides, glucocorticoids, thyroid drugs, oral contraceptives	10 min–1 h	UK	0.5–1 h	2–4 h	6–8 h
Semilente	A & C: SC: 100 U/mL; dose is individualized according to blood sugar	B	Same as all insulin	<13 h	UK	30–45 min	4–6 h	12–16 h

					Onset	Peak	Duration
Intermediate Acting							
Humulin L Insulin	B	Same as lente	13 h	UK	1–2 h	8–12 h	18–28 h
Humulin N Insulin	B	Same as NPH insulin	13 h	UK	1–2 h	6–12 h	18–24 h
Lente Insulin	B	A & C: SC: 100 U/mL; dose is individualized according to blood sugar	13 h	UK	1–2 h	8–12 h	18–28 h
NPH Insulin	B	See Prototype Drug Chart	13 h	UK	1–2 h	6–12 h	18–24 h
Long Acting							
PZI Insulin	B	Same as lente	13 h	UK	4–8 h	14–20 h	24–36 h
Ultralente Insulin	B	Same as lente	13 h	UK	5–8 h	14–20 h	30–36 h

KEY: For complete abbreviation key, see inside front cover.

Antidiabetics: Sulfonylurea

Acetohexamide

Acetohexamide
  (Dymelor)
Sulfonylurea, oral hypoglycemic
  drug
Pregnancy Category: C
Drug Forms:
Tab 250, 500 mg

Dosage

A: PO: 250–1,500 mg/d in 1 or 2
  divided doses

Contraindications

Diabetes mellitus (DM) type I; severe
  renal, hepatic, cardiac, or thyroid
  disease; unstable DM

Drug-Lab-Food Interactions

Increase hypoglycemic effect with
  aspirin, alcohol, anticoagulants,
  some NSAIDs, anticonvulsants,
  sulfonamides, oral contraceptives,
  MAOIs
Decrease hypoglycemic effect with
  glucocorticoids (cortisone),
  thiazide diuretics, estrogen,
  calcium channel blockers,
  phenytoin, thyroid drugs

Pharmacokinetics

Absorption: PO: Well absorbed
Distribution: PB: 90%
Metabolism: t 1/2: Drug: 1–1.5 h
  metabolite; 5–7 h
Excretion: Unchanged in urine

Pharmacodynamics

PO: Onset: 1 h
  Peak: 2–6 h
  Duration: 12–24 h

Therapeutic Effects/Uses: To control DM type II (maturity-onset diabetes); to lower
blood sugar.
Mode of Action: Stimulation of beta cells to secrete insulin.

Side Effects

Nausea, vomiting, diarrhea, rash,
  pruritus, headache,
  photosensitivity

Adverse Reactions

Hypoglycemic reaction
Life-threatening: Aplastic anemia,
  leukopenia, thrombocytopenia

KEY: For complete abbreviation key, see inside front cover.

■ NURSING PROCESS: Antidiabetics: Sulfonylurea

ASSESSMENT

• Assess the drugs the client is currently taking. Aspirin, alcohol, sulfonamides, oral contraceptives, and MAOIs increase the hypoglycemic effect; decrease in oral hypoglycemic drug may be needed. Glucocorticoids (cortisone),
thiazide diuretics, and estrogen increase blood sugar.
• Assess VS and blood sugar levels. Report abnormal findings.
• Assess the client's knowledge of diabetes mellitus and the use of oral antidiabetics (sulfonylurea).

POTENTIAL NURSING DIAGNOSES

High risk for impaired tissue integrity
Altered nutrition: more or less than body requirements

PLANNING

- Client's blood sugar will be within normal serum levels (70–100 mg/dL).
- Client will adhere to prescribed diet, blood testing, and drug.

NURSING INTERVENTIONS

- Monitor VS. Sulfonylureas increase cardiac function and oxygen consumption, which can lead to cardiac dysrhythmias.
- Administer oral antidiabetics with food to minimize gastric upset.
- Monitor blood glucose levels and report changes. The reference value is 60–100 mg/dL for blood glucose and 70–110 mg/dL for serum glucose.
- Prepare a teaching plan based on the client's knowledge of health problems, diet, and drug therapy.

CLIENT TEACHING

General

- Advise the client that hypoglycemic (insulin) reaction can occur when taking an oral hypoglycemic drug. This drug stimulates the release of insulin from the beta cells of the pancreas. Oral antidiabetics are *not* insulin. Normally, clients with diabetes mellitus type I do not have functioning beta cells and should *not* take oral antidiabetics, only insulin. Sulfonylureas are prescribed for clients with diabetes mellitus type II.
- Instruct the client to recognize symptoms of hypoglycemic reaction (headache, nervousness, sweating, tremors, rapid pulse), and symptoms of hyperglycemic reaction (thirst, increased urine output, sweet fruity breath odor).
- Explain that insulin might be needed instead of an oral antidiabetic drug during stress, surgery, or serious infection. Blood sugar levels are usually elevated during stressful times.
- Instruct the client about the necessity for compliance to diet and drug.
- Advise the client to obtain a medical alert card, tag, and/or bracelet indicating the health problem and insulin dosage.

Skill

- Instruct the client how to check the blood sugar level using a Chemstrip bG test. Client should record and report abnormal results.

Diet

- To avoid a hypoglycemic reaction, instruct the client not to ingest alcohol with sulfonylurea drugs. Food taken with oral antidiabetics will decrease gastric irritation.
- Advise the client taking sulfonylurea to eat the prescribed diet on schedule. Delaying or missing a meal can cause hypoglycemia.
- Explain the use of orange juice, sugar-containing drinks, and hard candy when a hypoglycemic reaction begins.

Side Effects

- Instruct the client to report side effects, such as vomiting, diarrhea, rash.

EVALUATION

- Evaluate the effectiveness of drug therapy by noting whether blood sugar levels are within the accepted range.

Antidiabetic: Sulfonylurea

Generic (Brand)	Route and Dosage	Preg Cat	Interaction	t 1/2	PB	Action		
						Onset	Peak	Duration
First Generation: Short Acting Tolbutamide (Orinase)	A: PO: 500–2,000 mg/d in 2–3 divided doses	C	*Increase* hypoglycemic effect with aspirin, NSAIDs, oral anticoagulants, insulin, cimetidine, sulfonamides, methyldopa *Decrease* effect with calcium channel blockers, glucocorticoids, estrogens, phenytoin, thyroid drugs, phenothiazines, thiazides	4–7 h	90–95%	1 h	3–5 h	6–12 h
First Generation: Intermediate Acting Acetohexamide (Dymelor)	See Prototype Drug Chart							
Tolazamide (Tolinase)	A: PO: 100–250 mg/d in 1–2 divided doses; max: 1 g/d	C	Similar to tolbutamide	7 h	90%	1–4 h	4–6 h	10–15 h

	Dosage	Pregnancy Category	Drug Interactions	t½	PB	Onset	Peak	Duration
First Generation: **Long Acting** Chlorpropamide (Diabinese)	A: PO: Initially: 100–250 mg/d; maint: 100–500 mg/d in 1–2 divided doses; max: 750 mg/d	C	Similar to tolbutamide *Decrease* digoxin level with digoxin	36 h	95%	1 h	3–6 h	24 h
Second Generation: Glipizide (Glucotrol)	A: PO: Initially: 2.5–5.0 mg a.c. q.d./b.i.d.; maint: 5–25 mg/d (dose should be divided if >15 mg), max: 40 mg/d	C	Similar to tolbutamide	2.5–5 h	90–95%	0.5–1 h	1–2 h	10–24 h
Glyburide (DiaBeta, Micronase)	A: PO: Initially: 1.25–5 mg/d; maint: 1.25–20 mg q.d./b.i.d.; max: 20 mg/d	B	Same as tolbutamide *Decrease* digoxin level with digoxin; *decrease* effect with cimetidine	3–10 h	90–95%	0.5–1 h	1–2 h	10–24 h

KEY: For complete abbreviation key, see inside front cover.

REPRODUCTIVE AND GENDER-RELATED AGENTS

Beta-Adrenergic Agonists

Oxytocins

Estrogen Replacements

Oral Contraceptives

Androgens

Ovulation Stimulants

Beta-Adrenergic Agonists: Ritodrine

Ritodrine HCl

Ritodrine HCl
   (Yutopar)
Adrenergic
Pregnancy Category: B
Drug Forms:
Tab 10 mg
Inj 10 mg/mL

Dosage

IV: Mix 150 mg in 500 mL D$_5$W and
   infuse at 10–20 mL/h; increase by
   10 mL/h q15 min until
   contractions >15 min apart; max:
   70 mL/h; decrease therapy as
   contractions taper off
Initiate PO therapy 10–20 mg 30 min
   before stopping IV drug; PO dose
   q1–6h until tocolysis not needed
Refer to specific protocol.

Contraindications

Before 20th week of gestation,
   condition in which maintenance of
   pregnancy is hazardous, e.g.,
   antepartal hemorrhage and
   intrauterine fetal death; selected
   preexisting maternal conditions,
   e.g., uncontrolled hypertension or
   diabetes

Drug-Lab-Food Interactions

Increase effects of ritodrine with
   diazoxide, meperidine, potent
   general anesthetics, magnesium
   sulfate; *increase* effects of
   sympathomimetic amines
Decrease effects of ritodrine with beta
   blockers

Pharmacokinetics

Absorption: PO: 30%
Distribution: PB: 32%, crosses
   placenta; probably crosses
   blood–brain barrier
Metabolism: t 1/2: 15 h
Excretion: In urine

Pharmacodynamics

PO: Onset: 30 min
   Peak: 30–60 min
   Duration: 4–6 h
IV: Onset: Within 5 min
   Peak: 50–60 min
   Duration: 30 min

Therapeutic Effects/Uses: To inhibit uterine contractions.

Mode of Action: Stimulation of receptors in smooth muscles of uterus, thereby decreasing intensity and frequency of contractions.

Side Effects

Malaise, weakness, dyspnea,
   tachycardia (maternal and fetal),
   palpitations, increased systolic
   pressure, chest pain, nausea,
   vomiting, diarrhea, hyperglycemia,
   hypokalemia

Adverse Reactions

Ketoacidosis
Life-threatening: Long term:
   pulmonary edema, anaphylactic
   shock

KEY: For complete abbreviation key, see inside front cover.

■ NURSING PROCESS: Beta-Adrenergic Agonists: Ritodrine

ASSESSMENT
- Identify clients at risk for preterm labor early in pregnancy.
- Obtain a history, complete physical assessment, VS, fetal heart rate (FHR), and urine specimen for infection screening.

POTENTIAL NURSING DIAGNOSES
High risk for activity intolerance
Altered health maintenance

PLANNING
- Client's preterm contractions will be eliminated by resting in left side lying position, increasing fluid intake, and tocolytic therapy as needed.

NURSING INTERVENTIONS
- Monitor and assess uterine activity and FHR before, during, and for 1 h after discontinuing IV infusion.
- Maintain client in left lateral position as much as possible.
- Monitor maternal and fetal VS every 15 min when the client is receiving IV dose. Report if systolic blood pressure drops to <90 mm Hg or is >140 mm Hg, if diastolic blood pressure is <50 mm Hg, or if pulse increases to >120 beats per minute. If any of these occur, place client in Trendelenburg position and increase the infusion rate of primary IV (*not* of the piggyback IV containing the drug).
- Report auscultated cardiac dysrhythmias. An ECG may be ordered.
- Auscultate breath sounds every 4 h. Notify health care provider if respirations are >30/min or there is a change in quality (wheezes, rales, coughing).
- Monitor daily weight to assess fluid overload; monitor strict input and output every 8 h.
- Provide passive range of motion of legs every 1–2 h.
- Report fetal baseline heart rate >180 beats per min.
- Report persistence of frequent contractions despite tocolytic therapy.
- Report rupture of membranes, vaginal bleeding, or sudden complaints of rectal pressure, suggesting impending delivery.
- Be alert to presence of hypoglycemia and hypokalemia in the newborn delivered within 5 h of discontinued beta-sympathomimetic drugs.
- Administer only clear solutions of drugs if using IV form.
- Assist clients on home tocolytic therapy plan for assistance with self-care and family responsibilities.

CLIENT TEACHING

General
- Teach client the signs and symptoms of impending preterm labor (menstrual type cramps, sensation of pelvic pressure, low backache, and increased vaginal discharge).
- Instruct client that if she experiences preterm labor contractions at home, she should void, recline on her left side to increase uterine blood flow, drink extra fluids to decrease the release of antidiuretic hormone (ADH) and oxytocin from the posterior pituitary, rest for 30 min, and then attempt to resume her activities if asymptomatic. Stress that she should notify her health care provider if the contractions do not end or if they return.

• Tell client that she may return to her normal activities after 36–48 h without contractions; check with health care provider.
• Explain the effects of beta-sympathomimetic drugs; the contractions should be arrested. Report heart palpitations or dizziness.
• Instruct client to take the drug as directed.
• Advise the client to contact the health care provider before taking any other drugs while on tocolysis.
• Instruct the client that if she misses a dose and <1 h has elapsed, she should take the missed dose. However, if >1 h has elapsed, she should wait until the next regularly scheduled dose.

EVALUATION

• Evaluate the effectiveness of the tocolytic drug by noting the absence of six or more contractions in 1 h.
• Evaluate the client's understanding of nonpharmacologic measures for decreasing preterm contractions, such as increasing fluid intake and resting on the left side.
• Continue monitoring the client's and fetal VS. Report any change immediately.

Beta-Adrenergic Agonists

Generic (Brand)	Route and Dosage	Preg Cat	Interaction	t 1/2	PB	Action		
						Onset	Peak	Duration
Ritodrine HCl (Yutopar)	See Prototype Drug Chart							
Terbutaline SO$_4$ (Brethine, Bricanyl, Brethaire)	SC: Initially: 0.25 mg (repeat as necessary); SC maint: 0.1 mg q4h followed with PO: 2.5 mg q4–6h starting with last SC dose	B	Hypertensive crises with MAOIs *Decrease* effects of beta blockers	10–15 h	25%	PO: 30–45 min SC: 5–15 min	1–2 h 0.5–1 h	4–8 h 1.5–4 h

KEY: For complete abbreviation key, see inside front cover.

Oxytocins

Oxytocin

Oxytocin
  (Pitocin, Syntocinon)
Oxytocic
Pregnancy Category: X
Drug Forms:
Nasal sol 40 U/mL
Inj 10 U/mL

Dosage

A: IV: 10 U (1 amp) diluted in
  1,000 mL lactated Ringer's to
  10 mU/mL; connect to control IV
  line at the needle site of main IV
  line, as a secondary line; start at
  0.5 mU/min (3 mL/h) and titrate
  at rate of 0.5–2.5 mU every
  15–30 min until contractions are
  approximately 3 min apart and
  adequate
IV: 10 U added to 1 L electrolyte or
  dextrose solution; infuse at rate to
  control atony
  (IM: 10 U after delivery of the
  placenta if no IV)
Nasal spray: 1 spray into 1 or both
  nostrils 2–3 min before nursing or
  pumping

Contraindications

Toxemia, cephalopelvic
  disproportionment, fetal distress,
  hypersensitivity, anticipated
  nonvaginal delivery, pregnancy
  (intranasal spray)

Drug-Lab-Food Interactions

Hypertension with vasopressors,
  cyclopropane anesthetics

Pharmacokinetics

Absorption: PO: Well absorbed
Distribution: PB: Low; widely
  distributed in extracellular fluid;
  minute amounts in fetal circulation
Metabolism: t 1/2: 1–9 min; rapidly
  metabolized by liver
Excretion: In urine

Pharmacodynamics

IM: Onset: 3–5 min
    Peak: UK
    Duration: 2–3 h
IV: Onset: Immediate
    Peak: UK
    Duration: 1 h
Intranasal: Onset: Few minutes
            Peak: UK
            Duration: 20 min

Therapeutic Effects/Uses: To induce/augment labor contractions; to treat uterine atony; milk letdown (intranasal spray).

Mode of Action: Action of myofibrils to stimulate letdown of milk and promote uterine contractions.

Side Effects

Maternal effects with IV use only:
  Hypotension, hypertension,
  nausea, vomiting, constipation,
  decreased uterine blood flow, rash,
  anorexia

Adverse Reactions

Seizures, water intoxication
Life-threatening: Intracranial
  hemorrhage, cardiac dysrhythmias,
  asphyxia; fetus: jaundice, hypoxia

KEY: For complete abbreviation key, see inside front cover.

■ NURSING PROCESS: Oxytocins

ASSESSMENT

For induction or augmentation of labor:
- Collect accurate baseline data before beginning infusion, including maternal pulse and blood pressure, uterine activity, and fetal heart rate (FHR).
- Record assessment results on FHR monitor graph paper in addition to other agency records.

POTENTIAL NURSING DIAGNOSIS

Knowledge deficit

PLANNING

- Oxytocin will enhance uterine contractions without adverse effects.
- Client's VS will be within acceptable ranges during the therapy.

NURSING INTERVENTIONS

- Have magnesium sulfate and/or other tocolytic agents and oxygen readily available in case hypertonicity occurs.
- Monitor input and output every 2 h. Fluids should not exceed 1,000 mL/ 8 h.
- Monitor maternal pulse and blood pressure, uterine activity, and FHR before increasing oxytocin infusion.
- Maintain the client in the lateral recumbent position or sitting to promote placental infusion.
- Be alert for signs of uterine rupture (very infrequent), which include sudden increased pain, loss of contractions and decreased or absent FHR, hemorrhage, and rapidly developing hypovolemic shock.

CLIENT TEACHING

- Explain to the client that the drug is given intravenously to adjust dosage in response to contraction pattern.
- For milk letdown: Teach client timing and method of nasal administration.

EVALUATION

- Evaluate the effectiveness of the drug. Labor progresses.
- Continue monitoring VS. Report changes in VS or vaginal bleeding.

Oxytocic Drugs Used to Enhance Uterine Motility

Generic (Brand)	Route and Dosage	Preg Cat	Interaction	t 1/2	PB	Onset	Peak	Duration
							Action	
						Onset	Peak	Duration
Ergonovine maleate (Ergotrate)	PO: 0.2–0.4 mg q6–12 h over 48 h IM: 0.2 mg q2–4h; max: 5 doses IV: 0.2 mg (only for severe bleeding) over 1 min while blood pressure and contractions are monitored	X	*Increase* vasoconstriction with other vasopressors, smoking	UK	UK	PO: 5–15 min IM: 2–5 min IV: <5 min	60–90 min UK UK	3 h 3 h 45 min
Methylergonovine maleate (Methergine)	PO: 0.2–0.4 mg q6–12 h; max: 1 wk IM: 0.2 mg, after delivery of placenta, or postpartum; repeat q2–4h; oral doses may follow parenteral IV: Same as for IM; but slowly over 1 min with careful monitoring of blood pressure	C	Similar to ergonovine maleate	Initially: 1–5 min Terminal: 30–120 min	UK	PO: 5–15 min IM: 2–5 min IV: Immediate	0.5–3 h UK UK	3 h 3 h 0.5–3 h

Oxytocin (Pitocin, Syntocinon)				1–5 min	30%	IV: 1 min IM: 3–5 min	UK	IV: <30 min IM: 30–60 min
IV: 10 U diluted in 1,000 mL lactated Ringer's to 10 mU/mL; connect to control IV at needle site of main IV as a secondary line; start at 0.5 mU/min (3 mL/h) and titrate at rate of 0.5–2.5 mU q15–30 min until contractions are q2–3 min and adequate IV: 10 U added to 1 L electrolyte or dextrose solution (10 mU/mL); infuse at rate to control atony (IM: 10 U after delivery of placenta if no IV)	X	*Increase vasoconstriction with other pressor drugs* Hypotension with cyclopropane						

KEY: For complete abbreviation key, see inside front cover.

Estrogen Replacements

Conjugated Estrogens	Dosage
Conjugated estrogens (Premarin, PMB, Milprem-400) Hormone replacement therapy (HRT) *Pregnancy Category:* X *Drug Forms:* Tab 0.3, 0.65, 0.9, 1.25, 2.5 mg Cream 0.0623% Inj 25 mg Patch	A: PO: 0.3–1.25 mg/d cyclically (with or without progestins); most often, 0.625 mg/d

Contraindications	Drug-Lab-Food Interactions
Breast or reproductive cancer, undiagnosed genital bleeding, pregnancy, lactation, thromboembolitic disorders, smoking *Caution:* Cardiovascular disease, severe renal or hepatic disease, smoking, diabetes mellitus	*Increase* effects with corticosteroids *Decrease* effects of anticoagulants, oral hypoglycemics; *decrease* effects with rifampin, anticonvulsants, barbiturates Toxicity with tricyclic antidepressants

Pharmacokinetics	Pharmacodynamics
Absorption: PO: Well absorbed *Distribution:* PB: Widely distributed; crosses placenta and enters breast milk *Metabolism:* t 1/2: UK *Excretion:* In urine and bile	PO/IV: Onset: Rapid Peak: UK Duration: UK IM: Onset: Delayed Peak: UK Duration: UK

Therapeutic Effects/Uses: To relieve vasodilation, hot flashes, and vaginal dryness; to prevent cardiovascular disease and osteoporosis.

Mode of Action: Development and maintenance of female genital system, breasts, and secondary sex characteristics; increased synthesis of protein.

Side Effects	Adverse Reactions
Nausea, vomiting, fluid retention, breast tenderness, leg cramps and breakthrough bleeding, chloasma	Jaundice, thromboembolic disorders, depression, hypercalcemia, gall bladder disease *Life-threatening:* Thromboembolism, cerebrovascular accident, pulmonary embolism, MI, endometrial cancer

KEY: For complete abbreviation key, see inside front cover.

■ **NURSING PROCESS: Estrogen Replacements**

ASSESSMENT

• Assess the client for baseline data, including height, weight, usual physical activity, diet, family history, and personal risk factors regarding osteoporosis,

family and personal risk of cardiovascular disease, and the nature of the family members' climacteric experience, the client's menstrual history, and current experience with the climacteric and the drugs the client is using.
- Assess the client's perception of menopause.
- Assess the client's attitude toward resumption of menstrual periods.

POTENTIAL NURSING DIAGNOSES
Sexual dysfunction
Body image disturbance
Health-seeking behaviors

PLANNING
- Client will know menopausal symptoms and the nonpharmacologic and pharmacologic measures that may aid in alleviating symptoms.

NURSING INTERVENTIONS
- Educate women about the nature of the climacteric, its potential effects, and nonpharmacologic as well as pharmacologic treatment. Place current educational materials in health and community sites.
- Indicate on the laboratory slip or specimen that the client is taking hormone replacement therapy (HRT).
- Administer IM route at bedtime to decrease adverse effects.
- Administer IV route slowly to avoid flushing reaction.

CLIENT TEACHING
General
- Review the risk-to-benefit ratio for deciding to use or not to use estrogen replacement therapy.
- Review the contraindications to this HRT.
- Advise the client to have a thorough breast examination, pelvic examination, Pap test, and endometrial biopsy before starting HRT.
- Tell the client that warm weather and stress exacerbate vasodilation/hot flashes.
- Advise the client to use a fan, drink cool liquids, wear layered cotton clothes, decrease intake of caffeine and spicy foods, and talk with her health care provider about the use of vitamin E to cope more comfortably with vasodilation. Individuals with diabetes, hypertension, or rheumatic heart disease should use vitamin E in low doses with the health care provider's approval.
- Encourage the client on HRT to have medical follow-up every 6–12 mo, including blood pressure check and breast and pelvic examinations.
- Suggest that the client carry sanitary pads or tampons for breakthrough bleeding or irregular periods.
- Stress the need to use nonhormonal birth control since irregular periods may create anxiety about pregnancy. Tell the client to plan to use birth control for 2 y. If she has progesterone-induced bleeding, the only way to determine whether she is truly menopausal is by hormone assay.
- Suggest to the client that she use a water-soluble vaginal lubricant to reduce painful intercourse (dyspareunia) and prevent trauma.
- Advise the client to decrease use of antihistamines and decongestants if she is experiencing vaginal dryness.
- Advise the client to wear cotton underwear and pantyhose with a cotton liner and to avoid douche and feminine hygiene products.

Estrogen Replacements

- Suggest that client take Premarin after meals together with progestin to avoid nausea and vomiting.
- Tell the client to report any heavy bleeding (flooding) and to have her hematocrit and hemoglobin evaluated for anemia.
- Tell the client to report bleeding that occurs between periods or return of bleeding after cessation of menstruation. A cancer work-up may be indicated.
- Advise the client starting on HRT that the withdrawal bleeding that occurs from days 25–30 is normal and not the same as the cyclic menstrual periods she had secondary to ovulation. Tell her that this bleeding will usually last only 2–3 d and that she will not experience the same degree of premenstrual symptoms she may have had with regular periods.
- Advise the client to report if bleeding occurs other than on days 25–30 once she has started on HRT.
- Tell her that the withdrawal bleeding does not signify that she can become pregnant (since she is not fertile).
- Advise the client that after HRT is discontinued, there may be a recurrence of menopausal signs and symptoms such as hot flashes.

Diet

- Discuss the use of yogurt containing *Acidophilus* or *Lactobacillus* as a way of maintaining normal bacterial flora in the vagina.
- Tell the client that she may experience an occasional hot flash on days 25–30 when she is going through withdrawal bleeding. Instruct the client to stop treatment and contact health care provider if she has headache, visual disturbances, signs of thrombophlebitis, heaviness in legs, chest pain, or breast lumps.
- Tell the client that if she wants to stop HRT, she should do so with guidance of her health care provider.
- Suggest that the client at risk for osteoporosis have consistent exercise such as walking or bicycling, eat a well-balanced diet (low in red meat and sugar) with 1,200 mg calcium/d if premenopausal or 1,200–1,500 mg/d if menopausal, and avoid smoking and alcohol.

Skill

- Teach the client to perform breast self-examination consistently.
- If the client is using vaginal cream, review the application procedure and suggest that she wear minipads.
- If the client is using the transdermal patch, tell her to open the package and apply it immediately, holding it in place for about 10 s; to check the edges to ensure adequate contact; to use the abdomen (except waistline) for the patch; to rotate the sites with at least 1 wk before reuse of a site; to not use the breast as a site; to not put the patch on an irritated or oily area; to reapply the patch if it loosens or put on a new one; and to follow the same cycle schedule.

EVALUATION

- Evaluate the effectiveness of the nonpharmacologic or pharmacologic measures for premenopausal symptoms.
- Determine whether side effects are occurring. Plan with the client alternative measures to control menopausal symptoms.

Estrogen Replacements

Estrogens and Progestins

Generic (Brand)	Route and Dosage	Preg Cat
Steroidal Estrogens		
Estradiol (Estrace, Estraderm)	*Menopausal/hypogonadism:* PO: 1–2 mg/d for 21 d; then, 7–10 d off cycle; may repeat cycle *Patch:* 10–20 cm² system 2×/wk, in above cycle *Breast cancer:* 10 mg t.i.d. *Prostate cancer:* 1–2 mg t.i.d. *Atrophic vaginitis:* Cream: 2–4 g/d for 1–2 wk; maint: 1 g 2×/wk	X
Estradiol cypionate (Depo-Estradiol Cypionate)	*Menopausal symptoms:* IM: 1–4 mg q3–4wk *Hypogonadism:* IM: 1.5–2 mg q mo	X
Esterified estrogens (Estratab, Menest)	*Menopausal symptoms:* PO: 0.3–1.25 mg/d for 3 wk; then 7–10 d off cycle *Breast cancer:* PO: 10 mg t.i.d. *Prostate cancer:* 1.25–2.5 mg t.i.d.	X
Estrone (Theelin, Kestrone 5)	*Hypogonadism:* 0.1–2 mg/wk *Prostate cancer:* 2–4 mg 3×/wk	X
Estropipate SO₄ (Ogen, Ortho-Est)	*Hypogonadism:* 1.25–7.5 mg/d for 3 wk; then 7–10 d off cycle	X
Nonsteroidal Estrogens		
Chlorotrianisene (Tace)	*Menopausal/hypogonadism:* 12–25 mg/d for 21 d; then, 10 d off cycle; repeat cycle *Prostate cancer:* 12–25 mg/d	X
Dienestrol (DV)	*Atrophic vaginitis:* Cream: Apply q.d./b.i.d. for 1–2 wk; maint: 1–3×/wk	X
Diethylstilbestrol	*Breast cancer:* 15 mg/d *Prostate cancer:* 1–3 mg t.i.d.	X
Quinestrol (Estrovis)	*Menopausal/hypogonadism:* 100 μg daily for 7 d; then 7 d off cycle; maint: q wk	X
Progestins		
Progesterone	*DUB:* IM: 5–10 mg/d for 7 d *Amenorrhea:* IM: 5–10 mg/d for 6–8 d	X
Medroxyprogesterone acetate (Amen, Curretab, Provera, Cycrin, Depo-Provera)	*DUB/amenorrhea:* 5–10 mg/d for 5–10 d *Endometriosis:* IM: 150 mg q3mon	X

431

continued

Estrogen Replacements

Generic (Brand)	Route and Dosage	Preg Cat
Megestrol acetate (Megace)	*Breast cancer:* PO: 40 mg q.i.d. *Endometrial cancer:* 40–320 mg/d in divided doses	X
Norethindrone (Norlutin)	*DUB/amenorrhea:* 5–20 mg/d on days 5–25 of menstrual cycle	X

KEY: For complete abbreviation key, see inside front cover.

Oral Contraceptives

Product	Amount of Estrogen (μg)	Amount of Progestin (mg)
Combination Products: Listed by Decreasing Estrogen Content		
Monophasic Products		
Norinyl 1 + 50 (21 d)	50 mestranol	1 norethindrone
Genora 1/50	50 mestranol	1 norethindrone
Ovcon 50	50 ethinyl estradiol	1 norethindrone
Norlestrin 1/50	50 ethinyl estradiol	1 norethindrone acetate
Demulen 1/50	50 ethinyl estradiol	1 ethynodiol diacetate
Norlestrin 21 2.5/50	50 ethinyl estradiol	2.5 norethindrone acetate
Ovral	50 ethinyl estradiol	0.5 norgestrel
Genora 1/35	35 ethinyl estradiol	1 norethindrone
Norcept-E 1/35	35 ethinyl estradiol	1 norethindrone
Ortho-Novum 1/35	35 ethinyl estradiol	1 norethindrone
N.E.E. 1/35	35 ethinyl estradiol	1 norethindrone
Norethin 1/35 E	35 ethinyl estradiol	1 norethindrone
Norinyl 1 + 35	35 ethinyl estradiol	1 norethindrone
Modicon	35 ethinyl estradiol	0.5 norethindrone
Brevicon	35 ethinyl estradiol	0.5 norethindrone
Nelova	35 ethinyl estradiol	0.5 norethindrone
Ovcon 35	35 ethinyl estradiol	0.4 norethindrone
Demulen 1/35	35 ethinyl estradiol	1 ethynodiol diacetate
Desogen	30 ethinyl estradiol	0.15 desogestrel
Loestrin 21 1.5/30	30 ethinyl estradiol	1.5 norethindrone acetate
Lo/Ovral	30 ethinyl estradiol	0.3 norgestrel
Levlen	30 ethinyl estradiol	0.15 levonorgestrel
Nordette	30 ethinyl estradiol	0.15 levonorgestrel
Loestrin 21 1/20	20 ethinyl estradiol	1 norethindrone acetate
Biphasic Products		
Jenest-28	*Phase I:* 7 d 35 ethinyl estradiol	0.5 norethindrone
	Phase II: 14 d 35 ethinyl estradiol	1.0 norethindrone
N.E.E. 10/11	*Phase I:* 10 d 35 ethinyl estradiol	0.5 norethindrone
	Phase II: 11 d 35 ethinyl estradiol	1.0 norethindrone

Estrogen Replacements

Product	Amount of Estrogen (μg)	Amount of Progestin (mg)
Nelova 10/11	*Phase I:*	
	10 d	
	35 ethinyl estradiol	0.5 norethindrone
	Phase II:	
	11 d	
	35 ethinyl estradiol	1 norethindrone
Ortho-Novum 10/11	Same formulation as above but different colors for tablets	
Triphasic Products		
Tri-Norinyl	*Phase I:*	
	7 d	
	35 ethinyl estradiol	0.5 norethindrone
	Phase II:	
	9 d	
	35 ethinyl estradiol	1 norethindrone
	Phase III:	
	5 d	
	35 ethinyl estradiol	0.5 norethindrone
Ortho Tri-Cyclen	*Phase I:*	
	7 d	
	35 ethinyl estradiol	0.18 norgestimate
	Phase II:	
	7 d	
	35 ethinyl estradiol	0.215 norgestimate
	Phase III:	
	7 d	
	35 ethinyl estradiol	0.25 norgestimate
Ortho-Novum 7/7/7	*Phase I:*	
	7 d	
	35 ethinyl estradiol	0.5 norethindrone
	Phase II:	
	7 d	
	35 ethinyl estradiol	0.75 norethindrone
	Phase III:	
	7 d	
	35 ethinyl estradiol	1 norethindrone
Tri-Levlen	*Phase I:*	
	6 d	
	30 ethinyl estradiol	0.05 levonorgestrel
	Phase II:	
	5 d	
	40 ethinyl estradiol	0.075 levonorgestrel
	Phase III:	
	10 d	
	30 ethinyl estradiol	0.125 levonorgestrel
Triphasil	Same as above	

Progestin-Only Products: Listed by Decreasing Progestin Content

Micronor		0.35 norethindrone
Nor-QD		0.35 norethindrone
Ovrette		0.075 norgestrel

Androgens

Testosterone

Testosterone
  (Andro 100, Andro-Cyp 100,
  depAndro 100, Depotest 100,
  Duratest 100, DEPO-Testosterone,
  Testred Cypionate 200, Virilon,
  depAndrogyn, Everone)
Pregnancy Category: X
Drug Forms:
Inj IM 25, 50, 100 mg/mL
Tab
CSS III

Dosage

Androgen Replacement:
PO: 10–40 mg daily
Buccal: 5–20 mg daily
SC: 150–450 mg q3–6mo
IM: 10–30 mg 2–3×/wk
Metastatic Carcinoma of the Breast:
PO: 200 mg daily
Buccal: 200 mg daily
IM: 100 mg 3×/wk

Contraindications

Pregnancy, nephrosis, hypercalcemia,
  pituitary insufficiency, hepatic
  dysfunction, benign prostatic
  hypertrophy, prostatic cancer,
  history of MI, prepubertal status,
  non–estrogen-dependent breast
  cancer
Caution: Hypertension,
  hypercholesteremia, coronary
  artery disease, gynecomastia, renal
  disease, seizure disorders, before
  puberty, older adults

Drug-Lab-Food Interactions

Increases effects of anticoagulants
Decreases effect with barbiturates,
  phenytoin, phenylbutazone
Antagonizes calcitonin, parathyroid
Corticosteroids exacerbate edema
Lab: Decreases blood glucose in
  diabetics; *increase* serum
  cholesterol, thyroid, liver function,
  hematocrit

Pharmacokinetics

Absorption: IM: Well absorbed
Distribution: PB: 98%
Metabolism: t 1/2: 10–100 min
Excretion: In urine and bile

Pharmacodynamics

IM: Onset: UK
  Peak: UK
  Duration: cypionate enanthate:
  2–4 wk
    base, propionate: 1–3 d

Therapeutic Effects/Uses: To achieve normal androgen levels; to slow progress of estrogen-dependent breast cancers.

Mode of Action: Development and maintenance of male sex organs and secondary sex characteristics.

Side Effects

Abdominal pain, nausea, diarrhea,
  constipation, hives, irritation at
  injection site, increased salivation,
  mouth soreness, increased or
  decreased libido, insomnia,
  aggressive behavior, weakness,
  dizziness, pruritus

Adverse Reactions

Acne, masculinization, irregular
  menses, urinary urgency,
  gynecomastia, priapism, red skin,
  jaundice, sodium and water
  retention, allergic reaction,
  depression
Life-threatening: Hepatic necrosis,
  hepatitis, hepatic tumors,
  respiratory distress

KEY: For complete abbreviation key, see inside front cover.

■ NURSING PROCESS: Androgens: Testosterone

ASSESSMENT

- Assess the reason for androgen therapy and the client's perception of it. If delayed puberty is the indication, assess the client's and family's attitudes about the condition.
- Assess the client's weight, blood pressure, liver and thyroid function, hemoglobin, hematocrit, creatinine, clotting factors, glucose tolerance, serum lipids and electrolytes, and blood count before and throughout drug therapy.
- Assess the pregnancy status of fertile women. Concomitant anticoagulation therapy is recommended. When a prepubertal child is treated, assess x-rays before treatment and every 6 mo during and after treatment to monitor growth.
- Assess the client's affect during therapy, particularly aggressiveness in clients taking large doses. Self-concept is an important consideration with the client on androgen therapy, particularly in women and in children in whom puberty is delayed.

POTENTIAL NURSING DIAGNOSES

Sexual dysfunction
High risk for body image disturbance
High risk for situational low self-esteem

PLANNING

- Client adheres to prescribed drug regimen and monitoring.
- Medication is effective for intended purpose, and preventable side effects are avoided.
- Client maintains positive self-concept.

NURSING INTERVENTIONS

- Use lowest effective dose.
- Shake vial and warm to room temperature to dissolve crystals, as needed.
- Administer the IM form in a large muscle mass, such as the upper outer quadrant of the gluteus.
- Record body weight several times each week.
- Monitor muscle strength.
- Monitor bone maturation every 6 mo with x-rays of wrists and hands.

CLIENT TEACHING

General

- Instruct the client and family on the proper administration of the medication and potential undesired effects.
- Inform the client of effects that warrant prompt medical attention, such as urinary problems, priapism, and respiratory distress.
- Advise the client who is having an intermittent approach to treatment of the need for monitoring the endocrine status between courses of androgen therapy.
- Instruct the client to record body weight several times each week. Sodium may need to be restricted if edema develops.
- Advise the client with tissue wasting to reduce environmental stressors and promote rest and relaxation, since stress hormones are catabolic.

Androgens

- Instruct the client to take oral androgens with food to decrease gastric distress.
- Advise the family of normal development if the client is receiving treatment for delayed puberty.
- Instruct both prepubertal and adult female clients on good skin hygiene to control the severity of the acne.
- Instruct men to report priapism promptly; the drug dose needs to be reduced.

Diet

- Encourage adequate nutritional support with adequate intake of calories, proteins, vitamins, iron, and other minerals.

Side Effects

- Instruct the client with elevated serum calcium of the need for 3–4 L of fluid per day to prevent kidney stones. Individuals on bedrest need range-of-motion exercises, and ambulatory clients need to engage in active weight bearing. Hypercalcemia needs prompt medical attention because it can lead to cardiac arrest.

EVALUATION

- Evaluate the client's ability to adhere to treatment regimen.
- Identify therapeutic and side effects of drug.
- Determine the client's ability to cope with virilizing effects or acne and to maintain a positive self-concept.

Generic (Brand)	Route and Dosage	Preg Cat	Interaction	t 1/2	PB	Onset	Peak	Duration
							Action	
Natural Androgens Testosterone (Andro 100) CSS III	*Replacement:* IM: 10–30 mg 2–3×wk PO: 10–40 mg daily Buccal: 5–20 mg daily SC: 150–450 mg q3–6 mo *Carcinoma of breast:* IM: 100 mg 3×wk PO: 200 mg daily Buccal: 100 mg daily See Prototype Drug Chart	X						
Testosterone cypionate (Andro-Cyp, depAndro, Depotest, DEPO-Testosterone, Duratest) CSS III	IM: 50–400 mg q2–6wk	X	*Increase* effects of oral hypoglycemics, insulin, glucocorticoids, anticoagulants *Lab:* May affect thyroid function tests	8 d	98%	UK	UK	2–4 wk
Testosterone enanthate (Andro L.A., Delatestryl, Everone) CSS III	IM: 50–400 mg q2–6wk	X	Similar to testosterone cypionate	UK	99%	UK	UK	2–4 wk
Testosterone propionate CSS III	*Replacement:* IM: 10–25 mg 2–4×wk *Carcinoma of breast:* IM: 100 mg 3×wk	X	Similar to testosterone cypionate	UK	99%	UK	UK	1–4 d
Synthetic Androgens Danazol (Danocrine)	PO: 100–800 mg daily divided in 2 doses initially	X	May need increase in insulin dose *Lab:* Altered liver function tests	4.5 h	UK	3–4 wk	3–4 wk	2–6 mo

continued

437

Generic (Brand)	Route and Dosage	Preg Cat	Interaction	t 1/2	PB	Onset	Peak	Duration
							Action	
Fluoxymesterone (Halotestin) CSS III	*Replacement:* PO: 2–10 mg daily divided into 1–4 doses *Carcinoma of breast:* PO: 15–30 mg daily in divided doses	X	*Increase* effects of anticoagulants, oral antidiabetics *Lab:* Alters GTT, cholesterol, T_3, T_4, serum potassium, and calcium	20–100 min	98%	UK	UK	UK
Methyltestosterone (Android, Metandren, Oreton-Methyl, Testred Cypionate, Virilon) CSS III	PO: Initially: 10–50 mg daily in divided doses; maint: reduced Buccal: Initially: 5–25 mg daily in divided doses; maint: reduced *Carcinoma of breast:* PO: 50–200 mg daily Buccal: 25–100 mg daily	X	*Decrease* effect of insulin, oral anticoagulants	UK	UK	UK	PO: 2 h Buccal: 1 h	UK
Nandrolone decanoate (Deca-Durabolin) CSS III	*Carcinoma of breast and osteoporosis:* IM: 50–200 mg q1–4wk C: IM: 25–50 mg q3–4wk	X	*Increase* effects of oral hypoglycemics, insulin, oral anticoagulants	UK	UK	UK	3–6 d	UK
Nandrolone phenpropionate (Durabolin) CSS III	*Carcinoma of breast and osteoporosis:* IM: 25–100 mg/wk C: IM: 12.5–25 mg q2–4wk	X	*Similar to* nandrolone decanoate	UK	UK	UK	1–3 d	UK
Oxandrolone (Anavar) (Oxandrin, Oxandrolone) CSS III	*Osteoporosis:* PO: 5–20 mg daily in divided doses C: PO: 0.25 mg/kg/d	X	Use with anticoagulants may *increase* PT *Decrease* need for insulin *Lab:* May alter urine, blood glucose	Phase I: 1 h Phase II: 9 h	UK	UK	UK	UK

Generic (Brand)	Route and Dosage	Preg Cat	Interaction	t 1/2	PB	Onset	Action Peak	Duration
							Action	
						Onset	Peak	Duration
Oxymetholone (Anadrol-50) CSS III	*Osteoporosis:* PO: 5–50 mg daily for 7–21 d *Erythropoiesis:* PO: 1–4 mg/kg/d; max: 100 mg	X	Similar to oxandrolone	9 h	UK	UK	UK	UK
Stanozolol (Winstrol) CSS III	*Aplastic anemia:* A: PO: 2 mg t.i.d. C: 6–12 y: PO: 2 mg t.i.d. C <6 y: PO: 2–3 mg daily	X	Similar to oxandrolone	UK	UK	UK	UK	UK
Testolactone (Teslac)	*Carcinoma of breast:* PO: 250 mg q.i.d.	C	*Increase effects of oral anticoagulants*	UK	UK	UK	UK	UK

KEY: For complete abbreviation key, see inside front cover.

Ovulation Stimulants

Clomiphene Citrate

Clomiphene Citrate
  (Clomid, Milophene, Serophene)
Ovulation stimulant
Pregnancy Category: X
Drug Forms:
Tab 50 mg

Dosage

A: PO: 50–250 mg/d for days 5–9 of
  cycle
If ovulation does not occur with
  50 mg/d, increase next course to
  100 mg/d.

Contraindications

Pregnancy, undiagnosed vaginal
  bleeding, depression, fibroids,
  hepatic dysfunction,
  thrombophlebitis, primary
  pituitary or ovarian failure

Drug-Lab-Food Interactions

None are significant; Danazol may
  inhibit response; *decrease* effects of
  ethinyl estradiol
Lab: Increase in serum thyroxine

Pharmacokinetics

Absorption: Readily absorbed from GI
  tract
Distribution: PB: UK
Metabolism: t 1/2: 5–8 d
Excretion: In feces

Pharmacodynamics

PO: Onset: 5–14 d
  Peak: UK
  Duration: UK

Therapeutic Effects/Uses: To stimulate ovarian follicle growth.

Mode of Action: Stimulates release of follicle-stimulating hormone (FSH) and lu-
teinizing hormone (LH).

Side Effects

Breast discomfort, fatigue, dizziness,
  depression, anxiety, nausea,
  vomiting, constipation, increased
  appetite, headache, hot flashes,
  fluid retention

Adverse Reactions

Visual disturbances, abdominal pain,
  weight gain, hair loss, major
  congenital anomalies, ovarian
  hyperstimulation, flatulence,
  multiple gestation, anxiety, ovarian
  cysts

KEY: For complete abbreviation key, see inside front cover.

■ NURSING PROCESS: Ovulation Stimulants: Clomiphene Citrate

ASSESSMENT
- Obtain general health history and physical examination of clients. Clients' reproductive and sexual histories are assessed, with attention to the timing and techniques of coitus.
- Perform pelvic exam for baseline data, including ovarian size.
- Assess liver function studies before start of drug therapy.
- Use an extensive series of diagnostic tests to assess the cause of infertility.
- Assess the couple's interpretation of their infertility and its impact on their relationship. Placing blame on each other or their families can be devastating.

POTENTIAL NURSING DIAGNOSES
Altered sexuality patterns
Body image disturbance
Situational low self-esteem

PLANNING
- Short term: Clients will adhere to drug therapy regimen with minimal adverse effects. Long term: Achievement of pregnancy or considerations of alternatives to pregnancy with the couple's self-esteem and relationship remaining intact.

NURSING INTERVENTIONS
- Interventions are aimed at helping clients to understand the interrelationships among and timing of menses, ovulation, and coitus as they relate to conception.

CLIENT TEACHING
General
- Advise the woman to take medication at the same time each day to maintain steady serum levels.
- Advise the woman to avoid driving motor vehicles and operating dangerous equipment until stabilized on medication.
- Notify health care provider immediately of suspected pregnancy.
- Alert clients that drug therapy increases the chance of multiple births.

Skill
- Instruct the clients how to evaluate and record basal body temperature and cervical mucus changes on a chart. The first day of menses is day 1 of the cycle. Ovulation is predicted by a 0.5°F drop in basal body temperature followed by a 1°F rise. In addition, OTC diagnostic kits for assessing ovulatory status can be used to time coitus. Coitus is recommended no more frequently than every other day from 4 d before to 3 d after ovulation to maximize the man's sperm count.

EVALUATION
- Client tolerates drug regimen.
- Client achieves pregnancy.

Generic (Brand)	Route and Dosage	Preg Cat	Interaction	t 1/2	PB	Onset	Peak	Duration
							Action	
Clomiphene citrate (Clomid)	See Prototype Drug Chart							
Human chorionic gonadotropin (hCG) (A.P.L., Chorex, Glukor, Follutein, Gonic, Preznyl, Profasi HP)	IM: 5,000–10,000 U/d in presence of mature follicle (after last dose of menotropins)	C	None significant reported	23 h	UK	2 h	6 h	UK
Human menopausal gonadotropin (menotropins, Pergonal)	FSH and LH: 75 IU each IM daily for 9–12 d, followed by hCG next day	X	None significant reported	UK	UK	UK	18 h	UK
Urofollitropin (Metrodin)	IM: 75 IU/d 7–12 d followed by 5,000–10,000 IU hCG next day. May repeat course twice	X	None significant reported	4 and 70 h	UK	UK	UK	UK

KEY: For complete abbreviation key, see inside front cover.

AGENTS FOR EMERGENCY TREATMENT

Cardiac States

Neurosurgical States

Poisoning

Shock

Hypertensive Crisis

Emergency Treatment of Cardiac States: Antidysrhythmic

Lidocaine HCl

Lidocaine HCl
  (Xylocaine)
Antiarrhythmic, class IC
Pregnancy Category: C
Drug Forms:
IV: 20 mg/mL in 5-mL syringe
  (100 mg)

Dosage

A: IV: ETT*: 1–1.5 mg/kg; may
  repeat 0.5 mg/kg q3–10 min up to
  3 mg/kg (max)
Drip: 1–4 mg/min
C : IV: ETT* or IO: Initially: 1 mg/kg;
  maint: 30–50 μg/kg/min is
  recommended after bolus
*Note: For *endotracheal* drug
  administration, dose should be 2 to
  2.5 times IV dose in adults and up
  to 10 times the IV dose for
  pediatric arrest.
Therapeutic Range: 1.5–5 μg/mL

Contraindications

Hypersensitivity, advanced
  atrioventricular block
Caution: Liver disease, congestive
  heart failure, elderly

Drug-Lab-Food Interactions

Increase effects with phenytoin,
  quinidine, procainamide,
  propranolol; *increase* risk of toxicity
  with cimetidine, beta-adrenergic
  blockers

Pharmacokinetics

Absorption:
Distribution: PB: 60–80%;
  concentrates in adipose tissue
Metabolism: t 1/2: Initial: 7–30 min;
  terminal: 9–120 min
Excretion: Through the liver

Pharmacodynamics

PO: Onset: 45–60 s
     Peak: 45–60 s
     Duration: 10–20 min

Therapeutic Effects/Uses: Primary drug to treat ventricular dysrhythmias such as premature ventricular contractions (PVCs), ventricular tachycardia, and ventricular fibrillation.

Mode of Action: Decreases automaticity; increases electrical threshold of ventricle.

Side Effects

Drowsiness, confusion, dyspnea,
  lethargy, hypotension, nausea,
  vomiting

Adverse Reactions

Life-threatening: Seizures, cardiac
  arrest

KEY: For complete abbreviation key, see inside front cover.

■ NURSING PROCESS: Emergency Treatment of Cardiac States: Lidocaine

ASSESSMENT
- Assess health history. In clients with hepatic impairment, CHF, shock, or advanced age, client's lidocaine dose may need to be reduced by as much as 50%.
- Assess for chest pain.
- Assess mental status: baseline and ongoing.
- Assess ECG findings.
- Assess VS.

POTENTIAL NURSING DIAGNOSIS
Decreased cardiac output

PLANNING
- Client will be free of ventricular dysrhythmias.

NURSING INTERVENTIONS
- Continuous cardiac monitoring.
- Assess pulse for strength, rate, and rhythm.
- Assess for signs and symptoms of lidocaine toxicity (confusion, drowsiness, hearing impairment, muscle twitching, and seizures). If overdose occurs, stop infusion and monitor client closely; notify primary health care provider.
- Monitor serum lidocaine levels throughout therapy; desired range is 1.5–5 μg/mL.
- Monitor intake and output.
- Do not mix in same syringe with amphotericin B or cefazolin.
- Have dopamine readily available in the event of circulatory depression.

CLIENT TEACHING
General
- Advise the client and family of drug action.

Side Effects
- Instruct the client to be accompanied when ambulating due to drowsiness and dizziness.
- Instruct the client and family in use of automatic lidocaine injection device, if prescribed.

EVALUATION
- Determine the effectiveness of drug.
- Evaluate decrease in or absence of ventricular dysrhythmias.

Agents for Emergency Treatment of Cardiac States

Generic (Brand)	Route and Dosage	Preg Cat	Interaction	t 1/2	PB	Onset	Peak	Duration
							Action	
						Onset	Peak	Duration
Adenosine (Adenocard)	IV: Initially: 6 mg; then 12 mg in 1–2 min if needed; may repeat 12 mg ×1	C	*Increase* effects with dipyridamole; may increase heart block with carbamazepine *Decrease* effects with theophylline, caffeine	<10 s	UK	3–5 s	UK	1–2 min
Atropine sulfate	IV: ETT: 0.5–1 mg; can repeat up to 0.03–0.04 mg/kg (max)	C	*Increase* cholinergic effects with tricyclic antidepressants, antihistamines	2–3 h	60–80%	Immediate	2–4 min	3–6 h
Bretylium tosylate (Bretylol)	IV: Initially: 5 mg/kg; then 10 mg/kg q10–30 min up to 30 mg/kg total (max) over 24 h	C	May *increase* hypotensive effects of beta blockers, other antihypertensives	4–18 h	1–6%	5 min	End of infusion	6–24 h
Epinephrine	IV: ETT: 0.5–1 mg; may be repeated q5min	C	Alkaline solutions inactivate catecholamines; do *not* push through an IV line containing sodium bicarbonate	UK	UK	Rapid	20 min	15–30 min
Lidocaine	See Prototype Drug Chart							
Morphine sulfate	IV: 2–5 mg q5–30 min	C	*Increase* CNS depression with alcohol, phenothiazines, antihistamines	2–2.5 h	35%	1–3 min	20 min	6–7 h

Drug	Dosage		Interactions					
Nitroglycerin (Nitrostat, Tridil)	SL: 0.3–0.4 mg IV: Drip: 10–20 μg/min, increased 5–10 μg/min q5–10 min (titrated)	C	*Increase* effects with alcohol, beta blockers, calcium blockers, antihypertensives *Decrease* effects with heparin	1–4 min	60%	SL: 1–3 min IV: 1–3 min	4 min UK	20–30 min 0.5–2 h
Procainamide HCl (Pronestyl)	IV: 20–30 mg/min; max: 17 mg/kg *Recognize end points:* • Hypotension • QRS widens > 50% • Total dose of 17 mg/kg given Drip: 1–4 mg/min	C	*Increase* effects with histamine₂ blockers; *increase* hypotensive effects with antihypertensives, nitrates *Decrease* effects with barbiturates	3–4 h	20%	1–2 min	30–60 min	3–4 h
Sodium bicarbonate	IV: Initially: 1 mEq/kg; then 0.5 mEq/kg if needed	C	Alkaline solutions inactivate catecholamines; do *not* push through same line	UK	UK	15 min	UK	1–2 h
Verapamil HCl (Isoptin, Calan)	IV: Age- and weight-dependent dosages; should not exceed 10 mg; repeat doses may be needed	C	*Increase* effects with cimetidine; *increase* effects of theophylline, beta blockers, antihypertensives *Decrease* effects of lithium	3–8 h	90%	1–5 min	2–5 min	2 h

KEY: For complete abbreviation key, see inside front cover.

447

Emergency Treatment of Neurosurgical States: Diuretic

Mannitol	Dosage

Mannitol
  (Osmitrol)
Osmotic diuretic
Pregnancy Category: C
Drug Forms:
Inj IV 5%, 10%, 15%, 20%, 25%
	A: IV: Initially: 0.5–1.0 g/kg of
	  15–25% sol as a bolus
	Highly individualized

Contraindications	Drug-Lab-Food Interactions

Hypersensitivity, severe dehydration
Caution: Pregnancy, breast-feeding,
  current intracranial bleeding
	May *decrease* effectiveness with
	  lithium

Pharmacokinetics	Pharmacodynamics

Absorption: IV
Distribution: PB: Confined to
  extracellular space
Metabolism: t 1/2: 100 min
Excretion: In urine
	Decrease in Intracranial Pressure:
	IV: Onset: 30–60 min
	         Peak: 1 h
	         Duration: 6–8 h
	
	Diuresis: Onset: 1–3 h
	         Peak: 1 h
	         Duration: 6–8 h

Therapeutic Effects/Uses: To treat increased intracranial pressure, cerebral edema.

Mode of Action: Inhibition of reabsorption of electrolytes and water by affecting pressure of glomerular filtrate.

Side Effects	Adverse Reactions

Temporary volume expansion,
  hypo/hypernatremia,
  hypo/hyperkalemia, dehydration,
  blurred vision, dry mouth
	Pulmonary congestion,
	  fluid/electrolyte imbalances
	Life-threatening: Convulsions

KEY: For complete abbreviation key, see inside front cover.

■ NURSING PROCESS: Emergency Treatment of Neurosurgical States: Mannitol

ASSESSMENT

- Assess VS, including intracranial pressure, level of consciousness, and neurologic function.
- Assess fluid and electrolyte balances.

POTENTIAL NURSING DIAGNOSES

Fluid volume excess
Fluid volume deficit

PLANNING

- Client's intracranial pressure will be reduced to the desired range.

NURSING INTERVENTIONS

- Monitor VS, output, and pulmonary artery (PA) pressures (if PA catheter is present) frequently during administration.
- Assess the client for signs and symptoms of dehydration or fluid overload.
- Maintain accurate intake and output records to assess fluid volume status because diuresis may be substantial.
- Monitor for signs and symptoms of electrolyte imbalance; notify health care provider of imbalances.
- Careful monitoring of IV line site; extravasation may cause tissue necrosis.
- Use a filter needle when administering drug as crystals may form in solution and be inadvertently injected. Do not administer solution if crystals remain undissolved after shaking bottle. Try warming bottle in warm water to dissolve crystals; cool to room temperature before administering drug.
- Monitor laboratory studies, especially serum osmolality. Administration of mannitol to clients with serum osmolality >310–320 mOsm/kg is contraindicated.
- Do not mix in solution or syringe with any other drug.
- Client should be reevaluated if urine is not >30–50 mL/h for 2–3 h after two doses.

CLIENT TEACHING

- Explain expected drug action to the client and family.

EVALUATION

- Evaluate the effectiveness of drug.
- Client will have reduction in intracranial pressure; level is within desired range.
- Client's urine output is >30–50 mL/h or established goal.
- Client's serum osmolality will be in the desired range (usually 290–310 mOsm/kg).

Agents for Emergency Treatment of Neurosurgical States

Generic (Brand)	Route and Dosage	Preg Cat	Interaction	t1/2	PB	Onset	Peak	Duration
							Action	
						Onset	*Peak*	*Duration*
Mannitol	See Prototype Drug Chart							
Methylprednisolone sodium succinate (Solu-Medrol)	*Acute spinal cord injury:* IV: Loading dose: 30 mg/kg in 10 mL NSS then 5.4 mg/kg/h ×23h	C	*Decrease* effects of oral hypoglycemics, anticoagulants, phenobarbital, immunizations; *decrease* effects of drug with rifampin, barbiturates, ephedrine, theophylline	2–4 h	80–90%	IV: Rapid	UK	UK

KEY: For complete abbreviation key, see inside front cover.

NOTES:

_____

_____

_____

_____

_____

_____

_____

_____

_____

_____

Emergency Treatment of Poisoning

Naloxone HCl	Dosage
Naloxone HCl (Narcan) Narcotic antagonist *Pregnancy Category:* B *Drug Forms:* Inj 0.4, 1 mg/mL	IV/IM/SC: 0.4–2 mg; repeat every 2–3 min, as indicated

Contraindications	Drug-Lab-Food Interactions
Hypersensitivity, respiratory depression *Caution:* Opiate-dependent clients, cardiac disease, breast-feeding, neonates	Verapamil can precipitate withdrawal in a client dependent on narcotic analgesics *Lab*: Urine VMA, 5-HIAA, urine glucose

Pharmacokinetics	Pharmacodynamics

Absorption: IM/SC: Well absorbed
Distribution: PB: UK
Metabolism: t 1/2: Adults: 1–2 h;
neonates: 1–3 h
Excretion: In urine as metabolites
	SC/IM: Onset: 2–5 min
	        Peak: UK
	        Duration: 1–4 h
	IV: Onset: 1–2 min
	        Peak: UK
	        Duration: 1–4 h

Therapeutic Effects/Uses: To treat respiratory depression caused by narcotics; to treat narcotic-induced depressant effects and narcotic overdose.

Mode of Action: Blocks effects of narcotics by competing for the receptor sites.

Side Effects	Adverse Reactions
Negligible pharmacologic effect without narcotics in body	Nausea, vomiting, tremulousness, sweating, tachycardia, elevated blood pressure *Life-threatening:* Atrioventricular fibrillation, pulmonary edema (with overdose of morphine)

KEY: For complete abbreviation key, see inside front cover.

Emergency Treatment of Poisoning

■ NURSING PROCESS: Emergency Treatment of Poisoning: Naloxone

ASSESSMENT
- Assess VS and level of consciousness.
- Assess level of pain before administering drug to a client experiencing respiratory depression.
- Assess for signs and symptoms of withdrawal.
- Assess for improvement of symptoms; if improvement is not evident, symptoms are due to cause other than narcotic.

POTENTIAL NURSING DIAGNOSES
Ineffective breathing pattern
Altered comfort
Coping, ineffective individual

PLANNING
- Client will have respiratory depression reversed and have respiratory rate within the desired range.

NURSING INTERVENTIONS
- Have resuscitation equipment readily available to augment drug therapy if needed.
- Do *not* mix in the same syringe with heparin or benzquanamide.
- Monitor client closely for signs and symptoms of recurrent opiate effects, such as respiratory depression and hypotension. Effects of opiate may outlast effects of naloxone; a continuous naloxone infusion may be necessary.

CLIENT TEACHING
General
- Advise the client and family of drug action.

EVALUATION
- Determine the effectiveness of drug.
- Client's respiratory rate and VS (specifically, blood pressure) are within the desired range.

Agents for Emergency Treatment of Poisoning

Generic (Brand)	Route and Dosage	Preg Cat	Interaction	t 1/2	PB	Action Onset	Action Peak	Action Duration
Activated charcoal	PO: 30 g (minimum dose)	C	*Decreases* absorption of laxatives, ipecac	NA	NA	<1 min	UK	4–12 h
Digoxin immune Fab (Digibind)	Highly individualized	C	*Decreases* or eliminates cardiac glycosides	12–20 h	UK	<30 min; variable	UK	2–6 h
Ipecac syrup	See Prototype Drug Chart for emetics							
Naloxone (Narcan)	See Prototype Drug Chart							

KEY: For complete abbreviation key, see inside front cover.

NOTES:

Emergency Treatment of Shock

Dopamine HCl

Dopamine HCl
  (Intropin)
Adrenergic
Pregnancy Category: C
Drug Forms:
Inj 0.8, 1.6 mg/mL

Dosage

A: IV: Drip: 1–20 μg/kg/min (>10 μg/kg/min may be ordered if lower doses are ineffective)

Contraindications

Hypersensitivity, tachydysrhythmias, ventricular fibrillation, pheochromocytomas
Caution: Safety in children is not known

Drug-Lab-Food Interactions

Use within 2 wk of MAOIs may result in hypertensive crisis; concurrent IV administration of phenytoin may result in hypotension and bradycardia; sodium bicarbonate solutions inactivate dopamine—do *not* administer through the same IV line

Pharmacokinetics

Absorption: IV
Distribution: PB: UK
Metabolism: t 1/2: 2 min
Excretion: In urine

Pharmacodynamics

IV: Onset: 1–2 min
      Peak: <5 min
      Duration: <10 min

Therapeutic Effects/Uses: To treat hypotension in shock states not due to hypovolemia; to increase heart rate in atropine-refractory bradycardia. To increase urine output at a "renal dose" (<5 μg/kg/min).

Mode of Action: Stimulation of receptors to cause cardiac stimulation and renal vasodilation. Increase systemic vascular resistance at higher dose ranges.

Side Effects

Palpitations, tachycardia, hypertension, ectopic beats, angina, IV line site irritation, piloerection, nausea, vomiting

Adverse Reactions

Cardiac dysrhythmias, azotemia, tissue sloughing (from extravasation)
Life-threatening: MI, gangrene in extremities (from vasoconstriction)

KEY: For complete abbreviation key, see inside front cover.

■ NURSING PROCESS: Emergency Treatment of Shock: Dopamine

ASSESSMENT
- Assess VS frequently.
- Assess ECG readings; monitor intake and output.

POTENTIAL NURSING DIAGNOSES
Shock
Altered tissue perfusion
Decreased cardiac output

PLANNING
- Client will have increase in blood pressure and/or hemodynamic parameters that are within the desired range.

NURSING INTERVENTIONS
- Monitor IV line site every 30–60 min for signs of infiltration. Extravasasation can necessitate surgical debridement and skin grafting. If infiltration does occur, inject affected areas with phentolamine (Regitine) 5–10 mg SC diluted in 10–15 mL NSS to reduce or prevent tissue damage. Multiple injections may be necessary.
- Administer IV through a large vein; the central vein is preferable.
- Use an electronic infusion pump to ensure accurate IV rate.
- Monitor central venous pressure (CVP) or pulmonary artery catheter pressure readings to evaluate cardiovascular system response.
- Be alert that the solution appears slightly yellow. Any other color is indicative of decomposition; the solution should be discarded.
- Do not interrupt infusion; profound hypotension may result. Dopamine dose must be titrated downward slowly to avoid hypotensive response.

CLIENT TEACHING
General
- Advise the client and family of drug action.
- Alert the client to immediately report pain at the IV line site.

EVALUATION
- Determine the effectiveness of drug therapy and the presence of any side effects. The client should have blood pressure and/or other hemodynamic parameters (heart rate, cardiac output, urine output, systemic vascular resistance, and so on) within the desired range.

Agents for Emergency Treatment of Shock

Generic (Brand)	Route and Dosage	Preg Cat	Interaction	t 1/2	PB	Onset	Peak	Duration
							Action	
						Onset	Peak	Duration
Dextrose 50%	IV: 50 mL	C	Alters insulin and oral antidiabetic requirements of diabetics	UK	UK	Rapid	Rapid	Brief
Diphenhydramine (Benadryl)	IM/IV: 10–50 mg	C	*Increase* anticholinergic effects with tricyclic antidepressants, MAOIs, quinidine; *increase* CNS depression with sedative-hypnotics, alcohol, analgesics, antihistamines	3–8 h	98–99%	IV: Rapid IM: 20–30 min	UK 1–4 h	4–7 h 4–8 h
Dobutamine (Dobutrex)	IV: Drip: 2.5–10 μg/kg/min	C	*Increase* dysrhythmias with general anesthetics, MAOIs, tricyclic antidepressants; effects are antagonized by beta blockers	2 min	UK	IV: Within 2 min	10–20 min	Shortly after infusion terminated

Drug	Route and Dosage	Pregnancy Category	Drug-Lab-Food Interactions			Onset	Peak	Duration
Dopamine HCl (Intropin)	See Prototype Drug Chart							
Epinephrine	SC/IM: 0.1–0.5 mg (1:1,000 sol) IV: 0.1–0.25 mg (1:10,000 sol) Intratracheal: 0.1 mg/kg (q3–5 min)	C	*Increase* effects with other adrenergics; hypertensive crises with MAOIs; *increase* dysrhythmias with cardiac glycosides, general anesthetics	UK	UK	Intratracheal: <1 min SC: 3–5 min IV: Rapid	20 min 20 min	1–3 h 20–30 min
Glucagon	SC/IM/IV: 0.5–1 mg; may repeat ×1	B	Negates effects of insulin and oral antidiabetics; may *increase* effects of oral anticoagulants (large doses)	3–10 min	UK	Hyperglycemic: 5–20 min GI musculature: 1 min	30 min UK	1–2 h 9–25 min
Norepinephrine (Levophed)	IV: Drip: 2–12 µg/min	D	*Increase* effects with ergot alkaloids, tricyclic antidepressants, antihistamines, MAOIs, methyldopa	UK	UK	IV: Rapid	UK	1–2 min after infusion terminated

KEY: For complete abbreviation key, see inside front cover.

Emergency Treatment of Hypertensive Crisis

Sodium Nitroprusside	Dosage
Sodium Nitroprusside (Nipride) *Pregnancy Category:* C *Drug Forms:* Inj IV 10 mg/mL in 5-mL vial	A: IV: Drip: 0.5–10 μg/kg/min; begin at 0.1 μg/kg/min and titrate to desired effect up to 10 μg/kg/min

Contraindications	Drug-Lab-Food Interactions
Hypersensitivity, hypertension (compensatory), decreased cerebral perfusion, coarctation of aorta *Caution:* Increased intracranial pressure	Antihypertensives, general anesthetics Do not mix with any other drug in syringe or solution. *Lab:* Decrease in carbonate, P_{CO_2}, pH

Pharmacokinetics	Pharmacodynamics
Absorption: IV only *Distribution:* PB: UK *Metabolism:* t 1/2: <10 min *Excretion:* In urine	IV: Onset: 1–2 min Peak: Rapid Duration: 1–10 min

Therapeutic Effects/Uses: To treat hypertensive crisis; to produce controlled hypotension to reduce surgical bleeding; and to decrease systemic vascular resistance to improve cardiac performance.

Mode of Action: Stimulation of smooth muscle of veins and arteries; produces peripheral vasodilation.

Side Effects	Adverse Reactions
Dizziness, headache, nausea, abdominal pain, sweating, palpitations, weakness, vomiting	Tinnitus, dyspnea, blurred vision *Life-threatening:* Severe hypotension, loss of consciousness, profound cardiovascular depression

KEY: For complete abbreviation key, see inside front cover.

■ NURSING PROCESS: Emergency Treatment of Hypertensive Crisis: Sodium Nitroprusside

ASSESSMENT
- Assess VS frequently.
- Assess serum thiocyanate and/or cyanide levels. Elevations are indicative of toxicity.

POTENTIAL NURSING DIAGNOSES
Altered tissue perfusion
Decreased cardiac output

PLANNING
- Client's hypertension and blood pressure will be controlled.

NURSING INTERVENTIONS
- Reconstitute drug using sterile water without preservative.
- Cover infusion bottle with aluminum foil immediately after reconstituting; do not cover IV tubing.
- Use drug within 24 h of preparation; new solution has slight brown color. Do not use solution if dark brown or blue.
- Administer via electronic infusion device to ensure accurate rate and dosage.
- Be attentive to avoiding extravasation (sloughing of tissue and severe pain).
- Do not interrupt infusion; alteration in blood pressure may result.
- If hypotension ensues, titrate drug downward; discontinuation of infusion may be necessary.

CLIENT TEACHING
General
- Alert the client to immediately report pain at the IV line site.

Side Effects
- Instruct client to immediately report dyspnea, dizziness, blurred vision, headache, or tinnitus.

EVALUATION
- Blood pressure is within desired range. Client is free of drug side effects.

Agents for Emergency Treatment of Hypertensive Crisis

Generic (Brand)	Route and Dosage	Preg Cat	Interaction	t 1/2	PB	Onset	Peak	Duration
							Action	
						Onset	Peak	Duration
Diazoxide (Hyperstat)	IV: 1–3 mg/kg; max: 150 mg; bolus q5–15 min until blood pressure is satisfactory	C	*Increase* side effects with hypotensive agents, diuretics; *increase* effects of anticoagulants	A: 21–45 h C: 10–24 h	90%	Rapid	<5 min	3–10 h
Sodium nitroprusside (Nipride)	See Prototype Drug Chart							

KEY: For complete abbreviation key, see inside front cover.

BIBLIOGRAPHY

American Heart Association (1994). *Textbook of Advanced Cardiac Life Support*. Dallas, TX: American Heart Association.

American Society of Hospital Pharmacists (1995). *AHFS Drug Information*. Bethesda, MD: American Society of Hospital Pharmacists.

Bobak, I.M. (1991). *Quick Reference for Maternity Nursing*. St. Louis: Mosby–Year Book, Inc.

Chernecky, C. (1991). *Cancer Diagnostics and Chemotherapy*. Philadelphia: W.B. Saunders Co.

Clark, J., and Longo, D. (1986). Biological response modifiers. *Mediguide to Oncology*, 6 (2), 1–5, 9, 10.

Davis, J.R., and Sherer, K. (1994). *Applied Nutrition and Diet Therapy for Nurses* (2nd ed.). Philadelphia: W.B. Saunders Co.

Drug Facts and Comparisons (1994, updated monthly). St. Louis: J.B. Lippincott Co.

Drug Information for Health Care Professionals, Vol 1 (14th ed.). Taunton, MA.

Formulary and Drug Therapy Guide: 1993–1994. Medical Center of Delaware. Newark, DE: Lexi-Comp Inc.

Gilman, A.G., Goodman, L.S., and Gilman, A. (1991). *Goodman and Gilman's The Pharmacologic Basis of Therapeutics* (8th ed). New York: Pergamon Press Inc.

Green, M.R. (1991). *The Role of Colony-Stimulating Factors in Chemotherapy-Induced Neutropenia*. Seattle, WA: Immunex Corp.

Haeuber, D., and Dijulio, J.E. (1989). Hematopoietic colony-stimulating factors: An overview. *Oncology Nursing Forum*. 16 (2), 247–255.

Hodgson, B.B., Kizior, R.J., and Kingdon, R.T. (1995). *Nurse's Drug Handbook* (2nd ed). Philadelphia: W.B. Saunders Co.

Hoechst-Roussel Pharmaceuticals, Inc. (1991). *Myeloid Growth Factors*. Somerville, NJ: Hoechst-Roussel Pharmaceuticals, Inc.

Kee, J.L., and Paulanka, B.J. (1994). *Fluids and Electrolytes with Clinical Applications* (5th ed). New York: Delmar Publishers Inc.

Kee, J.L. (1995). *Laboratory and Diagnostic Tests With Nursing Implications* (4th ed). Norwalk, CT: Appleton and Lange.

Kuhn, M.M. (1991). *Pharmacotherapeutics* (2nd ed). Philadelphia: F.A. Davis Co.

Lehne, R. (1994). *Pharmacology for Nursing Care* (2nd ed). Philadelphia: W.B. Saunders Co.

McKenry, L.M., and Salerno, E. (1992). *Mosby's Pharmacology in Nursing* (18th ed). St. Louis: C.V. Mosby Co.

(1994). *Physicians' Desk Reference* (48th ed). Montvale, NJ: Medical Economics Co, Inc.

Schwertz, D.W. (1991). Basic principles of pharmacologic action. *Nursing Clinics of North America*, 26 (2), 245–262.

Shannon, M.T., and Wilson, B.A. (1995). *Govoni and Hayes: Drugs and Nursing Implications* (8th ed). Norwalk, CT: Appleton and Lange.

Skidmore-Roth, L. (1995). *Mosby's 1995 Nursing Drug Reference*. St. Louis: Mosby–Year Book, Inc.

Spratto, G.R., and Woods, A.L. (1995). *Nurse's Drug Reference*. New York: Delmar Publishers, Inc.

Timmons, M.C. (1990). The use of estrogen replacement therapy. In R.C. Cefalo (ed), *Clinical Decisions in Obstetrics and Gynecology* (pp. 229–231). Rockville, MD: Aspen Publishers, Inc.

APPENDIX A

Generic Drug Names	Canadian Trade/Brand Names
Acebutolol	Monitan
Acetaminophen	Abenol, Atasol, Campain, Exdol, Robigesic, Rounox
Acetazolamide	Acetazolam, Apo-Acetazolamide
Acetohexamide	Dimelor
Acetylcysteine	Airbron
Albuterol	Novosalmol, Salbutamol
Allopurinol	Alloprin, Apo-Allopurinol, Novopurinol, Purinol
Aminophylline	Gorophyllin, Paladron
Aminosalicylate sodium	Parasal Sodium
Amitriptyline hydrochloride	Apo-Amitriptyline, Levate, Meravil, Novotriptyn, Rolavil
Amoxicillin	Apo-Amoxi, Amoxican
Amoxicillin clavulanate K	Clavulin
Ampicillin	Ampilean, Novo-Ampicillin, Penbritin
Ascorbic acid	Apo-C, Ce-Vi-Sol, Redoxon
Asparaginase	Kidrolase
Aspirin	Ancasal, Astrin, Entrophen, Novasen, Supasa, Triaphen-10
Atenolol	Apo-Atenolol
Atropine sulfate	Atropair
Bacampicillin hydrochloride	Penglobe
Benzalkonium chloride	Pharmatex
Benztropine mesylate	Apo-Benzotropine, Bensylate, PMS Benzotropine
Betamethasone	Beban, Betaderm, Betanelan, Betnesol, Betnovate, Celestoderm, Novobetamet
Bisacodyl	Apo-Bisacodyl, Bisco-Lax, Laxit
Bretylium tosylate	Bretylate
Carbamazepine	Apo-Carbamazepine, Mazepine, PMS Carbamazepine
Carbenicillin disodium	Pyopen
Cephalexin	Ceporex, Novolexin
Cephalothin sodium	Ceporacin
Chloral hydrate	Novochlorhydrate
Chloramphenicol	Novochorocap, Pentamycetin
Chlordiazepoxide hydrochloride	Medilium, Novopoxide, Solium
Chlorphenesin carbamate	Mycil
Chlorpheniramine maleate	Chlor-Tripolon, Novopheniram
Chlorpromazine hydrochloride	Chlorpromanyl, Largactil, Novochlorpromazine
Chlorpropamide	Apo-Chlorpropamide, Chloronase, Novopropamide
Chlorprothixene	Tarasan
Chlorthalidone	Novothalidone, Uridon
Cimetidine	Novocimetine, Peptol
Cisplatin	Abiplatin

continued

Generic Drugs with Corresponding Canadian Trade Drug Names*—*Continued*

Generic Drug Names	Canadian Trade/Brand Names
Clindamycin	Dalacin-C
Clofibrate	Claripen, Claripex, Novofibrate
Clonazepam	Rivotril
Clonidine hydrochloride	Dixarit
Clorazepate dipotassium	Novoclopate
Clotrimazole	Canesten
Cloxacillin sodium	Apo-Cloxi, Bactopen, Novocloxin, Orbenin
Codeine phosphate	Paveral
Colchicine	Novocolchine
Colestipol hydrochloride	Cholestabyl, Lestid
Co-trimoxazole	Apo-Sulfatrim
Cromolyn sodium	Fivent, Intal p, Rynacrom, Vistacrom
Cyanocobalamin	Anacobin, Bedoz, Cyanabin, Rubion
Cyclizine hydrochloride	Marzine
Cyclophosphamide	Procytox
Cyproheptadine hydrochloride	Vimicon
Danazol	Cyclomen
Dapsone	Avlosulfon
Dexamethasone	Deronil, Dexasone, Oradexon, Stress-Pam
Dextromethorphan	Balminil DM, Koffex, Ornex DM, Robidex, Sedatuss
Diazepam	Apo-Diazepam, Diazemuls, E-Pam, Meval, Novodipam, Vivol
Dicyclomine hydrochloride	Bentylol, Formulex, Lomine, Protylol, Viscerol
Diethylpropion hydrochloride	Nobesine
Diethylstilbestrol	Honval, Stilboestrol
Digitoxin	Digitaline, Purodigin
Dimenhydrinate	Apo-Dimenhydrinate, Gravol, Nauseatol, Novodimenate, Travamine
Dinoprostone	Prepidil Gel
Diphenhydramine hydrochloride	Allerdryl
Dipyridamole	Apo-Dipyridamole
Disopyramide	Rythmodan
Docusate sodium	Regulax
Dopamine hydrochloride	Revimine
Doxepin hydrochloride	Triadapin
Doxycycline hyclate	Doryx, Doxycin, Novodoxylin
Dyphylline	Protophylline
Econazole nitrate	Ecostatin
Epinephrine hydrochloride	SusPhrine, Eppy
Epinephrine racemic	Vaponefrin
Ergocalciferol	Ostoforte, Radiostol
Ergotamine tartrate	Gynergen
Erythromycin	Apo-Erythro Base, Erythromid, Novorythro, Ro-Mycin
Estradiol	Delestrogen
Estrogen, conjugated	C.E.S.
Estrogen, esterified	Climestrone, Neo-Estrone
Estrone	Femogen Forte
Ethambutol hydrochloride	Etibi
Ethopropazine hydrochloride	Parsitan
Fenfluramine hydrochloride	Ponderal
Ferrous fumarate	Neo-Fer-50, Novofumar, Palafer
Ferrous gluconate	Fertinic, Novoferrogluc
Ferrous sulfate	Novoferrosulfa
Flucytosine	Ancotil

Appendix A

**Generic Drugs with Corresponding Canadian Trade Drug Names*—*Continued*

Generic Drug Names	Canadian Trade/Brand Names
Fluocinolone acetonide	Fluoderm
Fluocinonide	Lidemol, Lyderm, Topsyn
Fluoxymesterone	Ora T Estryl
Fluphenazine decanoate	Decanoate
Fluphenazine enanthate	Enanthate
Fluphenazine hydrochloride	Moditen HCl
Flurandrenolide	Drenison
Flurazepam	Apo-Flurazepam, Novoflupam, Somnol
Folic acid	Apo-Folic, Novofolacid
Furosemide	Fumide, Furomide, Luramide, Uritol
Gentamicin sulfate	Alcomicin, Cidomycin, Novosemide
Glyburide	DiaBeta, Euglucon
Griseofulvin, microsize	Grisovin-FP
Guaifenesin	Balminil, Resyl
Guanethidine sulfate	Apo-Guanethidine
Haloperidol	Haldol LA, Peridol
Heparin calcium	Calcilean, Calciparine
Heparin sodium	Hepalean
Hydrochlorothiazide	Apo-Hydro, Hydrozide, Neo-Codema, Urozide
Hydrocodone bitartrate	Hycodan, Robidone
Hydrocortisone	Cortamed, Cortiment, Rectocort
Hydroxocobalamin	Acti-B$_{12}$
Ibuprofen	Amersol
Imipramine hydrochloride	Impril, Novopramine
Indapamide	Lozide
Indomethacin	Indocid
Isoniazid (INH)	Isotamine
Isosorbide dinitrate	Coronex, Novosorbide
Iodoquinol	Diodoquin
Kaolin/pectin	Donnagel-MB, Kao-Con
Ketoprofen	Rhodis, Orudis E
Lactulose	Lactulax
Levothyroxine sodium (T$_4$)	Eltroxin
Lidocaine hydrochloride	Xylocard
Lithium carbonate	Carbolith, Duralith, Lithizine
Lorazepam	Apo-Lorazepam, Novolorazepam
Loxapine hydrochloride	Loxapac
Magaldrate	Antiflux
Meclizine hydrochloride	Bonamine
Mefenamic acid	Ponstan
Meperidine hydrochloride	Pethadol, Pethidine Hydrochloride
Meprobamate	Apo-Meprobamate, Novomepro
Mesalamine	Salofalk
Methohexital	Brietal
Methotrimeprazine	Nozinan
Methylclothiazide	Duretic
Methyldopa	Apo-Methyldopa, Dopamet, Novomedopa
Methyltestosterone	Metandren
Metoclopramide	Maxeran
Metoprolol	Apo-Metoprolol, Betaloc, Novometoprol
Metronidazole	Neo-Metric, Novonidazol, PMS Metronidazole
Miconazole	Monistat
Mineral oil	Kondremul, Lansoyl
Morphine sulfate	Epimorph, Statex
Naphazoline	Vasocon

continued

Generic Drugs with Corresponding Canadian Trade Drug Names*—*Continued*

Generic Drug Names	Canadian Trade/Brand Names
Naproxen	Apo-Naproxen, Naxen, Novonaprox
Niacin (vitamin B_3, nicotinic acid)	Novo-Niacin, Tri-B3
Nifedipine	Adalat P.A., Apo-Nifed, Novo-Nifedin
Nitrofurantoin	Apo-Nitrofurantoin, Nephronex, Novofuran
Norethindrone acetate	Aygestin, Norlutate
Nylidrin hydrochloride	Arlidin Forte, PMS Nylidrin
Nystatin	Nadostine, Nyaderm
Omeprazole	Losec
Oxazepam	Ox-Pam, Zapex, Apo-Oxazepam, Novoxapam
Oxtriphylline	Apo-Oxtriphylline, Novotriphyl
Oxycodone	Supeudol
Oxymetazoline hydrochloride	Nafrine
Oxymetholone	Anapolon
Penicillin G potassium	Megacillin, NovoPen-G, P-50, Crystapen
Penicillin G procaine	Ayercillin
Penicillin G sodium	Crystapen
Penicillin V	Apo-Pen-VK, Nadopen-V, Novopen-VK
Pentamidine isethionate	Pentacarinat
Pentobarbital	Novopentobarb
Perphenazine	Apo-Perphenazine, Phenazine
Phenazopyridine hydrochloride	Phenazo, Pyronium
Phentolamine mesylate	Rogitine
Phenazopyridine	Phenazo, Pyronium
Phenylephrine, ophthalmic	Minims Phenylephrine
Pilocarpine hydrochloride	Pilocarpine, Milocarpine
Piroxicam	Apo-Piroxicant
Potassium chloride	Apo-K, Kalium Durules, Klong, Novolente K, Roychlor 10% and 20%, Slo-Pot
Potassium gluconate	Potassium Rougier, Royonate
Potassium iodide	Thyro-Block
Pramoxine hydrochloride	Tronothane
Prednisone	Apo-Prednisone, Winpred
Primidone	Apo-Primidone, Sertan
Probenecid	Benuryl
Procarbazine hydrochloride	Natulan
Prochlorperazine maleate	Stemetil
Procyclidine hydrochloride	Procyclid
Progesterone	Progestilin
Promethazine hydrochloride	Histantil
Propantheline bromide	Propanthel
Propoxyphene hydrochloride	642, Novopropoxyn
Propranolol hydrochloride	Apo-Propranolol, Detensol, Novopranol
Propylthiouracil (PTU)	Propyl-Thyracil
Protriptyline hydrochloride	Triptil
Pseudoephedrine hydrochloride	Eltor, Eltor 120, Pseudofrin, Robidrine
Psyllium hydrophilic muciloid	Karasil
Pyrantel pamoate	Combantrin
Pyrazinamide	Tebrazid, PMS Pyrazinamide
Pyridostigmine	Mestinon Supraspan
Quinidine sulfate	APO-Quinidine, Novoquinidin
Quinine sulfate	Novoquinine
Reserpine	Novoreseroine, Reserfia
Rifampin	Rofact
Scopolamine	Transderm-V
Secobarbital	Novosecobarb
Silver sulfadiazine	Flamazine

Generic Drugs with Corresponding Canadian Trade Drug Names*—*Continued*	
Generic Drug Names	**Canadian Trade/Brand Names**
Simethicone	Ovol
Sodium fluoride	Fluor-A-Day
Sotalol	Sotacor
Spironolactone	Novospiroton, Sincomen
Sucralfate	Sulcrate
Sulfasalazine	PMS Sulfasalazine, Salazopyrin, SAS-Enema, SAS Enteric-500, S.A.S.-500
Sulfinpyrazone	Antazone, Anturan, Apo-Sulfinpyrazone, Novopyrazone
Sulfisoxazole	Novosoxazole
Tamoxifen citrate	Nolvadex-D, Tamofen
Testosterone	Malogen
Testosterone enanthate	Malogex
Testosterone propionate	Malogen in oil
Tetracycline hydrochloride	Novotetra, Apo-Tetra, Tetralean
Theophylline	PMS Theophylline, Pulmopylline, Somophyllin-12
Thiamine HCl (vitamin B₁)	Bewon, Betaxin
Thioguanine (TG, 6-thioguanine)	Lanvis
Thioridazine hydrochloride	Novoridazine
Timolol maleate	Apo-Timol
Tolbutamide	Mobenol, Novobutamide
Tolnaftate	Pitrex
Trifluoperazine hydrochloride	Novoflurazine, Solazine, Terfluzine
Trihexyphenidyl hydrochloride	Aparkane, Apo-Trihex, Novohexidyl
Trimeprazine tartrate	Panectyl
Tripelennamine hydrochloride	Pyribenzamine
Valproic acid (divalproex sodium, sodium valproate)	Epival
Vinblastine sulfate	Velbe
Warfarin sodium	Warfilone

*Many of the trade or brand names are used in both the United States and Canada. This appendix lists selected trade or brand names that are specific to Canada.

APPENDIX B

Canadian Trade/Brand Names	Generic Drug Names
Abenol	Acetaminophen
Acetazolam	Acetazolamide
Acti-B$_{12}$	Hydroxocobalamin
Adalat P.A.	Nifedipine
Airbron	Acetylcysteine
Alcomicin	Gentamicin sulfate
Allerdryl	Diphenhydramine hydrochloride
Alloprin	Allopurinol
Amersol	Ibuprofen
Amoxican	Amoxicillin
Ampilean	Ampicillin
Anacobin	Cyanocobalamin
Anapolon	Oxymetholone
Ancasal	Aspirin
Ancotil	Flucytosine
Antazone	Sulfinpyrazone
Antiflux	Magaldrate
Anturan	Sulfinpyrazone
Aparkane	Trihexyphenidyl hydrochloride
Apo-Acetazolamide	Acetazolamide
Apo-Allopurinol	Allopurinol
Apo-Amitriptyline	Amitriptyline hydrochloride
Apo-Amoxi	Amoxicillin
Apo-Atenolol	Atenolol
Apo-Benzotropine	Benztropine mesylate
Apo-Bisacodyl	Bisacodyl
Apo-C	Ascorbic acid
Apo-Carbamazepine	Carbamazepine
Apo-Chlorpropamide	Chlorpropamide
Apo-Cloxi	Cloxacillin sodium
Apo-Diazepam	Diazepam
Apo-Dimenhydrinate	Dimenhydrinate
Apo-Dipyridamole	Dipyridamole
Apo-Erythro Base	Erythromycin
Apo-Flurazepam	Flurazepam
Apo-Folic	Folic acid
Apo-Guanethidine	Guanethidine sulfate
Apo-Hydro	Hydrochlorothiazide
Apo-Lorazepam	Lorazepam
Apo-Meprobamate	Meprobamate
Apo-Methyldopa	Methyldopa
Apo-Metoprolol	Metoprolol
Apo-Naproxen	Naproxen
Apo-Nifed	Nifedipine

continued

Canadian Trade Drug Names with Corresponding Generic Drugs—*Continued*

Canadian Trade/Brand Names	Generic Drug Names
Apo-Nitrofurantoin	Nitrofurantoin
Apo-Oxazepam	Oxazepam
Apo-Oxtriphylline	Oxtriphylline
Apo-PenVK	Penicillin V
Apo-Perphenazine	Perphenazine
Apo-Piroxicant	Piroxicam
Apo-Prednisone	Prednisone
Apo-Primidone	Primidone
Apo-Propranolol	Propranolol hydrochloride
Apo-Quinidine	Quinidine sulfate
Apo-Sulfatrim	Co-trimoxazole
Apo-Timol	Timolol maleate
Apo-Trihex	Trihexyphenidyl hydrochloride
Arlidin Forte	Nylidrin hydrochloride
Astrin	Aspirin
Atasol	Acetaminophen
Atropair	Atropine sulfate
Avlosulfon	Dapsone
Ayercillin	Penicillin G procaine
Aygestin	Norethindrone acetate
Bactopen	Cloxacillin sodium
Balminil	Guaifenesin
Beben	Betamethasone
Bedoz	Cyanocobalamin
Bensylate	Benztropine mesylate
Benuryl	Probenecid
Betaderm	Betamethasone
Betaloc	Metoprolol
Betanelan	Betamethasone
Betaxin	Thiamine hydrochloride
Betnesol	Betamethasone
Betnovate	Betamethasone
Bewon	Thiamine hydrochloride
Bisco-Lax	Bisacodyl
Bonamine	Meclizine hydrochloride
Bretylate	Bretylium tosylate
Brietal	Methohexital
Calcilean	Heparin calcium
Calciparine	Heparin calcium
Campain	Acetaminophen
Canesten	Clotrimazole
Carbolith	Lithium carbonate
Celestoderm	Betamethasone
Ceporacin	Cephalothin sodium
Ceporex	Cephalexin
C.E.S.	Estrogen, conjugated
Ce-Vi-Sol	Ascorbic acid
Chloronase	Chlorpropamide
Chlorpromanyl	Chlorpromazine hydrochloride
Chlor-Tripolon	Chlorpheniramine maleate
Cholestabyl	Colestipol hydrochloride
Cidomycin	Gentamicin sulfate
Claripen	Clofibrate
Claripex	Clofibrate
Clavulin	Amoxicillin clavulanate K
Climestrone	Estrogen, esterified

Canadian Trade Drug Names with Corresponding Generic Drugs—*Continued*	
Canadian Trade/Brand Names	**Generic Drug Names**
Combantrin	Pyrantel pamoate
Coronex	Isosorbide dinitrate
Cortamed	Hydrocortisone
Cortiment	Hydrocortisone
Crystapen	Penicillin G sodium, penicillin G potassium
Cyanabin	Cyanocobalamin
Cyclomen	Danazol
Dalacin-C	Clindamycin
Decanoate	Fluphenazine decanoate
Delestrogen	Estradiol
Deronil	Dexamethasone
Detensol	Propranolol hydrochloride
Dexasone	Dexamethasone
DiaBeta	Glyburide
Diazemuls	Diazepam
Digitaline	Digitoxin
Dimelor	Acetohexamide
Diodoquin	Iodoquinol
Dixarit	Clonidine hydrochloride
Donnagel-MB	Kaolin/pectin
Doryx	Doxycycline hyclate
Doxycin	Doxycycline hyclate
Drenison	Flurandrenolide
Duralith	Lithium carbonate
Duretic	Methylclothiazide
Ecostatin	Econazole nitrate
Eltor, Eltor 120	Pseudoephedrine hydrochloride
Eltroxin	Levothyroxine sodium
Enanthate	Fluphenazine enanthate
E-Pam	Diazepam
Epimorph	Morphine sulfate
Epival	Valproic acid
Eppy	Epinephrine hydrochloride
Erythromid	Erythromycin
Etibi	Ethambutol hydrochloride
Euglucon	Glyburide
Exdol	Acetaminophen
Femogen Forte	Estrone
Fertinic	Ferrous gluconate
Flamazine	Silver sulfadiazine
Fluoderm	Fluocinolone acetonide
Fluor-A-Day	Sodium fluoride
Formulex	Dicyclomine hydrochloride
Fumide	Furosemide
Furomide	Furosemide
Gorophyllin	Aminophylline
Gravol	Dimenhydrinate
Grisovin-FP	Griseofulvin, microsize
Gynergen	Ergotamine tartrate
Haldol LA	Haloperidol
Hepalean	Heparin sodium
Histantil	Promethazine hydrochloride
Honval	Diethylstilbestrol
Hycodan	Hydrocodone bitartrate

continued

Canadian Trade Drug Names with Corresponding Generic Drugs—*Continued*

Canadian Trade/Brand Names	Generic Drug Names
Hydrozide	Hydrochlorothiazide
Impril	Imipramine hydrochloride
Indocid	Indomethacin
Isotamine	Isoniazid
Kalium Durules	Potassium chloride
Kao-Con	Kaolin/pectin
Karasil	Psyllium hydrophilic muciloid
Kidrolase	Asparaginase
Klong	Potassium chloride
Koffex	Dextromethorphan
Kondremul	Mineral oil
Lactulax	Lactulose
Lansoyl	Mineral oil
Lanvis	Thioguanine
Largactil	Chlorpromazine hydrochloride
Lestid	Colestipol hydrochloride
Lidemol	Fluocinonide
Lithizine	Lithium carbonate
Lomine	Dicyclomine hydrochloride
Losec	Omeprazole
Loxapac	Loxapine hydrochloride
Lozide	Indapamide
Lyderm	Fluocinonide
Malogen	Testosterone
Malogen in oil	Testosterone propionate
Malogex	Testosterone enanthate
Marzine	Cyclizine hydrochloride
Maxeran	Metoclopramide
Mazepine	Carbamazepine
Medilium	Chlordiazepoxide hydrochloride
Megacillin	Penicillin G potassium
Meravil	Amitriptyline hydrochloride
Mestinon Supraspan	Pyridostigmine
Metandren	Methyltestosterone
Meval	Diazepam
Milocarpine	Pilocarpine hydrochloride
Minims Phenylephrine	Phenylephrine, ophthalmic
Mobenol	Tolbutamide
Moditen HCl	Fluphenazine hydrochloride
Monistat	Miconazole
Monitan	Acebutolol
Mycil	Chlorphenesin carbamate
Nadopen V	Penicillin V
Nadostine	Nystatin
Nafrine	Oxymetazoline hydrochloride
Nauseatol	Dimenhydrinate
Naxen	Naproxen
Neo-Codema	Hydrochlorothiazide
Neo-Estrone	Estrogen, esterified
Neo-Fer-50	Ferrous fumarate
Neo-Metric	Metronidazole
Nephronex	Nitrofurantoin
Nobesine	Diethylproprion hydrochloride
Nolvadex-D	Tamoxifen citrate
Norlutate	Norethindrone acetate
Novasen	Aspirin

Canadian Trade Drug Names with Corresponding Generic Drugs—*Continued*	
Canadian Trade/Brand Names	**Generic Drug Names**
Novo-Ampicillin	Ampicillin
Novobetamet	Bethamethasone
Novobutamide	Tolbutamide
Novochlorhydrate	Chloral hydrate
Novochlorpromazine	Chlorpromazine hydrochloride
Novochorocap	Chloramphenicol
Novocimetine	Cimetidine
Novoclopate	Clorazepate dipotassium
Novocloxin	Cloxacillin sodium
Novocolchine	Colchicine
Novodimenate	Dimenhydrinate
Novodipam	Diazepam
Novodoxylin	Doxycycline hyclate
Novoferrogluc	Ferrous gluconate
Novoferrosulfa	Ferrous sulfate
Novofibrate	Clofibrate
Novoflupam	Flurazepam
Novoflurazine	Trifluoperazine hydrochloride
Novofolacid	Folic acid
Novofumar	Ferrous fumarate
Novofuran	Nitrofurantoin
Novohexidyl	Trihexyphenidyl hydrochloride
Novolente K	Potassium chloride
Novolexin	Cephalexin
Novolorazepam	Lorazepam
Novomedopa	Methyldopa
Novomepro	Meprobamate
Novometoprol	Metoprolol
Novonaprox	Naproxen
Novo-Niacin	Niacin
Novonidazol	Metronidazole
Novo-Nifedin	Nifedipine
Novopentobarb	Pentobarbital
Novopen-VK	Penicillin V
Novopheniram	Chlorpheniramine maleate
Novopoxide	Chlordiazepoxide hydrochloride
Novopramine	Imipramine hydrochloride
Novopranol	Propranolol hydrochloride
Novopropoxyn	Propoxyphene hydrochloride
Novopurinol	Allopurinol
Novoquinidin	Quinidine sulfate
Novoquinine	Quinine sulfate
Novoreseroine	Reserpine
Novoridazine	Thioridazine hydrochloride
Novorythro	Erythromycin
Novosalmol	Albuterol
Novosecobarb	Secobarbital
Novosemide	Gentamicin sulfate
Novosorbide	Isosorbide dinitrate
Novosoxazole	Sulfisoxazole
Novospiroton	Spironolactone
Novotetra	Tetracycline hydrochloride
Novothalidone	Chlorthalidone
Novotriphyl	Oxtriphylline
Novotriptyn	Amitriptyline hydrochloride

continued

Canadian Trade Drug Names with Corresponding Generic Drugs—*Continued*

Canadian Trade/Brand Names	Generic Drug Names
Novoxapam	Oxazepam
Nyaderm	Nystatin
Ora T Estryl	Fluoxymesterone
Orbenin	Cloxacillin sodium
Ostoforte	Ergocalciferol
Ovol	Simethicone
Ox-Pam	Oxazepam
Paladron	Aminophylline
Palafer	Ferrous fumarate
Panectyl	Trimeprazine tartrate
Parasal Sodium	Aminosalicylate sodium
Parsitan	Ethoproprazine hydrochloride
Paveral	Codeine phosphate
Penbritin	Ampicillin
Penglobe	Bacampicillin hydrochloride
Pentacarinat	Pentamidine isethionate
Pentamycetin	Chloramphenicol
Peptol	Cimetidine
Pethadol	Meperidine hydrochloride
Pethidine Hydrochloride	Meperidine hydrochloride
Pharmatex	Benzalkonium chloride
Phenazine	Perphenazine
Phenazo	Phenazopyridine hydrochloride
Pilocarpine	Pilocarpine hydrochloride
Pitrex	Tolnaftate
PMS Carbamazepine	Carbamazepine
PMS Metronidazole	Metronidazole
PMS Nylidrin	Nylidrin hydrochloride
PMS Pyrazinamide	Pyrazinamide
PMS Sulfasalazine	Sulfasalazine
PMS Theophylline	Theophylline
Ponderal	Fenfluramine hydrochloride
Ponstan	Mefenamic acid
Potassium Rougier	Potassium gluconate
Prepidil Gel	Dinoprostone
Procyclid	Procyclidine hydrochloride
Procytox	Cyclophosphamide
Progestilin	Progesterone
Propanthel	Propantheline bromide
Propyl-Thyracil	Propylthiouracil
Protophylline	Dyphylline
Protylol	Dicyclomine hydrochloride
Pseudofrin	Pseudoephedrine hydrochloride
Pulmophylline	Theophylline hydrochloride
Purinol	Allopurinol
Purodigin	Digitoxin
Pyopen	Carbenicillin disodium
Pyronium	Phenazopyridine
Radiostol	Ergocalciferol
Rectocort	Hydrocortisone
Redoxon	Ascorbic acid
Regulax	Docusate sodium
Resyl	Guaifenesin
Revimine	Dopamine hydrochloride
Rhodis	Ketoprofen
Robidex	Dextromethorphan

Canadian Trade Drug Names with Corresponding Generic Drugs—*Continued*

Canadian Trade/Brand Names	Generic Drug Names
Robigesic	Acetaminophen
Rofact	Rifampin
Rogitine	Phentolamine mesylate
Rolavil	Amitriptyline hydrochloride
Rounox	Acetaminophen
Royonate	Potassium gluconate
Rubion	Cyanocobalamin
Rythmodan	Disopyramide
Salbutamol	Albuterol
Salofalk	Mesalamine
SAS Enteric-500	Sulfasalazine
Sedatuss	Dextromethorphan
Sincomen	Spironolactone
Solazine	Trifluoperazine hydrochloride
Solium	Chlordiazepoxide hydrochloride
Somnol	Flurazepam
Somophyllin-12	Theophylline
Sotacor	Sotalol
Statex	Morphine sulfate
Stemetil	Prochlorperazine maleate
Stilboestrol	Diethylstilbestrol
Stress-Pam	Dexamethasone
Sulcrate	Sucralfate
Supasa	Aspirin
Supeudol	Oxycodone
SusPhrine	Epinephrine hydrochloride
Tamofen	Tamoxifen citrate
Tarasan	Chlorprothixene
Tebrazid	Pyrazinamide
Terfluzine	Trifluoperazine hydrochloride
Tetralean	Tetracycline hydrochloride
Thyro-Block	Potassium iodide
Travamine	Dimenhydrinate
Triadapin	Doxepin hydrochloride
Triaphen-10	Aspirin
Triptil	Protriptyline hydrochloride
Tronothane	Pramoxine hydrochloride
Uritol	Furosemide
Vaponefrin	Epinephrine racemic
Vasocon	Naphazoline
Velbe	Vinblastine sulfate
Vimicon	Cyproheptadine hydrochloride
Vistacrom	.Cromolyn sodium
Warfilone	Warfarin sodium
Xylocard	Lidocaine hydrochloride

Index

Note: Page numbers followed by t refer to tables.

485

PROTOTYPES

Minerals and Electrolytes
Vitamin A: fat-soluble
Antianemia, mineral: iron
Electrolyte:
potassium
calcium

Central Nervous System Stimulants and Depressants
CNS stimulant: methylphenidate HCl (Ritalin)
Sedative-hypnotic, barbiturate: pentobarbital (Nembutal)
Benzodiazepine: flurazepam HCl (Dalmane)
Analgesic:
aspirin
acetaminophen (Tylenol)
Narcotic:
opiate: morphine sulfate (Duramorph)
synthetic: meperidine HCl (Demerol)
agonist-antagonist: pentazocine lactate (Talwin)

Anticonvulsants
Hydantoin: phenytoin (Dilantin)

Antipsychotics, Anxiolytics, and Antidepressants
Antipsychotic,
phenothiazine: chlorpromazine (Thorazine)
nonphenothiazine: haloperidol (Haldol)
Anxiolytic, benzodiazepine: diazepam (Valium)
Antidepressant, tricyclic: amoxapine (Asendin)
Antimanic: lithium carbonate (Eskalith)

Neurologic and Neuromuscular Agents
Sympathomimetic: epinephrine HCl (Adrenalin Chloride)
Adrenergic blocker: propranolol HCl (Inderal)
Parasympathomimetic: bethanechol chloride (Urecholine)
Parasympatholytic: atropine sulfate
Anticholinergic: trihexyphenidyl HCl (Artane)
Dopaminergic: carbidopa-levodopa (Sinemet)
Cholinesterase inhibitor: pyridostigmine bromide (Mestinon)
Skeletal muscle relaxant: carisoprodol (Soma)

Anti-inflammatory Agents
Anti-inflammatory,
nonsteroidal antiinflammatory drugs (NSAIDs): ibuprofen (Motrin)
gold: auranofin (Ridaura)
antigout: allopurinol (Zyloprim)

Anti-infective Agents
Antibacterial,
penicillin: amoxicillin trihydrate (Amoxil)
cephalosporin: cefaclor (Ceclor)
macrolide: erythromycin (E-Mycin)
tetracycline (Achromycin)
aminoglycoside: gentamicin sulfate (Garamycin)
quinolone: ciprofloxacin HCl (Cipro)
sulfonamide: (Bactrim)
Antitubercular, isoniazid (INH)
Antifungal, nystatin (Mycostatin)
Antiviral, acyclovir sodium (Zovirax)
Antiinfective, topical: mafenide acetate (Sulfamylon)

Urinary Agents
Antibacterial: nitrofurantoin (Furadantin)
Antipruritic: phenazopyridine (Pyridium)

Antineoplastic Agents
Aklylating: cyclophosphamide (Cytoxan)